Immunology: Principles and Practice

Immunology: Principles and Practice

Olivia Hooper

Larsen & Keller
www.larsen-keller.com

Immunology: Principles and Practice
Olivia Hooper
ISBN: 978-1-64172-615-3 (Hardback)

☐ Larsen & Keller

Published by Larsen and Keller Education,
5 Penn Plaza,
19th Floor,
New York, NY 10001, USA

Cataloging-in-Publication Data

Immunology : principles and practice / Olivia Hooper.
    p. cm.
Includes bibliographical references and index.
ISBN 978-1-64172-615-3
1. Immunology. 2. Life sciences. 3. Serology. I. Hooper, Olivia.
QR181 .I46 2022
616.079--dc23

For more information regarding Larsen and Keller Education and its products, please visit the publisher's website www.larsen-keller.com

TABLE OF CONTENTS

It is with great pleasure that I present this book. It has been carefully written after numerous discussions with my peers and other practitioners of the field. I would like to take this opportunity to thank my family and friends who have been extremely supporting at every step in my life.

The branch of biology which deals with the study of immune system in all organisms is referred to as immunology. It measures and contextualizes the physiological functioning of the immune system in terms of both health and diseases. It also observes the malfunctions of the immune system in immunological disorders such as autoimmune disease, hypersensitivities, immune deficiency and transplant rejection. Immunology studies the physical, chemical and physiological characteristics of the components of the immune system. It is applied in various disciplines of medicine, including organ transplantation, oncology, virology, rheumatology, bacteriology, parasitology, psychiatry and dermatology. This book is a valuable compilation of topics, ranging from the basic to the most complex theories and principles in the field of immunology. It brings forth some of the most innovative concepts and elucidates the unexplored aspects of this field. This book aims to serve as a resource guide for students and experts alike and contribute to the growth of the discipline.

The chapters below are organized to facilitate a comprehensive understanding of the subject:

Chapter – Introduction

The biological branch which deals with the study of immune systems in all organisms is referred to as immunology. One of its major branches is immunopathology. This is an introductory chapter which will introduce briefly all the significant aspects of immunology and immunopathology.

Chapter – Immune System

The host defense system which consists of various biological structures and processes that protects an organism against diseases is known as the immune system. There are two major subsystems within immune system, namely, innate immune system and adaptive immune system. The topics elaborated in this chapter will help in gaining a better perspective about immune system, its components and its types.

Chapter – Immune System Receptors

Receptors that bind to a substance and cause a response in the immune system are termed as immune system receptors. Some of these receptors are cytokine receptors, killer-cell immunoglobulin-like receptors, leukocyte immunoglobulin-like receptors and chemokine receptors. This chapter discusses in detail these receptors of the immune system.

Chapter – Concepts of Immunology

Some of the fundamental concepts of immunology are immune tolerance, antigen presentation, intrinsic immunity, immunoglobulin class switching, immune repertoire and immunological synapse. This chapter has been carefully written to provide an easy understanding of these key concepts of immunology.

Chapter – Sub-disciplines of Immunology

Immunology is a broad field that is divided into various sub-disciplines. Some of them are immunoproteomics, cancer immunology, computational immunology, immunomics, psychoneuroimmunology, systems immunology and Immunotoxicology. All the diverse aspects of these sub-disciplines of immunology have been carefully analyzed in this chapter.

Chapter – Immunologic Tests

Immunologic tests are used to detect the presence of substances and pathogens. Some of the common immunologic tests are epitope mapping, chromatin immunoprecipitation, complement fixation test, skin allergy test and radioallergosorbent test. This chapter discusses in detail these types of immunologic tests.

Olivia Hooper

Introduction

- **Immunology**
- **Immunopathology**

The biological branch which deals with the study of immune systems in all organisms is referred to as immunology. One of its major branches is immunopathology. This is an introductory chapter which will introduce briefly all the significant aspects of immunology and immunopathology.

Immunology

Immunology is the study of the immune system and is a very important branch of the medical and biological sciences. The immune system protects us from infection through various lines of defence. If the immune system is not functioning as it should, it can result in disease, such as auto-immunity, allergy and cancer. It is also now becoming clear that immune responses contribute to the development of many common disorders not traditionally viewed as immunologic, including metabolic, cardiovascular, and neurodegenerative conditions such as Alzheimer's.

Importance of Immunology

From Edward Jenner's pioneering work in the 18th Century that would ultimately lead to vaccination in its modern form (an innovation that has likely saved more lives than any other medical advance), to the many scientific breakthroughs in the 19th and 20th centuries that would lead to, amongst other things, safe organ transplantation, the identification of blood groups, and the now ubiquitous use of monoclonal antibodies throughout science and healthcare, immunology has changed the face of modern medicine. Immunological research continues to extend horizons in our understanding of how to treat significant health issues, with ongoing research efforts in immunotherapy, autoimmune diseases, and vaccines for emerging pathogens, such as Ebola. Advancing our understanding of basic immunology is essential for clinical and commercial application and has facilitated the discovery of new diagnostics and treatments to manage a wide array of diseases. In addition, coupled with advancing technology, immunological research has provided critically important research techniques and tools, such as flow cytometry and antibody technology. An immunologist is a scientist and/or clinician who specialises in immunology. Many immunologists work in a laboratory focusing on research, either in academia or private industry (e.g. in the pharmaceutical industry). Other immunologists – "clinical immunologists" – are clinicians who focus on the diagnosis and management of diseases of the immune system, such as autoimmune diseases and allergies.

Immune System

The immune system is a complex system of structures and processes that has evolved to protect us from disease. Molecular and cellular components make up the immune system. The function of these components is divided up into nonspecific mechanisms, those which are innate to an organism, and responsive responses, which are adaptive to specific pathogens. Fundamental or classical immunology involves studying the components that make up the innate and adaptive immune system.

Innate immunity is the first line of defence and is non-specific. That is, the responses are the same for all potential pathogens, no matter how different they may be. Innate immunity includes physical barriers (e.g. skin, saliva etc) and cells (e.g. macrophages, neutrophils, basophils, mast cells etc). These components 'are ready to go' and protect an organism for the first few days of infection. In some cases, this is enough to clear the pathogen, but in other instances the first defence becomes overwhelmed and a second line of defence kicks in.

Adaptive immunity is the second line of defence which involves building up memory of encountered infections so can mount an enhanced response specific to the pathogen or foreign substance. Adaptive immunity involves antibodies, which generally target foreign pathogens roaming free in the bloodstream. Also involved are T cells, which are directed especially towards pathogens that have colonised cells and can directly kill infected cells or help control the antibody response.

Immune Dysfunction and Clinical Immunology

The immune system is a highly regulated and balanced system and when the balance is disturbed, disease can result. Research in this area involves studying disease that is caused by immune system dysfunction. Much of this work has significance in the development of new therapies and treatments that can manage or cure the condition by altering the way the immune system is working or, in the case of vaccines, priming the immune system and boosting the immune reaction to specific pathogens.

Immunodeficiency disorders involve problems with the immune system that impair its ability to mount an appropriate defence. As a result, these are almost always associated with severe infections that persist, recur and/or lead to complications, making these disorders severely debilitating and even fatal. There are two types of immunodeficiency disorders: primary immunodeficiencies are typically present from birth, are generally hereditary and are relatively rare. Such an example is common variable immunodeficiency (CVID). Secondary immunodeficiencies generally develop later in life and may result following an infection, as is the case with AIDS following HIV infection.

Autoimmune diseases occur when the immune system attacks the body it is meant to protect. People suffering from autoimmune diseases have a defect that makes them unable to distinguish 'self' from 'non-self' or 'foreign' molecules. The principles of immunology have provided a wide variety of laboratory tests for the detection of autoimmune diseases. Autoimmune diseases may be described as 'primary' autoimmune diseases, like type-1 diabetes, which may be manifested from birth or during early life; or as 'secondary' autoimmune diseases, which manifest later in life due to various factors. Rheumatoid arthritis and multiple sclerosis are thought to belong to this type of autoimmunity. Also, autoimmune diseases can be localised, such as Crohn's Disease affecting the GI tract, or systemic, such as systemic lupus erythematosus (SLE).

Allergies are hypersensitivity disorders that occur when the body's immune system reacts against harmless foreign substances, resulting in damage to the body's own tissues. Almost any substance can cause allergies (an allergen), but most commonly, allergies arise after eating certain types of food, such as peanuts, or from inhaling airborne substances, such as pollen, or dust. In allergic reactions, the body believes allergens are dangerous and immediately produces substances to attack them. This causes cells of the immune system to release potent chemicals like histamine, which causes inflammation and many of the symptoms associated with allergies. Immunology strives to understand what happens to the body during an allergic response and the factors responsible for causing them. This should lead to better methods of diagnosing, preventing and controlling allergic diseases.

Asthma is a debilitating and sometimes fatal disease of the airways. It generally occurs when the immune system responds to inhaled particles from the air, and can lead to thickening of the airways in patients over time. It is a major cause of illness and is particularly prevalent in children. In some cases it has an allergic component, however in a number of cases the origin is more complex and poorly understood.

Cancer is a disease of abnormal and uncontrolled cell growth and proliferation and is defined by a set of hallmarks, one of which is the capacity for cancer cells to avoid immune destruction. With the knowledge that evasion of the immune system can contribute to cancer, researchers have turned to manipulating the immune system to defeat cancer (immunotherapy). Cancer immunotherapy seeks to stimulate the immune system's innate powers to fight cancerous tissue and has shown extraordinary promise as a new weapon in our arsenal against the disease. Other applications of immunological knowledge against cancer include the use of monoclonal antibodies (proteins that seek and directly bind to a specific target protein called an antigen. An example is Herceptin, which is a monoclonal antibody used to treat breast and stomach cancer). Moreover, a number of successful cancer vaccines have been developed, most notably the HPV vaccine.

Transplants involve transferring cells, tissues or organs from a donor to a recipient. The most formidable barrier to transplants is the immune system's recognition of the transplanted organs as foreign. Understanding the mechanisms and clinical features of rejection is important in determining a diagnosis, advising treatment and is critical for developing new strategies and drugs to manage transplants and limit the risk of rejection.

Vaccines are agents that teach the body to recognise and defend itself against infections from harmful pathogens, such as bacteria, viruses and parasites. Vaccines provide a sneak 'preview' of a specific pathogen, which stimulates the body's immune system to prepare itself in the event that infection occurs. Vaccines contain a harmless element of the infectious agent that stimulate the immune system to mount a response, beginning with the production of antibodies. Cells responsive to the vaccine proliferate both in order to manufacture antibodies specific to the provoking agent and also to form 'memory cells'. Upon encountering the infectious agent a second time, these memory cells are quickly able to deal with the threat by producing sufficient quantities of antibody. Pathogens inside the body are eventually destroyed, thereby thwarting further infection. Several infectious diseases including smallpox, measles, mumps, rubella, diphtheria, tetanus, whooping cough, tuberculosis and polio are no longer a threat in Europe due to the successful application of vaccines.

Veterinary Immunology

Veterinary immunology is a branch of Immunology dedicated to improving animal health. Like humans, animals also suffer from diseases caused either when organisms try to invade their body, or when their immune system does not function properly. Wild, domestic, and farm animals are commonly exposed to a whole range of dangerous bacteria, viruses and parasites, which threaten their welfare. Animal infections can have widespread effects on human working sectors, like food and agriculture. Moreover, many animal infections can be naturally transmitted across the species barrier to infect humans and vice-versa, a process termed zoonosis. For example, well-studied infections including swine and avian influenza, as well as, malaria and Lyme disease are due to transmission from animals and insects to humans. It is therefore extremely important that these types of diseases are effectively controlled. These measures not only prevent any further transmission to other animals and humans, but also reduce any potentially devastating social and economic consequences.

Immunopathology

Immunopathology (often abbreviated to IP) is what patients experience when they fight an infection. In the context of the Marshall Protocol, immunopathology refers to an increase in one's present symptoms of inflammation, or a return of previous inflammatory symptoms. This is caused by cytokines and endotoxins being released from dying bacteria. Occasionally, immunopathology will consist of a new symptom or abnormal lab value due to the occurrence of subclinical inflammation that has been revealed by the Marshall Protocol (MP). Immunopathology is a necessary part of recovery for most patients. The amount of immunopathology a patient experiences on the Marshall Protocol (MP) is correlated with disease severity. Patients who are less sick will have comparatively less strong immunopathology.

Immunopathology is sometimes used synonymously with "herx" or the "Jarisch-Herxheimer reaction."

Note that three forms of immunopathology are particularly life-threatening and should be handled with an abundance of caution: Cardiac immunopathology, neurological immunopathology, and respiratory immunopathology.

Immunopathology is one's immune system reaction. Symptoms of immunopathology are unique to a patient and can include: fatigue, muscle weakness, rash, headache, photosensitivity, pain anywhere, numbness, nausea, diarrhea, constipation, ringing in the ears, toothache, sinus congestion, nasal stuffiness, fever/chills, flu-like bodyache, cough, irritability, depression, sleep disturbances and "brain fog."

Any symptom, including abnormal lab results, that correlates with MP therapy is most likely due to immunopathology. Patients who are less sick will have comparatively less strong immunopathology.

The increase in symptoms due to immunopathology typically begins 1-24 hours after the minocycline dose and usually dissipates 12-24 hours before the next antibiotic dose. Many patients find that the reaction is strongest on the second day.

As opposed to the disease itself, which progresses over the course of decades, immunopathology symptoms usually flare quickly. However, dramatic waxing and waning of immunopathology does not always happen. An increase in symptoms may be constant.

Immunopathology is sometimes mistaken for an allergy to a MP antibiotic. A number of strategies are available for managing immunopathology.

Expected Symptoms of Immunopathology

When bacteria are killed, endotoxins and cytokines are released at the site of the infection. This contributes to a sense that one's original disease is getting worse. In fact, the increase in symptoms is only temporary. Although these symptoms may be similar to one's disease, unlike disease symptoms, they are a sign that something is being accomplished: the Th1 pathogens are being killed.

As evidenced by high rates of depression and anxiety in the population at large, the brain itself is a frequent site of chronic bacterial infection. One of the challenges of having neurological immunopathology is a lack of awareness about the role infection and immunopathology play in one's mood, cognitive abilities, and ability to think clearly. It is very common for patients with neurological immunopathology not to recognize that their recovery will involve the temporary exacerbation of these types of symptoms. One's life events play a role in, say, depression, but often enough they are not the driving force behind it.

Along with neurological immunopathology, cardiac immunopathology and respiratory immunopathology are potentially life-threatening. Patients who have, or worry that they may have, these symptoms should work particularly closely with their physician and proceed on the MP cautiously.

Unexpected Symptoms of Immunopathology

The MP can't create new inflammation because it can't make bacteria appear where there weren't any before. The presence of new symptoms is a clear indication that bacteria are being targeted in areas of the body not known to be infected. In the absence of undergoing some kind of curative therapy like the MP, it seems probable that these sites of sub-clinical infection would in time be part of the disease process.

If extra Benicar reduces a symptom, one can be sure it is due to immunopathology. But, lack of response to Benicar does not rule out immunopathology. Palliative medication may reduce symptoms of immunopathology also.

Necessity of Immunopathology

Immunopathology is not a "side effect" of the MP – not in the traditional sense anyway. Also, the MP does not "cause" an exacerbation of disease symptoms. Patients are hardwired to equate symptoms with disease, but what many do not realize is that all disease symptoms are the result of an immune system response.

A rise in intensity of symptoms is not a sign that the disease process is advancing, but an indication that the immune system is active and killing bacteria. If a person gets infected with a virus, the rise in symptoms he or she displays is not caused by the virus, but the response of the immune system to the virus. The symptoms of food poisoning including diarrhea and vomiting are very unpleasant, but are extremely effective in rapidly eliminating toxins.

The Jarisch-Herxheimer response, a term which is sometimes used interchangeably with immunopathology, has been documented as necessary to recovery in over 10 diseases, to say nothing of evidence supporting the MP's effectiveness.

A potent anti-inflammatory, Benicar should palliate negative symptoms and minimize any tissue damage caused by the disease process.

Assessing Immunopathology

Immunopathology is necessary for making progress on the MP. Throughout the course of one's treatment, the goal is to generate a tolerable level of immunopathology. But how does one determine if immunopathology is tolerable or intolerable?

Using Lab Tests to Track Immunopathology

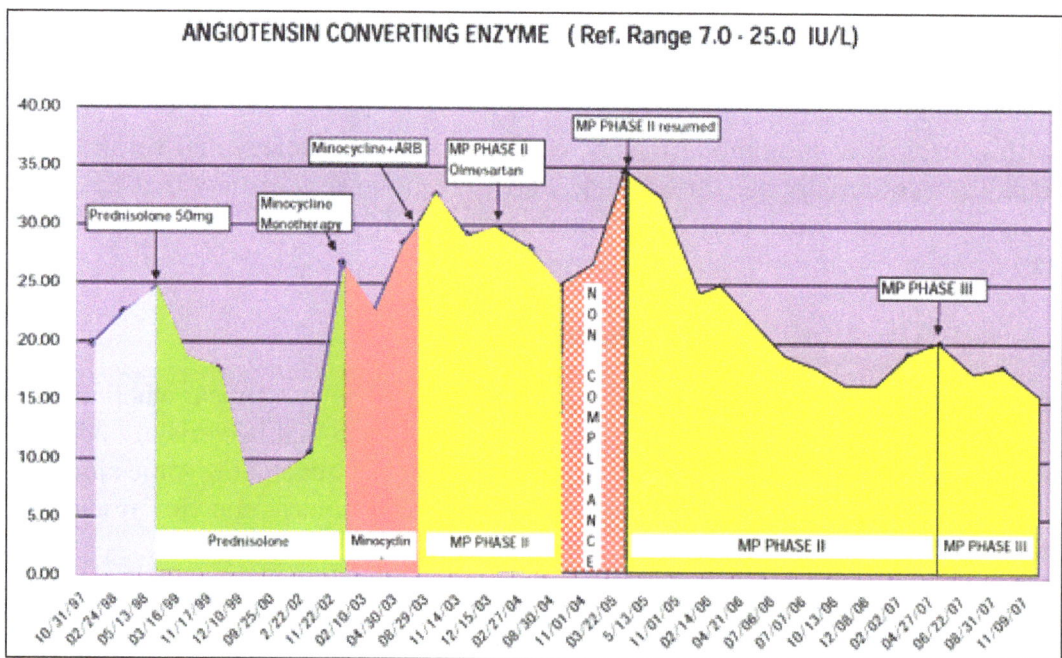

ACE (Angiotensin Converting Enzyme) is a marker, which reflects
the severity of inflammatory diseases such as sarcoidosis.

In this graphic, taken from a patient interview on Bacteriality, it's possible to see how one patient's ACE, waxed and waned over the course of the MP. Note that the ACE continued to fall.

Abnormal lab work or ECG tracing may reveal unacceptable "silent" immunopathology. In that case, monitor these signs regularly and use them as a guide to gauge pace of therapy.

Other ways to Assess Immunopathology

Even for diseases that have ideal measures for tracking immunopathology, it is sometimes possible to have a flare in symptoms and not know why. This is particularly true for patients whose diseases have a strong mental component and have trouble thinking critically about their illness. Sometimes the onset of uncomfortable symptoms simply cannot be explained, only managed. Other times though, it is a factor within a patient's control. These questions might help patients gain insight into why they feel worse.

Immune System 2

- **Innate Immune System**
- **Adaptive Immune System**
- **Complement System**
- **Lymphatic System**
- **White Blood Cell**
- **Innate Lymphoid Cell**
- **Cytokine**

The host defense system which consists of various biological structures and processes that protects an organism against diseases is known as the immune system. There are two major subsystems within immune system, namely, innate immune system and adaptive immune system. The topics elaborated in this chapter will help in gaining a better perspective about immune system, its components and its types.

The immune system is made up of special organs, cells and chemicals that fight infection (microbes). The main parts of the immune system are: white blood cells, antibodies, the complement system, the lymphatic system, the spleen, the thymus, and the bone marrow. These are the parts of your immune system that actively fight infection.

Immune System and Microbial Infection

The immune system keeps a record of every microbe it has ever defeated, in types of white blood cells (B- and T-lymphocytes) known as memory cells. This means it can recognise and destroy the microbe quickly if it enters the body again, before it can multiply and make you feel sick.

Some infections, like the flu and the common cold, have to be fought many times because so many different viruses or strains of the same type of virus can cause these illnesses. Catching a cold or flu from one virus does not give you immunity against the others.

Parts of the Immune System

The main parts of the immune system are:

- White blood cells;

- Antibodies;

- Complement system;

- Lymphatic system;

- Spleen;

- Bone marrow;

- Thymus.

White Blood Cells

White blood cells are the key players in your immune system. They are made in your bone marrow and are part of the lymphatic system.

White blood cells move through blood and tissue throughout your body, looking for foreign invaders (microbes) such as bacteria, viruses, parasites and fungi. When they find them, they launch an immune attack.

White blood cells include lymphocytes (such as B-cells, T-cells and natural killer cells), and many other types of immune cells.

Antibodies

Antibodies help the body to fight microbes or the toxins (poisons) they produce. They do this by recognising substances called antigens on the surface of the microbe, or in the chemicals they produce, which mark the microbe or toxin as being foreign. The antibodies then mark these antigens for destruction. There are many cells, proteins and chemicals involved in this attack.

Complement System

The complement system is made up of proteins whose actions complement the work done by antibodies.

Lymphatic System

The lymphatic system is a network of delicate tubes throughout the body. The main roles of the lymphatic system are to:

- Manage the fluid levels in the body;

- React to bacteria;

- Deal with cancer cells;

- Deal with cell products that otherwise would result in disease or disorders;

- Absorb some of the fats in our diet from the intestine.

The lymphatic system is made up of:

- Lymph nodes (also called lymph glands) - which trap microbes;
- Lymph vessels - tubes that carry lymph, the colourless fluid that bathes your body's tissues and contains infection-fighting white blood cells;
- White blood cells (lymphocytes).

Spleen

The spleen is a blood-filtering organ that removes microbes and destroys old or damaged red blood cells. It also makes disease-fighting components of the immune system (including antibodies and lymphocytes).

Bone Marrow

Bone marrow is the spongy tissue found inside your bones. It produces the red blood cells our bodies need to carry oxygen, the white blood cells we use to fight infection, and the platelets we need to help our blood clot.

Thymus

The thymus filters and monitors your blood content. It produces the white blood cells called T-lymphocytes.

Body's other Defences Against Microbes

As well as the immune system, the body has several other ways to defend itself against microbes, including:

- Skin: A waterproof barrier that secretes oil with bacteria-killing properties;
- Lungs: Mucous in the lungs (phlegm) traps foreign particles, and small hairs (cilia) wave the mucous upwards so it can be coughed out;
- Digestive tract: The mucous lining contains antibodies, and the acid in the stomach can kill most microbes;
- Other defences: Body fluids like skin oil, saliva and tears contain anti-bacterial enzymes that help reduce the risk of infection. The constant flushing of the urinary tract and the bowel also helps.

Fever is an Immune System Response

A rise in body temperature, or fever, can happen with some infections. This is actually an immune system response. A rise in temperature can kill some microbes. Fever also triggers the body's repair process.

Common Disorders of the Immune System

It is common for people to have an over- or underactive immune system.

Overactivity of the immune system can take many forms, including:

- Allergic diseases: Where the immune system makes an overly strong response to allergens. Allergic diseases are very common. They include allergies to foods, medications or stinging insects, anaphylaxis (life-threatening allergy), hay fever (allergic rhinitis), sinus disease, asthma, hives (urticaria), dermatitis and eczema.

- Autoimmune diseases: Where the immune system mounts a response against normal components of the body. Autoimmune diseases range from common to rare. They include multiple sclerosis, autoimmune thyroid disease, type 1 diabetes, systemic lupus erythematosus, rheumatoid arthritis and systemic vasculitis.

Underactivity of the immune system, also called immunodeficiency, can:

- Be inherited: Examples of these conditions include primary immunodeficiency diseases such as common variable immunodeficiency (CVID), x-linked severe combined immunodeficiency (SCID) and complement deficiencies.

- Arise as a result of medical treatment: This can occur due to medications such as corticosteroids or chemotherapy.

- Be caused by another disease: Such as HIV/AIDS or certain types of cancer.

An underactive immune system does not function correctly and makes people vulnerable to infections. It can be life threatening in severe cases.

People who have had an organ transplant need immunosuppression treatment to prevent the body from attacking the transplanted organ.

Immunoglobulin Therapy

Immunoglobulins (commonly known as antibodies) are used to treat people who are unable to make enough of their own, or whose antibodies do not work properly. This treatment is known as immunoglobulin therapy.

Until recently, immunoglobulin therapy in Australia mostly involved delivery of immunoglobulins through a drip into the vein – known as intravenous immunoglobulin (IVIg) therapy. Now, subcutaneous immunoglobulin (SCIg) can be delivered into the fatty tissue under the skin, which may offer benefits for some patients. This is known as subcutaneous infusion or SCIg therapy.

Subcutaneous immunoglobulin is similar to intravenous immunoglobulin. It is made from plasma – the liquid part of blood containing important proteins like antibodies.

Many health services are now offering SCIg therapy to eligible patients with specific immune conditions.

Immunisation

Immunisation works by copying the body's natural immune response. A vaccine (a small amount of a specially treated virus, bacterium or toxin) is injected into the body. The body then makes antibodies to it.

If a vaccinated person is exposed to the actual virus, bacterium or toxin, they won't get sick because their body will recognise it and know how to attack it successfully. Vaccinations are available against many diseases, including measles and tetanus.

The immunisations you may need are decided by your health, age, lifestyle and occupation. Together, these factors are referred to as HALO, which is defined as:

- Health: Some health conditions or factors may make you more vulnerable to vaccine-preventable diseases. For example, premature birth, asthma, diabetes, heart, lung, spleen or kidney conditions, Down syndrome and HIV will mean you may benefit from additional or more frequent immunisations.

- Age: At different ages you need protection from different vaccine-preventable diseases. Australia's National Immunisation Program sets out recommended immunisations for babies, children, older people and other people at risk, such as Aboriginal and Torres Strait Islanders. Most recommended vaccines are available at no cost to these groups.

- Lifestyle: Lifestyle choices can have an impact on your immunisation needs. Travelling overseas to certain places, planning a family, sexual activity, smoking, and playing contact sport that may expose you directly to someone else's blood, will mean you may benefit from additional or more frequent immunisations.

- Occupation: You are likely to need extra immunisations, or need to have them more often, if you work in an occupation that exposes you to vaccine-preventable diseases or puts you into contact with people who are more susceptible to problems from vaccine-preventable diseases (such as babies or young children, pregnant women, the elderly, and people with chronic or acute health conditions). For example, if you work in aged care, childcare, healthcare, emergency services or sewerage repair and maintenance, discuss your immunisation needs with your doctor.

Innate Immune System

Innate immunity refers to nonspecific defense mechanisms that come into play immediately or within hours of an antigen's appearance in the body. These mechanisms include physical barriers such as skin, chemicals in the blood, and immune system cells that attack foreign cells in the body. The innate immune response is activated by chemical properties of the antigen. Innate immune responses are not specific to a particular pathogen in the way that the adaptive immune responses are. They depend on a group of proteins and phagocytic cells that recognize conserved features of pathogens and become quickly activated to help destroy invaders. Whereas the adaptive immune system arose in evolution less than 500 million years ago and is confined to vertebrates, innate immune responses have been found among both vertebrates and invertebrates, as well as in plants, and the basic mechanisms that regulate them are conserved. The innate immune responses in vertebrates are also required to activate adaptive immune responses.

Epithelial Surfaces Help Prevent Infection

In vertebrates, the skin and other epithelial surfaces, including those lining the lung and gut provide a physical barrier between the inside of the body and the outside world. Tight junctions between neighboring cells prevent easy entry by potential pathogens. The interior epithelial surfaces are also covered with a mucus layer that protects these surfaces against microbial, mechanical, and chemical insults; many amphibians and fish also have a mucus layer covering their skin. The slimy mucus coating is made primarily of secreted mucin and other glycoproteins, and it physically helps prevent pathogens from adhering to the epithelium. It also facilitates their clearance by beating cilia on the epithelial cells.

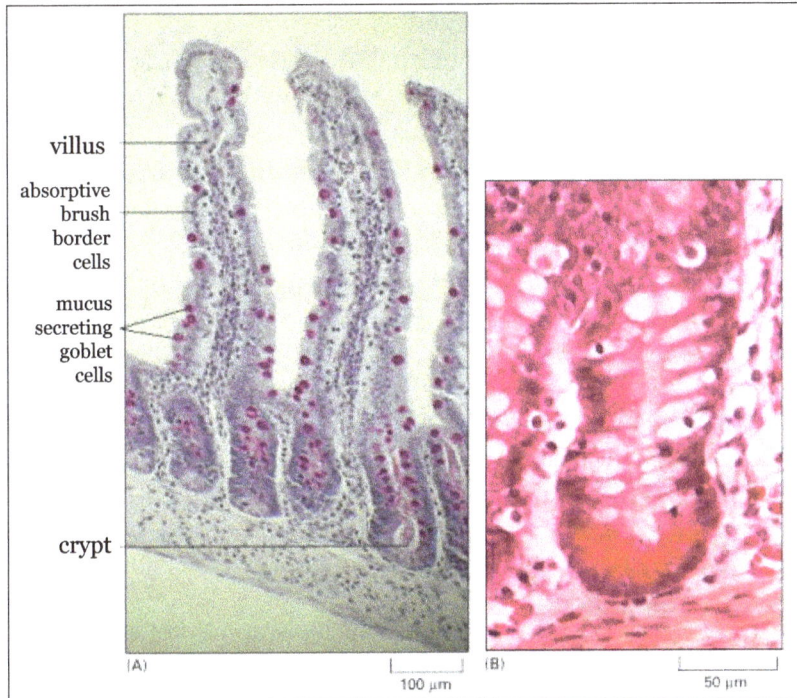

Figure: Epithelial defenses against microbial invasion.

(A) Cross section through the wall of the human small intestine, showing three villi. Goblet cells secreting mucus are stained magenta. The protective mucus layer covers the exposed surfaces of the villi. At the base of the villi lie the crypts where the epithelial cells proliferate. (B) Close-up view of a crypt, stained using a method that renders the granules in the Paneth cells scarlet. These cells secrete large quantities of antimicrobial peptides and defensins into the intestinal lumen.

The mucus layer also contains substances that kill pathogens or inhibit their growth. Among the most abundant of these are antimicrobial peptides, called defensins, which are found in all animals and plants. They are generally short (12–50 amino acids), positively charged, and have hydrophobic or amphipathic domains in their folded structure. They constitute a diverse family with a broad spectrum of antimicrobial activity, including the ability to kill or inactivate Gram-negative and Gram-positive bacteria, fungi (including yeasts), parasites (including protozoa and nematodes), and even enveloped viruses like HIV. Defensins are also the most abundant protein type in neutrophils, which use them to kill phagocytosed pathogens.

It is still uncertain how defensins kill pathogens. One possibility is that they use their hydrophobic or amphipathic domains to insert into the membrane of their victims, thereby disrupting membrane integrity. Some of their selectivity for pathogens over host cells may come from their preference for membranes that do not contain cholesterol. After disrupting the membrane of the pathogen, the positively-charged peptides may also interact with various negatively-charged targets within the microbe, including DNA. Because of the relatively nonspecific nature of the interaction between defensins and the microbes they kill, it is difficult for the microbes to acquire resistance to the defensins. Thus, in principle, defensins might be useful therapeutic agents to combat infection, either alone or in combination with more traditional drugs.

Human Cells Recognize Conserved Features of Pathogens

Microorganisms do occasionally breach the epithelial barricades. It is then up to the innate and adaptive immune systems to recognize and destroy them, without harming the host. Consequently, the immune systems must be able to distinguish self from nonself. The innate immune system relies on the recognition of particular types of molecules that are common to many pathogens but are absent in the host. These pathogen-associated molecules (called pathogen-associated immunostimulants) stimulate two types of innate immune responses—inflammatory responses and phagocytosis by cells such as neutrophils and macrophages. Both of these responses can occur quickly, even if the host has never been previously exposed to a particular pathogen.

The pathogen-associated immunostimulants are of various types. Procaryotic translation initiation differs from eucaryotic translation initiation in that formylated methionine, rather than regular methionine, is generally used as the first amino acid. Therefore, any peptide containing formylmethionine at the N-terminus must be of bacterial origin. Formylmethionine-containing peptides act as very potent chemoattractants for neutrophils, which migrate quickly to the source of such peptides and engulf the bacteria that are producing them.

In addition, the outer surface of many microorganisms is composed of molecules that do not occur in their multicellular hosts, and these molecules also act as immunostimulants. They include the peptidoglycan cell wall and flagella of bacteria, as well as lipopolysaccharide (LPS) on Gram-negative bacteria and teichoic acids on Gram-positive bacteria. They also include molecules in the cell walls of fungi such as zymosan, glucan, and chitin. Many parasites also contain unique membrane components that act as immunostimulants, including glycosylphosphatidylinositol in Plasmodium.

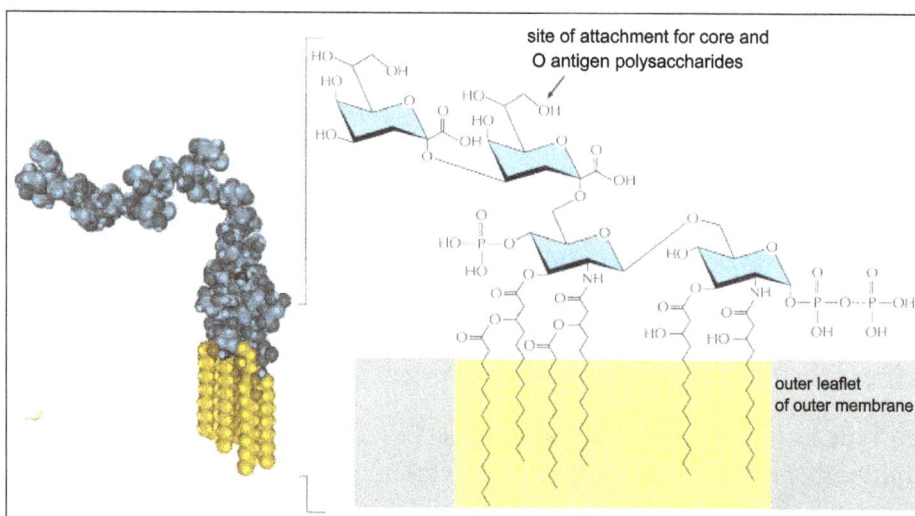

Figure: Structure of lipopolysaccharide (LPS).

The 3-dimensional structure of a molecule of LPS with the fatty acids shown in yellow and the sugars in blue. The molecular structure of the base of LPS is shown on the right. The hydrophobic membrane anchor is made up of two linked glucosamine sugars attached to three phosphates and six fatty acid tails. This basic structure is elaborated by attachment of a long, usually highly branched, chain of sugars. This drawing shows the simplest type of LPS that will allow E. coli to live; it has just two sugar molecules in the chain, both 3-deoxy-D-manno-octulosonic acid. At the position marked by the arrow, wild-type Gram-negative bacteria also attach a core saccharide made up of eight to twelve linked sugars and a long O antigen, which is made up of an oligosaccharide unit that is repeated many (up to 40) times. The sugars making up the core saccharide and O antigen vary from one bacterial species to another and even among different strains of the same species. All forms of LPS are highly immunogenic.

Short sequences in bacterial DNA can also act as immunostimulants. The culprit is a "CpG motif", which consists of the unmethylated dinucleotide CpG flanked by two 5′ purine residues and two 3′ pyrimidines. This short sequence is at least twenty times less common in vertebrate DNA than in bacterial DNA, and it can activate macrophages, stimulate an inflammatory response, and increase antibody production by B cells.

The various classes of pathogen-associated immunostimulants often occur on the pathogen surface in repeating patterns. They are recognized by several types of dedicated receptors in the host, that are collectively called pattern recognition receptors. These receptors include soluble receptors in the blood (components of the complement system) and membrane-bound receptors on the surface of host cells (members of the Toll-like receptor family). The cell-surface receptors have two functions: they initiate the phagocytosis of the pathogen, and they stimulate a program of gene expression in the host cell for stimulating innate immune responses. The soluble receptors also aid in the phagocytosis and, in some cases, the direct killing of the pathogen.

Complement Activation Targets Pathogens for Phagocytosis or Lysis

The complement system consists of about 20 interacting soluble proteins that are made mainly by the liver and circulate in the blood and extracellular fluid. Most are inactive until they are triggered by an infection. They were originally identified by their ability to amplify and "complement" the action of antibodies, but some components of complement are also pattern recognition receptors that can be activated directly by pathogen-associated immunostimulants.

The early complement components are activated first. There are three sets of these, belonging to three distinct pathways of complement activation—the classical pathway, the lectin pathway, and the alternative pathway. The early components of all three pathways act locally to activate C3, which is the pivotal component of complement. Individuals with a deficiency in C3 are subject to repeated bacterial infections. The early components and C3 are all proenzymes, which are activated sequentially by proteolytic cleavage. The cleavage of each proenzyme in the series activates the next component to generate a serine protease, which cleaves the next proenzyme in the series, and so on. Since each activated enzyme cleaves many molecules of the next proenzyme in the chain, the activation of the early components consists of an amplifying, proteolytic cascade.

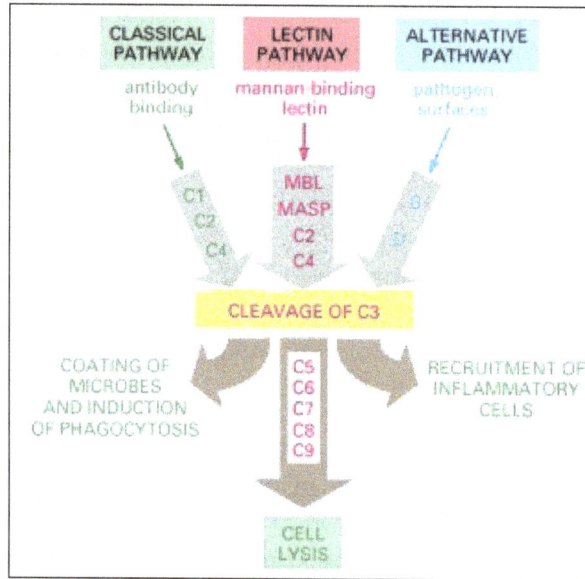

Figure: The principal stages in complement activation by the classical, lectin, and alternative pathways.

In all three pathways, the reactions of complement activation usually take place on the surface of an invading microbe, such as a bacterium. C1–C9 and factors B and D are the reacting components of the complement system; various other components regulate the system. The early components are shown within gray arrows, while the late components are shown within a brown arrow.

Many of these cleavages liberate a biologically active small peptide fragment and a membrane-binding larger fragment. The binding of the large fragment to a cell membrane, usually the surface of a pathogen, helps to carry out the next reaction in the sequence. In this way, complement activation is confined largely to the particular cell surface where it began. The larger fragment of C3, called C3b, binds covalently to the surface of the pathogen. Once in place, it not only acts as a protease to catalyze the subsequent steps in the complement cascade, but it also is recognized by specific receptors on phagocytic cells that enhance the ability of these cells to phagocytose the pathogen. The smaller fragment of C3 (called C3a), as well as fragments of C4 and C5, act independently as diffusible signals to promote an inflammatory response by recruiting phagocytes and lymphocytes to the site of infection.

The classical pathway is activated by IgG or IgM antibody molecules bound to the surface of a microbe. Mannan-binding lectin, the protein that initiates the second pathway of complement activation, is a serum protein that forms clusters of six carbohydrate-binding heads around a central collagen-like stalk. This assembly binds specifically to mannose and fucose residues in bacterial cell walls that have the correct spacing and orientation to match up perfectly with the six carbohydrate-binding sites, providing a good example of a pattern recognition receptor. These initial binding events in the classical and lectin pathways cause the recruitment and activation of the early complement components. In the alternative pathway, C3 is spontaneously activated at low levels, and the resulting C3b covalently attaches to both host cells and pathogens. Host cells produce a series of proteins that prevent the complement reaction from proceeding on their cell surfaces. Because pathogens lack these proteins, they are singled out for destruction. Activation of the classical or lectin pathways also activates the alternative pathway through a positive feedback loop, amplifying their effects.

Membrane-immobilized C3b, produced by any of the three pathways, triggers a further cascade of reactions that leads to the assembly of the late components to form membrane attack complexes. These complexes assemble in the pathogen membrane near the site of C3 activation and have a characteristic appearance in negatively stained electron micrographs, where they are seen to form aqueous pores through the membrane. For this reason, and because they perturb the structure of the bilayer in their vicinity, they make the membrane leaky and can, in some cases, cause the microbial cell to lyse, much like the defensins mentioned earlier.

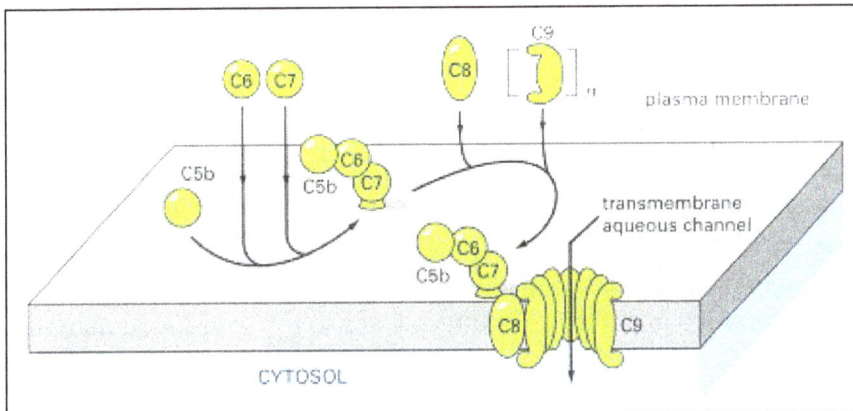

Figure: Assembly of the late complement components to form a membrane attack complex.

When C3b is produced by any of the three activation pathways, it is immobilized on a membrane, where it causes the cleavage of the first of the late components, C5, to produce C5a and C5b. C5b remains loosely bound to C3b and rapidly assembles with C6 and C7 to form C567, which then binds firmly via C7 to the membrane, as illustrated. To this complex is added one molecule of C8 to form C5678. The binding of a molecule of C9 to C5678 induces a conformational change in C9 that exposes a hydrophobic region and causes C9 to insert into the lipid bilayer of the target cell. This starts a chain reaction in which the altered C9 binds a second molecule of C9, where it can bind another molecule of C9, and so on. In this way, a large transmembrane channel is formed by a chain of C9 molecules.

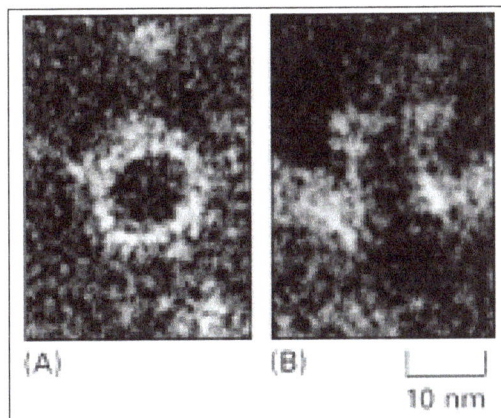

Figure: Electron micrographs of negatively stained complement lesions in the plasma membrane of a red blood cell.

The lesion in (A) is seen en face, while that in (B) is seen from the side as an apparent transmembrane channel. The negative stain fills the channels, which therefore look black.

The self-amplifying, inflammatory, and destructive properties of the complement cascade make it essential that key activated components be rapidly inactivated after they are generated to ensure that the attack does not spread to nearby host cells. Deactivation is achieved in at least two ways. First, specific inhibitor proteins in the blood or on the surface of host cells terminate the cascade, by either binding or cleaving certain components once they have been activated by proteolytic cleavage. Second, many of the activated components in the cascade are unstable; unless they bind immediately to either an appropriate component in the cascade or to a nearby membrane, they rapidly become inactive.

Toll-like Proteins are an Ancient Family of Pattern Recognition Receptors

Many of the mammalian cell-surface pattern recognition receptors responsible for triggering host cell gene expression in response to pathogens are members of the Toll-like receptor (TLR) family. Drosophila Toll is a transmembrane protein with a large extracellular domain consisting of a series of leucine-rich repeats. It was originally identified as a protein involved in the establishment of dorso-ventral polarity in developing fly embryos. It is also involved, however, in the adult fly's resistance to fungal infections. The intracellular signal transduction pathway activated downstream of Toll when a fly is exposed to a pathogenic fungus leads to the translocation of the NF-κB protein into the nucleus, where it activates the transcription of various genes, including those encoding antifungal defensins. Another member of the Toll family in Drosophila is activated by exposure to pathogenic bacteria, leading to the production of an antibacterial defensin.

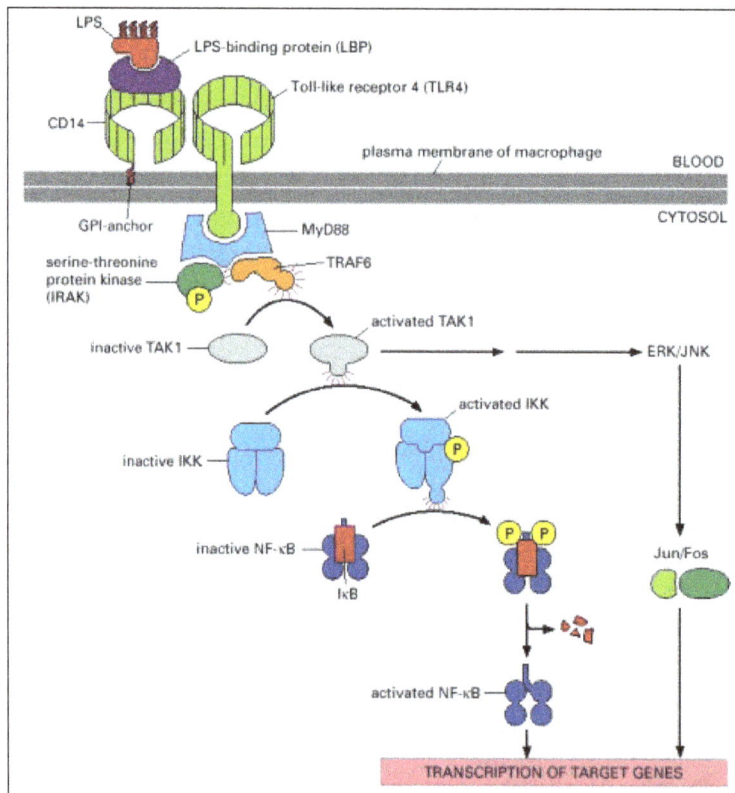

Figure: The activation of a macrophage by lipopolysaccharide (LPS).

LPS is bound by LPS-binding protein (LBP) in the blood, and the complex binds to the GPI-anchored receptor CD14 on the macrophage surface. The ternary complex then activates Toll-like receptor 4

(TLR4). Activated TLR4 recruits the adaptor protein MyD88, which interacts with the serine-threonine protein kinase IRAK. Recruitment of IRAK to the activated receptor complex results in its autophosphorylation and association with another adaptor protein, TRAF6. TRAF6, in turn, associates with and activates a MAP kinase kinase kinase, TAK1. Via several intermediate steps, TAK1 activation leads to the phosphorylation and activation of the IκB kinase (IKK). IKK phosphorylates the NF-κB inhibitor, IκB, inducing its degradation and releasing NF-κB. By way of additional MAP kinases (ERK and JNK), TAK1 also activates the AP-1 transcription family members Jun and Fos, which, together with NF-κB, activate the transcription of genes that promote immune and inflammatory responses.

Humans have at least ten TLRs, several of which have been shown to play important parts in innate immune recognition of pathogen-associated immunostimulants, including lipopolysaccharide, peptidoglycan, zymosan, bacterial flagella, and CpG DNA. As with Drosophila Toll family members, the different human TLRs are activated in response to different ligands, although many of them use the NF-κB signaling pathway. In mammals, TLR activation stimulates the expression of molecules that both initiate an inflammatory response and help induce adaptive immune responses. TLRs are abundant on the surface of macrophages and neutrophils, as well as on the epithelial cells lining the lung and gut. They act as an alarm system to alert both the innate and adaptive immune systems that an infection is brewing.

Molecules related to Toll and TLRs are apparently involved in innate immunity in all multicellular organisms. In plants, proteins with leucine-rich repeats and with domains homologous to the cytosolic portion of the TLRs are required for resistance to fungal, bacterial, and viral pathogens. Thus, at least two parts of the innate immune system—the defensins and the TLRs—seem to be evolutionarily very ancient, perhaps predating the split between animals and plants over a billion years ago. Their conservation during evolution indicates the importance of these innate responses in the defense against microbial pathogens.

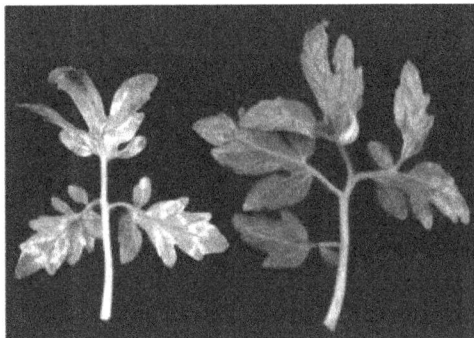

Figure: Microbial disease in a plant.

These tomato leaves are infected with the leaf mold fungus Cladosporium fulvum. Resistance to this type of infection depends on recognition of a fungal protein by a host receptor that is structurally related to the TLRs.

Phagocytic Cells Seek, Engulf and Destroy Pathogens

In all animals, invertebrate as well as vertebrate, the recognition of a microbial invader is usually quickly followed by its engulfment by a phagocytic cell. Plants, however, lack this type of innate immune response. In vertebrates, macrophages reside in tissues throughout the body and are especially abundant in areas where infections are likely to arise, including the lungs and gut. They are also present in large numbers in connective tissues, the liver, and the spleen. These long-lived cells patrol the tissues of the body and are among the first cells to encounter invading microbes. The second major family of phagocytic cells in vertebrates, the neutrophils, are short-lived cells, which are abundant in blood but are not present in normal, healthy tissues. They are rapidly recruited to sites of infection both by activated macrophages and by molecules such as formylmethionine-containing peptides released by the microbes themselves.

Macrophages and neutrophils display a variety of cell-surface receptors that enable them to recognize and engulf pathogens. These include pattern recognition receptors such as TLRs. In addition, they have cell-surface receptors for the Fc portion of antibodies produced by the adaptive immune system, as well as for the C3b component of complement. Ligand binding to any of these receptors induces actin polymerization at the site of pathogen attachment, causing the phagocyte's plasma membrane to surround the pathogen and engulf it in a large membrane-enclosed phagosome.

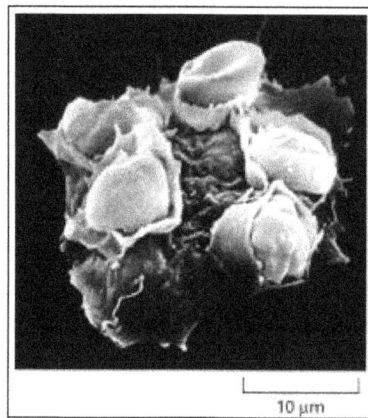

Phagocytosis

This scanning electron micrograph shows a macrophage in the midst of consuming five red blood cells that have been coated with an antibody against a surface glycoprotein.

Once the pathogen has been phagocytosed, the macrophage or neutrophil unleashes an impressive armory of weapons to kill it. The phagosome is acidified and fuses with lysosomes, which contain lysozyme and acid hydrolases that can degrade bacterial cell walls and proteins. The lysosomes also contain defensins, which make up about 15% of the total protein in neutrophils. In addition, the phagocytes assemble an NADPH oxidase complex on the phagosomal membrane that catalyzes the production of a series of highly toxic oxygen-derived compounds, including superoxide (O_2^-), hypochlorite (HOCl, the active ingredient in bleach), hydrogen peroxide, hydroxyl radicals, and nitric oxide (NO). The production of these toxic compounds is accompanied by a transient increase in oxygen consumption by the cells, called the respiratory burst. Whereas macrophages will generally survive this killing frenzy and continue to patrol tissues for other pathogens, neutrophils usually die. Dead and dying neutrophils are a major component of the pus that forms in acutely infected wounds. The distinctive greenish tint of pus is due to the abundance in neutrophils of the copper-containing enzyme myeloperoxidase, which is one of the components active in the respiratory burst.

If a pathogen is too large to be successfully phagocytosed (if it is a large parasite such as a nematode, for example), a group of macrophages, neutrophils, or eosinophils will gather around the invader. They will secrete their defensins and other lysosomal products by exocytosis and will also release the toxic products of the respiratory burst. This barrage is generally sufficient to destroy the pathogen.

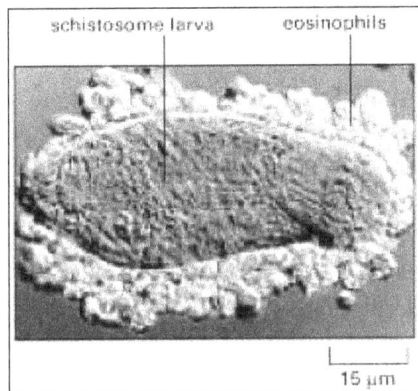

Figure: Eosinophils attacking a schistosome larva.

Large parasites, such as worms, cannot be ingested by phagocytes. When the worm is coated with antibody or complement, however, eosinophils and other white blood cells can recognize and attack it.

Many pathogens have developed strategies that allow them to avoid being ingested by phagocytes. Some Gram-positive bacteria coat themselves with a very thick, slimy polysaccharide coat, or capsule, that is not recognized by complement or any phagocyte receptor. Other pathogens are phagocytosed but avoid being killed; Mycobacterium tuberculosis prevents the maturation of the phagosome and thereby survives. Some pathogens escape the phagosome entirely, and yet others secrete enzymes that detoxify the products of the respiratory burst. For such wily pathogens, these first lines of defense are insufficient to clear the infection, and adaptive immune responses are required to contain them.

Activated Macrophages Recruit Additional Phagocytic Cells to Sites of Infection

When a pathogen invades a tissue, it almost always elicits an inflammatory response. This response is characterized by pain, redness, heat, and swelling at the site of infection, all caused by changes in local blood vessels. The blood vessels dilate and become permeable to fluid and proteins, leading to local swelling and an accumulation of blood proteins that aid in defense, including the components of the complement cascade. At the same time, the endothelial cells lining the local blood vessels are stimulated to express cell adhesion proteins that facilitate the attachment and extravasation of white blood cells, including neutrophils, lymphocytes, and monocytes (the precursors of macrophages).

The inflammatory response is mediated by a variety of signaling molecules. Activation of TLRs results in the production of both lipid signaling molecules such as prostaglandins and protein (or peptide) signaling molecules such as cytokines, all of which contribute to the inflammatory response. The proteolytic release of complement fragments also contribute. Some of the cytokines produced by activated macrophages are chemoattractants (known as chemokines). Some of these attract neutrophils, which are the first cells recruited in large numbers to the site of the new infection. Others later attract monocytes and dendritic cells. The dendritic cells pick up antigens from the invading pathogens and carry them to nearby lymph nodes, where they present the antigens to lymphocytes to marshal the forces of the adaptive immune system. Other cytokines trigger fever, a rise in body temperature. On balance, fever helps the immune system in the fight against infection, since most bacterial and viral pathogens grow better at lower temperatures, whereas adaptive immune responses are more potent at higher temperatures.

Some proinflammatory signaling molecules stimulate endothelial cells to express proteins that trigger blood clotting in local small vessels. By occluding the vessels and cutting off blood flow, this response can help prevent the pathogen from entering the bloodstream and spreading the infection to other parts of the body.

The same inflammatory responses, however, which are so effective at controlling local infections, can have disastrous consequences when they occur in a disseminated infection in the bloodstream, a condition called sepsis. The systemic release of proinflammatory signaling molecules into the blood causes dilation of blood vessels, loss of plasma volume, and widespread blood clotting, which is an often fatal condition known as septic shock. Inappropriate or overzealous inflammatory responses are also associated with some chronic conditions, such as asthma.

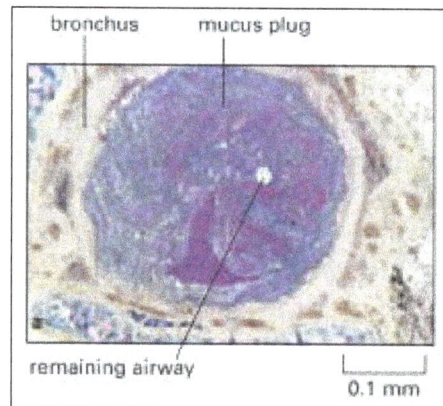

Figure: Inflammation of the airways in chronic asthma restricts breathing.

Light micrograph of a section through the bronchus of a patient who died of asthma. There is almost total occlusion of the airway by a mucus plug. The mucus plug is a dense inflammatory infiltrate that includes eosinophils, neutrophils, and lymphocytes.

Just as with phagocytosis, some pathogens have developed mechanisms to either prevent the inflammatory response or, in some cases, take advantage of it to spread the infection. Many viruses, for example, encode potent cytokine antagonists that block aspects of the inflammatory response. Some of these are simply modified forms of cytokine receptors, encoded by genes acquired by the viral genome from the host. They bind the cytokines with high affinity and block their activity. Some bacteria, such as Salmonella, induce an inflammatory response in the gut at the initial site of infection, thereby recruiting macrophages and neutrophils that they then invade. In this way, the bacteria hitch a ride to other tissues in the body.

Virus-infected Cells take Drastic Measures to Prevent Viral Replication

The pathogen-associated immunostimulants on the surface of bacteria and parasites that are so important in eliciting innate immune responses are generally not present on the surface of viruses. Viral proteins are constructed by the host cell ribosomes, and the membranes of enveloped viruses are composed of host cell lipids. The only unusual molecule associated with viruses is the double-stranded RNA (dsRNA) that is an intermediate in the life cycle of many viruses. Host cells can detect the presence of dsRNA and initiate a program of drastic responses in attempt to eliminate it.

The program occurs in two steps. First, the cells degrade the dsRNA into small fragments (about 21–25 nucleotide pairs in length). These fragments bind to any single-stranded RNA (ssRNA) in the host cell with the same sequence as either strand of the dsRNA fragment, leading to the destruction of the ssRNA. This dsRNA-directed ssRNA destruction is the basis of the technique of RNA interference (RNAi) that is used by researchers to block specific gene expression. Second, the dsRNA induces the host cell to produce and secrete two cytokines—interferon α (IFN-α) and interferon β (IFN-β), which act in both an autocrine fashion on the infected cell and a paracrine fashion on uninfected neighbors. The binding of the interferons to their cell-surface receptors stimulates specific gene transcription by the Jak/STAT intracellular signaling pathway, leading to the activation of a latent ribonuclease, which nonspecifically degrades ssRNA. It also leads to the activation of a protein kinase that phosphorylates and inactivates the protein synthesis initiation factor eIF-2, shutting down most protein synthesis in the embattled host cell. Apparently, by destroying most of the RNA it contains and transiently halting most protein synthesis, the cell inhibits viral replication without killing itself. In some cases, however, a cell infected with a virus is persuaded by white blood cells to destroy itself to prevent the virus from replicating.

Natural Killer Cells Induce Virus-infected Cells to Kill Themselves

Another way that the interferons help vertebrates defend themselves against viruses is by stimulating both innate and adaptive cellular immune responses. Here, we consider how interferons enhance the activity of natural killer cells (NK cells), which are part of the innate immune system. Like cytotoxic T cells, NK cells destroy virus-infected cells by inducing the infected cell to kill itself by undergoing apoptosis. Unlike T cells, however, NK cells do not express antigen-specific receptors. How, then, do they distinguish virus-infected cells from uninfected cells.

NK cells monitor the level of class I MHC proteins, which are expressed on the surface of most vertebrate cells. The presence of high levels of these proteins inhibits the killing activity of NK cells, so that the NK cells selectively kill cells expressing low levels, including both virally-infected cells and some cancer cells. Many viruses have developed mechanisms to inhibit the expression of class I MHC molecules on the surface of the cells they infect, in order to avoid detection by cytotoxic T lymphocytes. Adenovirus and HIV, for example, encode proteins that block class I MHC gene transcription. Herpes simplex virus and cytomegalovirus block the peptide translocators in the ER membrane that transport proteasome-derived peptides from the cytosol into the lumen of the ER; such peptides are required for newly-made class I MHC proteins to assemble in the ER membrane and be transported through the Golgi apparatus to the cell surface.

Cytomegalovirus causes the retrotranslocation of class I MHC proteins from the ER membrane into the cytosol, where they are rapidly degraded by proteasomes. Proteins encoded by still other viruses prevent the delivery of assembled class I MHC proteins from the ER to the Golgi apparatus, or from the Golgi apparatus to the plasma membrane. By evading recognition by cytotoxic T cells in these ways, however, a virus incurs the wrath of NK cells. The local production of IFN-α and IFN-β activates the killing activity of NK cells and also increases the expression of class I MHC proteins in uninfected cells. The cells infected with a virus that blocks class I MHC expression are thereby exposed and become the victims of the activated NK cells. Thus, it is difficult or impossible for viruses to hide from both the innate and adaptive immune systems simultaneously.

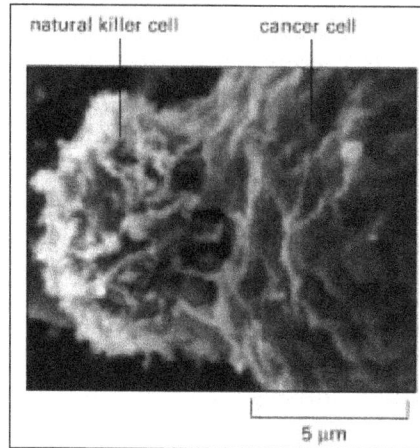

Figure: Natural killer (NK) cell attacking a cancer cell.

The NK cell is the smaller cell on the left. This scanning electron micrograph was taken shortly after the NK cell attached, but before it induced the cancer cell to kill itself.

Both NK cells and cytotoxic T lymphocytes kill infected target cells by inducing them to undergo apoptosis before the virus has had a chance to replicate. It is not surprising, then, that many viruses have acquired mechanisms to inhibit apoptosis, particularly early in infection. apoptosis depends on an intracellular proteolytic cascade, which the cytotoxic cell can trigger either through the activation of cell-surface death receptors or by injecting a proteolytic enzyme into the target cell. Viral proteins can interfere with nearly every step in these pathways. In some cases, however, viruses encode proteins that act late in their replication cycle to induce apoptosis in the host cell, thereby releasing progeny virus that can infect neighboring cells.

The battle between pathogens and host defenses is remarkably balanced. At present, humans seem to be gaining a slight advantage, using public sanitation measures, vaccines, and drugs to aid the efforts of our innate and adaptive immune systems. However, infectious and parasitic diseases are still the leading cause of death worldwide, and new epidemics such as AIDS continue to emerge. The rapid evolution of pathogens and the almost infinite variety of ways that they can invade the human body and elude immune responses will prevent us from ever winning the battle completely.

Adaptive Immune System

The adaptive immune system, also known as the acquired immune system or, more rarely, as the specific immune system, is a subsystem of the overall immune system that is composed of highly specialized, systemic cells and processes that eliminate pathogens or prevent their growth. The acquired immune system is one of the two main immunity strategies found in vertebrates (the other being the innate immune system).

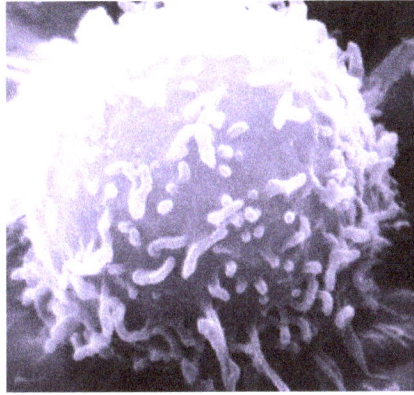

A scanning electron microscope image of a single human lymphocyte.

Acquired immunity creates immunological memory after an initial response to a specific pathogen, and leads to an enhanced response to subsequent encounters with that pathogen. This process of acquired immunity is the basis of vaccination. Like the innate system, the acquired system includes both humoral immunity components and cell-mediated immunity components.

The term "adaptive" was first used by Robert Good in reference to antibody responses in frogs as a synonym for "acquired immune response" in 1964. Good acknowledged he used the terms as synonyms but explained only that he "preferred" to use the term "adaptive". He might have been thinking of the then not implausible theory of antibody formation in which antibodies were plastic and could adapt themselves to the molecular shape of antigens, and/or to the concept of "adaptive enzymes" as described by Monod in bacteria, that is, enzymes whose expression could be induced by their substrates. The phrase was used almost exclusively by Good and his students and a few other immunologists working with marginal organisms until the 1990s when it became widely used in tandem with the term "innate immunity" which became a popular subject after the discovery of the Toll receptor system in *Drosophila*, a previously marginal organism for the study of immunology. The term "adaptive" as used in immunology is problematic as acquired immune responses can be both adaptive and maladaptive in the physiological sense. Indeed, both acquired and innate immune responses can be both adaptive and maladaptive in the evolutionary sense. Most textbooks today, following the early use by Janeway, use "adaptive" almost exclusively and noting in glossaries that the term is synonymous with "acquired".

The classic sense of "acquired immunity" came to mean, since Tonegawas's discovery, "antigen-specific immunity mediated by somatic gene rearrangements that create clone-defining antigen receptors". In the last decade, the term "adaptive" has been increasingly applied to another class of immune response not so-far associated with somatic gene rearrangements. These include expansion of natural killer (NK) cells with so-far unexplained specificity for antigens, expansion of NK cells expressing germ-line encoded receptors, and activation of other innate immune cells to an activated state that confers a short-term "immune memory". In this sense, "adaptive immunity" more closely resembles the concept of "activated state" or "heterostasis", thus returning in sense to the physiological sense of "adaptation" to environmental changes.

Google Ngram of "acquired immunity " vs. "adaptive immunity". The peak for "adaptive" in the 1960s reflects its introduction to immunology by Robert A. Good and use by colleagues; the explosive increase in the 1990s was correlated with the use of the phrase "innate immunity".

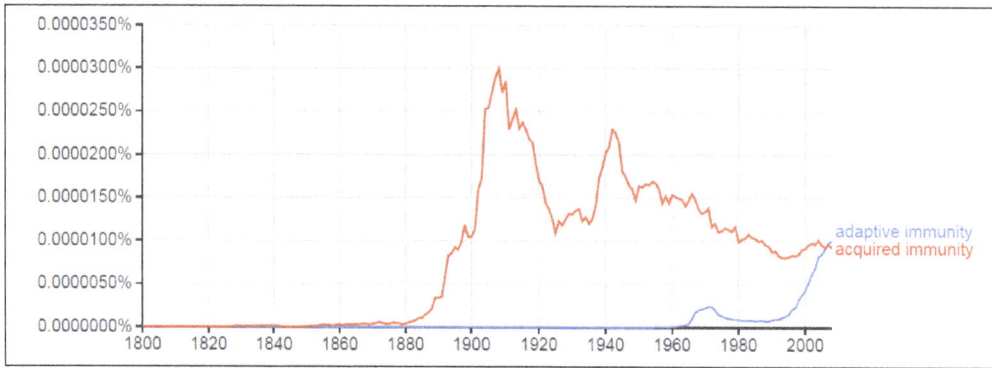

Unlike the innate immune system, the acquired immune system is highly specific to a particular pathogen. Acquired immunity can also provide long-lasting protection; for example, someone who recovers from measles is now protected against measles for their lifetime. In other cases it does not provide lifetime protection; for example, chickenpox. The acquired system response destroys invading pathogens and any toxic molecules they produce. Sometimes the acquired system is unable to distinguish harmful from harmless foreign molecules; the effects of this may be hayfever, asthma or any other allergy. Antigens are any substances that elicit the acquired immune response (whether adaptive or maladaptive to the organism). The cells that carry out the acquired immune response are white blood cells known as lymphocytes. Two main broad classes—antibody responses and cell mediated immune response—are also carried by two different lymphocytes (B cells and T cells). In antibody responses, B cells are activated to secrete antibodies, which are proteins also known as immunoglobulins. Antibodies travel through the bloodstream and bind to the foreign antigen causing it to inactivate, which does not allow the antigen to bind to the host.

In acquired immunity, pathogen-specific receptors are "acquired" during the lifetime of the organism (whereas in innate immunity pathogen-specific receptors are already encoded in the germline). The acquired response is called "adaptive" because it prepares the body's immune system for future challenges (though it can actually also be maladaptive when it results in autoimmunity).

The system is highly adaptable because of somatic hypermutation (a process of accelerated somatic mutations), and V(D)J recombination (an irreversible genetic recombination of antigen receptor gene segments). This mechanism allows a small number of genes to generate a vast number of different antigen receptors, which are then uniquely expressed on each individual lymphocyte. Since the gene rearrangement leads to an irreversible change in the DNA of each cell, all progeny (offspring) of that cell inherit genes that encode the same receptor specificity, including the memory B cells and memory T cells that are the keys to long-lived specific immunity.

A theoretical framework explaining the workings of the acquired immune system is provided by immune network theory. This theory, which builds on established concepts of clonal selection, is being applied in the search for an HIV vaccine.

Functions

Acquired immunity is triggered in vertebrates when a pathogen evades the innate immune system and generates a threshold level of antigen and generates "stranger" or "danger" signals activating dendritic cells.

The major functions of the acquired immune system include:

- Recognition of specific "non-self" antigens in the presence of "self", during the process of antigen presentation.

- Generation of responses that are tailored to maximally eliminate specific pathogens or pathogen-infected cells.

- Development of immunological memory, in which pathogens are "remembered" through memory B cells and memory T cells.

Lymphocytes

The cells of the acquired immune system are T and B lymphocytes; lymphocytes are a subset of leukocyte. B cells and T cells are the major types of lymphocytes. The human body has about 2 trillion lymphocytes, constituting 20–40% of white blood cells (WBCs); their total mass is about the same as the brain or liver. The peripheral blood contains 2% of circulating lymphocytes; the rest move within the tissues and lymphatic system.

B cells and T cells are derived from the same multipotent hematopoietic stem cells, and are morphologically indistinguishable from one another until after they are activated. B cells play a large role in the humoral immune response, whereas T cells are intimately involved in cell-mediated immune responses. In all vertebrates except Agnatha, B cells and T cells are produced by stem cells in the bone marrow.

T progenitors migrate from the bone marrow to the thymus where they are called thymocytes and where they develop into T cells. In humans, approximately 1–2% of the lymphocyte pool recirculates each hour to optimize the opportunities for antigen-specific lymphocytes to find their specific antigen within the secondary lymphoid tissues. In an adult animal, the peripheral lymphoid organs contain a mixture of B and T cells in at least three stages of differentiation:

- Naive B and naive T cells (cells that have not matured), left the bone marrow or thymus, have entered the lymphatic system, but have yet to encounter their cognate antigen.

- Effector cells that have been activated by their cognate antigen, and are actively involved in eliminating a pathogen.

- Memory cells – the survivors of past infections.

Antigen Presentation

Acquired immunity relies on the capacity of immune cells to distinguish between the body's own cells and unwanted invaders. The host's cells express "self" antigens. These antigens are different from those on the surface of bacteria or on the surface of virus-infected host cells ("non-self" or "foreign" antigens). The acquired immune response is triggered by recognizing foreign antigen in the cellular context of an activated dendritic cell.

With the exception of non-nucleated cells (including erythrocytes), all cells are capable of presenting antigen through the function of major histocompatibility complex (MHC) molecules. Some cells are specially equipped to present antigen, and to prime naive T cells. Dendritic cells, B-cells, and macrophages are equipped with special "co-stimulatory" ligands recognized by co-stimulatory receptors on T cells, and are termed professional antigen-presenting cells (APCs).

Several T cells subgroups can be activated by professional APCs, and each type of T cell is specially equipped to deal with each unique toxin or microbial pathogen. The type of T cell activated, and the type of response generated, depends, in part, on the context in which the APC first encountered the antigen.

Exogenous Antigens

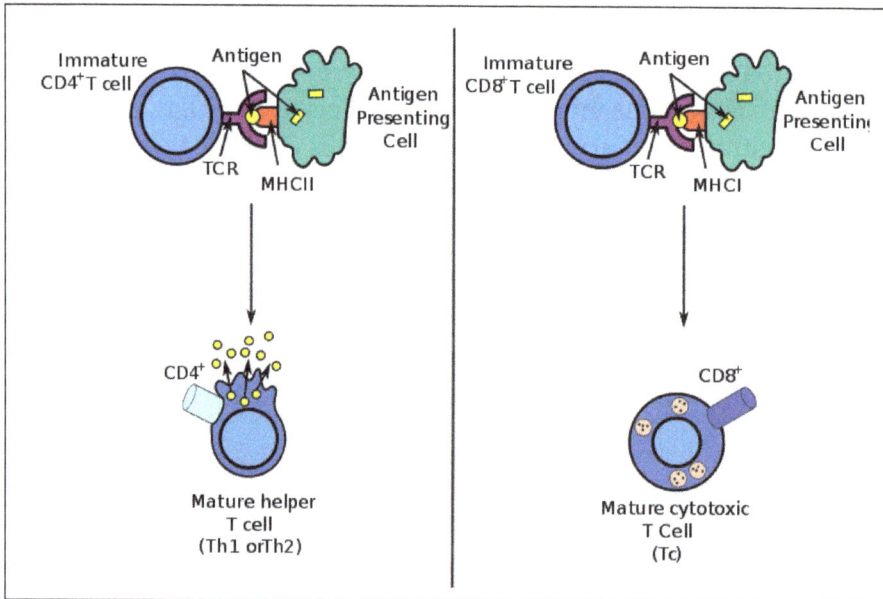

Antigen presentation stimulates T cells to become
either "cytotoxic" CD8+ cells or "helper" CD4+ cells.

Dendritic cells engulf exogenous pathogens, such as bacteria, parasites or toxins in the tissues and then migrate, via chemotactic signals, to the T cell-enriched lymph nodes. During migration, dendritic cells undergo a process of maturation in which they lose most of their ability to engulf other pathogens, and develop an ability to communicate with T-cells. The dendritic cell uses enzymes to chop the pathogen into smaller pieces, called antigens. In the lymph node, the dendritic cell displays these non-self antigens on its surface by coupling them to a receptor called the major histocompatibility complex, or MHC (also known in humans as human leukocyte antigen (HLA)). This MHC: antigen complex is recognized by T-cells passing through the lymph node. Exogenous antigens are usually displayed on MHC class II molecules, which activate CD4+T helper cells.

Endogenous Antigens

Endogenous antigens are produced by intracellular bacteria and viruses replicating within a host cell. The host cell uses enzymes to digest virally associated proteins, and displays these pieces on its surface to T-cells by coupling them to MHC. Endogenous antigens are typically displayed on MHC class I molecules, and activate CD8+ cytotoxic T-cells. With the exception of non-nucleated cells (including erythrocytes), MHC class I is expressed by all host cells.

T lymphocytes

CD8+ T Lymphocytes and Cytotoxicity

Cytotoxic T cells (also known as TC, killer T cell, or cytotoxic T-lymphocyte (CTL)) are a sub-group of T cells that induce the death of cells that are infected with viruses (and other pathogens), or are otherwise damaged or dysfunctional.

Naive cytotoxic T cells are activated when their T-cell receptor (TCR) strongly interacts with a peptide-bound MHC class I molecule. This affinity depends on the type and orientation of the antigen/MHC complex, and is what keeps the CTL and infected cell bound together. Once activated, the CTL undergoes a process called clonal selection, in which it gains functions and divides rapidly to produce an army of "armed" effector cells. Activated CTL then travels throughout the body searching for cells that bear that unique MHC Class I + peptide.

When exposed to these infected or dysfunctional somatic cells, effector CTL release perforin and granulysin: cytotoxins that form pores in the target cell's plasma membrane, allowing ions and water to flow into the infected cell, and causing it to burst or lyse. CTL release granzyme, a serine protease encapsulated in a granule that enters cells via pores to induce apoptosis (cell death). To limit extensive tissue damage during an infection, CTL activation is tightly controlled and in general requires a very strong MHC/antigen activation signal, or additional activation signals provided by "helper" T-cells.

On resolution of the infection, most effector cells die and phagocytes clear them away—but a few of these cells remain as memory cells. On a later encounter with the same antigen, these memory cells quickly differentiate into effector cells, dramatically shortening the time required to mount an effective response.

Helper T-cells

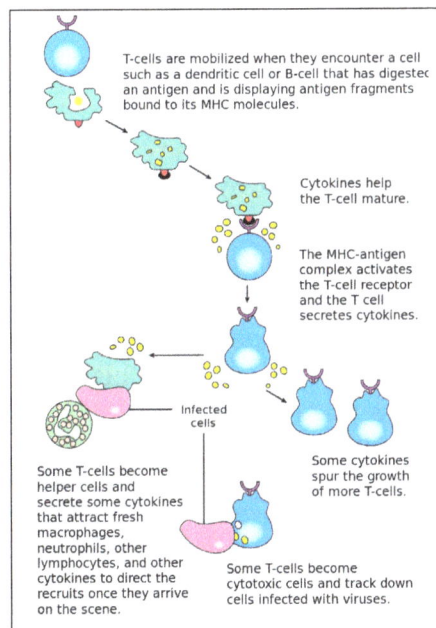

T-cells are mobilized when they encounter a cell such as a dendritic cell or B-cell that has digested an antigen and is displaying antigen fragments bound to its MHC molecules.

Cytokines help the T-cell mature.

The MHC-antigen complex activates the T-cell receptor and the T cell secretes cytokines.

Infected cells

Some T-cells become helper cells and secrete some cytokines that attract fresh macrophages, neutrophils, other lymphocytes, and other cytokines to direct the recruits once they arrive on the scene.

Some cytokines spur the growth of more T-cells.

Some T-cells become cytotoxic cells and track down cells infected with viruses.

The T lymphocyte activation pathway. T cells contribute to immune defenses in two major ways: some direct and regulate immune responses; others directly attack infected or cancerous cells.

CD4+ lymphocytes, also called "helper" T cells, are immune response mediators, and play an important role in establishing and maximizing the capabilities of the acquired immune response. These cells have no cytotoxic or phagocytic activity; and cannot kill infected cells or clear pathogens, but, in essence "manage" the immune response, by directing other cells to perform these tasks.

Helper T cells express T cell receptors (TCR) that recognize antigen bound to Class II MHC molecules. The activation of a naive helper T-cell causes it to release cytokines, which influences the activity of many cell types, including the APC (Antigen-Presenting Cell) that activated it. Helper T-cells require a much milder activation stimulus than cytotoxic T cells. Helper T cells can provide extra signals that "help" activate cytotoxic cells.

Th1 and Th2: Helper T Cell Responses

Classically, two types of effector CD4+ T helper cell responses can be induced by a professional APC, designated Th1 and Th2, each designed to eliminate different types of pathogens. The factors that dictate whether an infection triggers a Th1 or Th2 type response are not fully understood, but the response generated does play an important role in the clearance of different pathogens.

The Th1 response is characterized by the production of Interferon-gamma, which activates the bactericidal activities of macrophages, and induces B cells to make opsonizing (marking for phagocytosis) and complement-fixing antibodies, and leads to *cell-mediated immunity*. In general, Th1 responses are more effective against intracellular pathogens (viruses and bacteria that are inside host cells).

The Th2 response is characterized by the release of Interleukin 5, which induces eosinophils in the clearance of parasites. Th2 also produce Interleukin 4, which facilitates B cell isotype switching. In general, Th2 responses are more effective against extracellular bacteria, parasites including helminths and toxins. Like cytotoxic T cells, most of the CD4+ helper cells die on resolution of infection, with a few remaining as CD4+ memory cells.

Increasingly, there is strong evidence from mouse and human-based scientific studies of a broader diversity in CD4+ effector T helper cell subsets. Regulatory T (Treg) cells, have been identified as important negative regulators of adaptive immunity as they limit and suppresses the immune system to control aberrant immune responses to self-antigens; an important mechanism in controlling the development of autoimmune diseases. Follicular helper T (Tfh) cells are another distinct population of effector CD4+ T cells that develop from naive T cells post-antigen activation. Tfh cells are specialized in helping B cell humoral immunity as they are uniquely capable of migrating to follicular B cells in secondary lymphoid organs and provide them positive paracrine signals to enable the generation and recall production of high-quality affinity-matured antibodies. Similar to Tregs, Tfh cells also play a role in immunological tolerance as an abnormal expansion of Tfh cell numbers can lead to unrestricted autoreactive antibody production causing severe systemic autoimmune disorders.

The relevance of CD4+ T helper cells is highlighted during an HIV infection. HIV is able to subvert the immune system by specifically attacking the CD4+ T cells, precisely the cells that could drive the clearance of the virus, but also the cells that drive immunity against all other pathogens encountered during an organism's lifetime.

Gamma Delta T Cells

Gamma delta T cells (γδ T cells) possess an alternative T cell receptor (TCR) as opposed to CD4+ and CD8+ αβ T cells and share characteristics of helper T cells, cytotoxic T cells and natural killer cells. Like other 'unconventional' T cell subsets bearing invariant TCRs, such as CD1d-restricted natural killer T cells, γδ T cells exhibit characteristics that place them at the border between innate and acquired immunity. On one hand, γδ T cells may be considered a component of adaptive immunity in that they rearrange TCR genes via V(D)J recombination, which also produces junctional diversity, and develop a memory phenotype. On the other hand, however, the various subsets may also be considered part of the innate immune system where a restricted TCR or NK receptors may be used as a pattern recognition receptor. For example, according to this paradigm, large numbers of Vγ9/Vδ2 T cells respond within hours to common molecules produced by microbes, and highly restricted intraepithelial Vδ1 T cells respond to stressed epithelial cells.

B Lymphocytes and Antibody Production

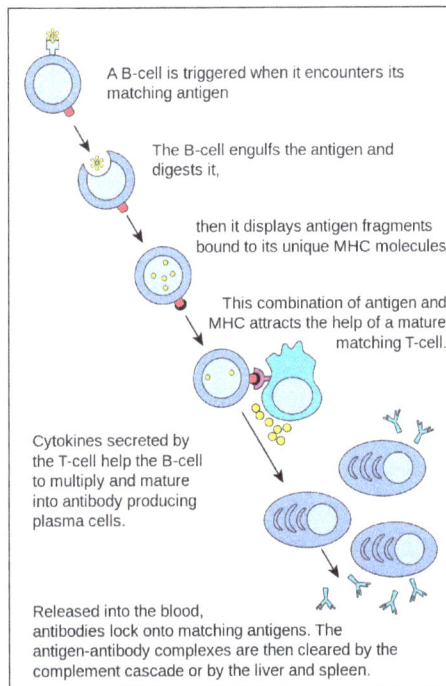

The B lymphocyte activation pathway. B cells function to protect the host by producing antibodies that identify and neutralize foreign objects like bacteria and viruses.

B Cells are the major cells involved in the creation of antibodies that circulate in blood plasma and lymph, known as humoral immunity. Antibodies (also known as immunoglobulin, Ig), are large Y-shaped proteins used by the immune system to identify and neutralize foreign objects. In mammals, there are five types of antibody: IgA, IgD, IgE, IgG, and IgM, differing in biological properties; each has evolved to handle different kinds of antigens. Upon activation, B cells produce antibodies, each of which recognize a unique antigen, and neutralizing specific pathogens.

Antigen and antibody binding would cause five different protective mechanisms:

- Agglutination: Reduces number of infectious units to be dealt with;

- Activation of complement: Cause inflammation and cell lysis;

- Opsonization: Coating antigen with antibody enhances phagocytosis;

- Antibody-dependent cell-mediated cytotoxicity: Antibodies attached to target cell cause destruction by macrophages, eosinophils, and NK cells;

- Neutralization: Blocks adhesion of bacteria and viruses to mucosa.

Like the T cell, B cells express a unique B cell receptor (BCR), in this case, a membrane-bound antibody molecule. All the BCR of any one clone of B cells recognizes and binds to only one particular antigen. A critical difference between B cells and T cells is how each cell "sees" an antigen. T cells recognize their cognate antigen in a processed form – as a peptide in the context of an MHC molecule, whereas B cells recognize antigens in their native form. Once a B cell encounters its cognate (or specific) antigen (and receives additional signals from a helper T cell (predominately Th2 type)), it further differentiates into an effector cell, known as a plasma cell.

Plasma cells are short-lived cells (2–3 days) that secrete antibodies. These antibodies bind to antigens, making them easier targets for phagocytes, and trigger the complement cascade. About 10% of plasma cells survive to become long-lived antigen-specific memory B cells. Already primed to produce specific antibodies, these cells can be called upon to respond quickly if the same pathogen re-infects the host, while the host experiences few, if any, symptoms.

Alternative Systems

In Jawless Vertebrates

Primitive jawless vertebrates, such as the lamprey and hagfish, have an adaptive immune system that shows 3 different cell lineages, each sharing a common origin with B cells, αβ T cells, and innate-like γΔ T cells. Instead of the classical antibodies and T cell receptors, these animals possess a large array of molecules called variable lymphocyte receptors (VLRs for short) that, like the antigen receptors of jawed vertebrates, are produced from only a small number (one or two) of genes. These molecules are believed to bind pathogenic antigens in a similar way to antibodies, and with the same degree of specificity.

In Insects

For a long time it was thought that insects and other invertebrates possess only innate immune system. However, in recent years some of the basic hallmarks of adaptive immunity have been discovered in insects. Those traits are immune memory and specificity. Although the hallmarks are present the mechanisms are different from those in vertebrates.

Immune memory in insects was discovered through the phenomenon of priming. When insects are exposed to non-lethal dose or heat killed bacteria they are able to develop a memory of that infection that allows them to withstand otherwise lethal dose of the same bacteria they were exposed to before. Unlike in vertebrates, insects do not possess cells specific for adaptive immunity. Instead those mechanisms are mediated by hemocytes. Hemocytes function similarly to phagocytes and after priming they are able to more effectively recognize and engulf the pathogen. It was also shown that it is possible to transfer the memory into offspring. For example, in honeybees if the queen is infected with bacteria then the newly born workers have enhanced abilities in fighting with the same bacteria. Other experimental model based on red flour beetle also showed pathogen specific primed memory transfer into offspring from both mothers and fathers.

Most commonly accepted theory of the specificity is based on *Dscam* gene. *Dscam* gene also known as Down syndrome cell adhesive molecule is a gene that contains 3 variable Ig domains. Those domains can be alternatively spliced reaching high numbers of variations. It was shown that after exposure to different pathogens there are different splice forms of dscam produced. After the animals with different splice forms are exposed to the same pathogen only the individuals with the splice form specific for that pathogen survive.

Other mechanisms supporting the specificity of insect immunity is RNA interference (RNAi). RNAi is a form of antiviral immunity with high specificity. It has several different pathways that all end with the virus being unable to replicate. One of the pathways is siRNA in which long double stranded RNA is cut into pieces that serve as templates for protein complex Ago2-RISC that finds and degrades complementary RNA of the virus. MiRNA pathway in cytoplasm binds to Ago1-RISC complex and functions as a template for viral RNA degradation. Last one is piRNA where small RNA binds to the Piwi protein family and controls transposones and other mobile elements. Despite the research the exact mechanisms responsible for immune priming and specificity in insects are not well described.

Immunological Memory

When B cells and T cells are activated some become memory B cells and some memory T cells. Throughout the lifetime of an animal these memory cells form a database of effective B and T lymphocytes. Upon interaction with a previously encountered antigen, the appropriate memory cells are selected and activated. In this manner, the second and subsequent exposures to an antigen produce a stronger and faster immune response. This is "adaptive" in the sense that the body's immune system prepares itself for future challenges, but is "maladaptive" of course if the receptors are autoimmune. Immunological memory can be in the form of either passive short-term memory or active long-term memory.

Passive Memory

Passive memory is usually short-term, lasting between a few days and several months. Newborn infants have had no prior exposure to microbes and are particularly vulnerable to infection. Several layers of passive protection are provided by the mother. *In utero*, maternal IgG is transported directly across the placenta, so that, at birth, human babies have high levels of antibodies, with the same range of antigen specificities as their mother. Breast milk contains antibodies (mainly IgA) that are transferred to the gut of the infant, protecting against bacterial infections, until the newborn can synthesize its own antibodies.

This is passive immunity because the fetus does not actually make any memory cells or antibodies: It only borrows them. Short-term passive immunity can also be transferred artificially from one individual to another via antibody-rich serum.

Active Memory

In general, active immunity is long-term and can be acquired by infection followed by B cells and T cells activation, or artificially acquired by vaccines, in a process called immunization.

Immunization

Historically, infectious disease has been the leading cause of death in the human population. Over the last century, two important factors have been developed to combat their spread: sanitation and immunization. Immunization (commonly referred to as vaccination) is the deliberate induction of an immune response, and represents the single most effective manipulation of the immune system that scientists have developed. Immunizations are successful because they utilize the immune system's natural specificity as well as its inducibility.

The principle behind immunization is to introduce an antigen, derived from a disease-causing organism, that stimulates the immune system to develop protective immunity against that organism, but that does not itself cause the pathogenic effects of that organism. An antigen (short for antibody generator), is defined as any substance that binds to a specific antibody and elicits an adaptive immune response.

Most viral vaccines are based on live attenuated viruses, whereas many bacterial vaccines are based on acellular components of microorganisms, including harmless toxin components. Many antigens derived from acellular vaccines do not strongly induce an adaptive response, and most bacterial vaccines require the addition of *adjuvants* that activate the antigen-presenting cells of the innate immune system to enhance immunogenicity.

Immunological Diversity

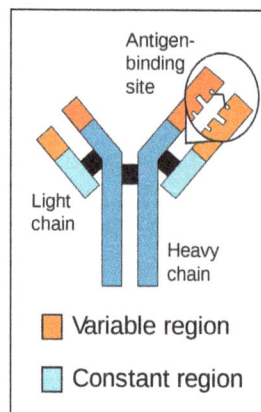

An antibody is made up of two heavy chains and two light chains.
The unique variable region allows an antibody to recognize its matching antigen.

Most large molecules, including virtually all proteins and many polysaccharides, can serve as antigens. The parts of an antigen that interact with an antibody molecule or a lymphocyte receptor, are called epitopes, or antigenic determinants. Most antigens contain a variety of epitopes and can stimulate the production of antibodies, specific T cell responses, or both. A very small proportion (less than 0.01%) of the total lymphocytes are able to bind to a particular antigen, which suggests that only a few cells respond to each antigen.

For the acquired response to "remember" and eliminate a large number of pathogens the immune system must be able to distinguish between many different antigens, and the receptors that recognize antigens must be produced in a huge variety of configurations, in essence one receptor (at least) for each different pathogen that might ever be encountered. Even in the absence of antigen stimulation, a human can produce more than 1 trillion different antibody molecules. Millions of genes would be required to store the genetic information that produces these receptors, but, the entire human genome contains fewer than 25,000 genes.

Myriad receptors are produced through a process known as clonal selection. According to the clonal selection theory, at birth, an animal randomly generates a vast diversity of lymphocytes (each bearing a unique antigen receptor) from information encoded in a small family of genes. To generate each unique antigen receptor, these genes have undergone a process called V(D)J recombination, or combinatorial diversification, in which one gene segment recombines with other gene segments to form a single unique gene. This assembly process generates the enormous diversity of receptors and antibodies, before the body ever encounters antigens, and enables the immune system to respond to an almost unlimited diversity of antigens. Throughout an animal's lifetime, lymphocytes that can react against the antigens an animal actually encounters are selected for action—directed against anything that expresses that antigen.

Note that the innate and acquired portions of the immune system work together, not in spite of each other. The acquired arm, B, and T cells couldn't function without the innate system' input. T cells are useless without antigen-presenting cells to activate them, and B cells are crippled without T cell help. On the other hand, the innate system would likely be overrun with pathogens without the specialized action of the adaptive immune response.

Acquired Immunity during Pregnancy

The cornerstone of the immune system is the recognition of "self" versus "non-self". Therefore, the mechanisms that protect the human fetus (which is considered "non-self") from attack by the immune system, are particularly interesting. Although no comprehensive explanation has emerged to explain this mysterious, and often repeated, lack of rejection, two classical reasons may explain how the fetus is tolerated. The first is that the fetus occupies a portion of the body protected by a non-immunological barrier, the uterus, which the immune system does not routinely patrol. The second is that the fetus itself may promote local immunosuppression in the mother, perhaps by a process of active nutrient depletion. A more modern explanation for this induction of tolerance is that specific glycoproteins expressed in the uterus during pregnancy suppress the uterine immune response.

During pregnancy in viviparous mammals (all mammals except Monotremes), endogenous retroviruses (ERVs) are activated and produced in high quantities during the implantation of the embryo. They are currently known to possess immunosuppressive properties, suggesting a role in protecting the embryo from its mother's immune system. Also, viral fusion proteins cause the formation of the placental syncytium to limit exchange of migratory cells between the developing embryo and the body of the mother (something an epithelium can't do sufficiently, as certain blood cells specialize to insert themselves between adjacent epithelial cells). The immunodepressive action was the initial normal behavior of the virus, similar to HIV. The fusion proteins were a way to spread the infection to other cells by simply merging them with the infected one (HIV does this too). It is believed that the ancestors of modern viviparous mammals evolved after an infection by this virus, enabling the fetus to survive the immune system of the mother.

The human genome project found several thousand ERVs classified into 24 families.

Immune Network Theory

A theoretical framework explaining the workings of the acquired immune system is provided by immune network theory, based on interactions between idiotypes (unique molecular features of one clonotype, i.e. the unique set of antigenic determinants of the variable portion of an antibody) and 'anti-idiotypes' (antigen receptors that react with the idiotype as if it were a foreign antigen). This theory, which builds on the existing clonal selection hypothesis and since 1974 has been developed mainly by Niels Jerne and Geoffrey W. Hoffmann, is seen as being relevant to the understanding of the HIV pathogenesis and the search for an HIV vaccine.

Stimulation of Adaptive Immunity

One of the most interesting developments in biomedical science during the past few decades has been elucidation of mechanisms mediating innate immunity. One set of innate immune mechanisms is humoral, such as complement activation. Another set comprises pattern recognition receptors such as toll-like receptors, which induce the production of interferons and other cytokines increasing resistance of cells such as monocytes to infections. Cytokines produced during innate immune responses are among the activators of adaptive immune responses. Antibodies exert additive or synergistic effects with mechanisms of innate immunity. Unstable HbS clusters Band-3, a major integral red cell protein; antibodies recognize these clusters and accelerate their removal by phagocytic cells. Clustered Band 3 proteins with attached antibodies activate complement, and complement C3 fragments are opsonins recognized by the CR1 complement receptor on phagocytic cells.

A population study has shown that the protective effect of the sickle-cell trait against falciparum malaria involves the augmentation of acquired as well as innate immune responses to the malaria parasite, illustrating the expected transition from innate to acquired immunity.

Repeated malaria infections strengthen acquired immunity and broaden its effects against parasites expressing different surface antigens. By school age most children have developed efficacious adaptive immunity against malaria. These observations raise questions about mechanisms that favor the survival of most children in Africa while allowing some to develop potentially lethal infections.

In malaria, as in other infections, innate immune responses lead into, and stimulate, adaptive immune responses. The genetic control of innate and acquired immunity is now a large and flourishing discipline.

Humoral and cell-mediated immune responses limit malaria parasite multiplication, and many cytokines contribute to the pathogenesis of malaria as well as to the resolution of infections.

Evolution

The acquired immune system, which has been best-studied in mammals, originated in jawed fish approximately 500 million years ago. Most of the molecules, cells, tissues, and associated mechanisms of this system of defense are found in cartilaginous fishes. Lymphocyte receptors, Ig and TCR, are found in all jawed vertebrates. The most ancient Ig class, IgM, is membrane-bound and then secreted upon stimulation of cartilaginous fish B cells. Another isotype, shark IgW, is related to mammalian IgD. TCRs, both α/β and γ/δ, are found in all animals from gnathostomes to mammals.

The organization of gene segments that undergo gene rearrangement differs in cartilaginous fishes, which have a cluster form as compared to the translocon form in bony fish to mammals. Like TCR and Ig, the MHC is found only in jawed vertebrates. Genes involved in antigen processing and presentation, as well as the class I and class II genes, are closely linked within the MHC of almost all studied species.

Lymphoid cells can be identified in some pre-vertebrate deuterostomes (i.e., sea urchins). These bind antigen with pattern recognition receptors (PRRs) of the innate immune system. In jawless fishes, two subsets of lymphocytes use variable lymphocyte receptors (VLRs) for antigen binding. Diversity is generated by a cytosine deaminase-mediated rearrangement of LRR-based DNA segments. There is no evidence for the recombination-activating genes (RAGs) that rearrange Ig and TCR gene segments in jawed vertebrates.

The evolution of the AIS, based on Ig, TCR, and MHC molecules, is thought to have arisen from two major evolutionary events: The transfer of the RAG transposon (possibly of viral origin) and two whole genome duplications. Though the molecules of the AIS are well-conserved, they are also rapidly evolving. Yet, a comparative approach finds that many features are quite uniform across taxa. All the major features of the AIS arose early and quickly. Jawless fishes have a different AIS that relies on gene rearrangement to generate diverse immune receptors with a functional dichotomy that parallels Ig and TCR molecules. The innate immune system, which has an important role in AIS activation, is the most important defense system of invertebrates and plants.

Types of Acquired Immunity

Immunity can be acquired either actively or passively. Immunity is acquired actively when a person is exposed to foreign substances and the immune system responds. Passive immunity is when antibodies are transferred from one host to another. Both actively acquired and passively acquired immunity can be obtained by natural or artificial means.

- Naturally Acquired Active Immunity: When a person is naturally exposed to antigens, becomes ill, then recovers.

- Naturally Acquired Passive Immunity: Involves a natural transfer of antibodies from a mother to her infant. The antibodies crosses the woman's placenta to the fetus. Antibodies can also be transferred through breast milk with the secretions of colostrum.

- Artificially Acquired Active Immunity: Is done by vaccination (introducing dead or weakened antigen to the host's cell).

- Artificially Acquired Passive Immunity: This involves the introduction of antibodies rather than antigens to the human body. These antibodies are from an animal or person who is already immune to the disease.

Naturally acquired	Artificially acquired
Active- Antigen enters the body naturally.	Active- Antigens are introduced in vaccines.
Passive-Antibodies pass from mother to fetus via placenta or infant via the mother's milk.	Passive- Preformed antibodies in immune serum are introduced by injection.

Complement System

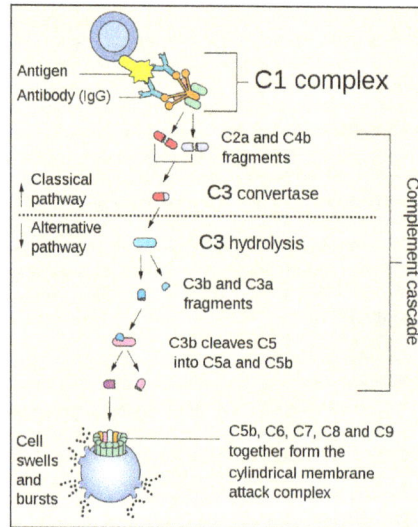

The complement system is a part of the immune system that enhances (complements) the ability of antibodies and phagocytic cells to clear microbes and damaged cells from an organism, promote inflammation, and attack the pathogen's cell membrane. It is part of the innate immune system, which is not adaptable and does not change during an individual's lifetime. The complement system can, however, be recruited and brought into action by antibodies generated by the adaptive immune system.

The complement system consists of a number of small proteins that are synthesized by the liver, and circulate in the blood as inactive precursors. When stimulated by one of several triggers, proteases in the system cleave specific proteins to release cytokines and initiate an amplifying cascade of further cleavages. The end result of this complement activation or complement fixation cascade is stimulation of phagocytes to clear foreign and damaged material, inflammation to attract additional phagocytes, and activation of the cell-killing membrane attack complex. Over 30 proteins and protein fragments make up the complement system, including serum proteins, and cell membrane receptors. They account for about 10% of the globulin fraction of blood serum.

Three biochemical pathways activate the complement system: The classical complement pathway, the alternative complement pathway, and the lectin pathway.

In 1888, George Nuttall found that sheep blood serum had mild killing activity against the bacterium that causes anthrax. The killing activity disappeared when he heated the blood. In 1891, Hans Ernst August Buchner, noting the same property of blood in his experiments, named the killing property "alexin", which means "to ward off" in Greek. By 1894, several laboratories had demonstrated that serum from guinea pigs that had recovered from cholera killed the cholera bacterium in vitro. Heating the serum destroyed its killing activity. Nevertheless, the heat-inactivated serum, when injected into guinea pigs exposed to the cholera bacteria, maintained its ability to protect the animals from illness. Jules Bordet, a young Belgian scientist in Paris at the Pasteur Institute, concluded that this principle has two components, one that maintained a "sensitizing" effect after being heated and one (alexin) whose toxic effect was lost after being heated. The heat-stable component was responsible for immunity against specific microorganisms, whereas the heat-sensitive component was responsible for the non-specific antimicrobial activity conferred by all normal sera. In 1899, Paul Ehrlich renamed the heat-sensitive component "complement."

Ehrlich introduced the term "complement" as part of his larger theory of the immune system. According to this theory, the immune system consists of cells that have specific receptors on their surface to recognize antigens. Upon immunisation with an antigen, more of these receptors are formed, and they are then shed from the cells to circulate in the blood. Those receptors, which we now call "antibodies", were called by Ehrlich "amboceptors" to emphasise their bifunctional binding capacity: They recognise and bind to a specific antigen, but they also recognise and bind to the heat-labile antimicrobial component of fresh serum. Ehrlich, therefore, named this heat-labile component "complement", because it is something in the blood that "complements" the cells of the immune system. Ehrlich believed that each antigen-specific amboceptor has its own specific complement, whereas Bordet believed that there is only one type of complement. In the early 20th century, this controversy was resolved when it became understood that complement can act in combination with specific antibodies, or on its own in a non-specific way.

Functions

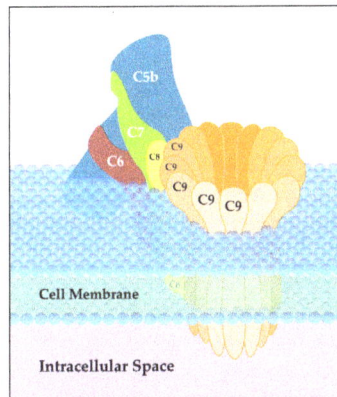

Membrane Attack Complex (Terminal Complement Complex C5b-9).

Complement triggers the following immune functions:

1. Phagocytosis – By opsonizing antigens. C3b has most important opsonizing activity.

2. Inflammation – By attracting macrophages and neutrophils.

3. Membrane attack – By rupturing cell wall of bacteria.

Classical Pathway

The classical pathway is triggered by activation of the C1-complex. The C1-complex is composed of 1 molecule of C1q, 2 molecules of C1r and 2 molecules of C1s, or *C1qr$_2$s$_2$*. This occurs when C1q binds to IgM or IgG complexed with antigens. A single pentameric IgM can initiate the pathway, while several, ideally six, IgGs are needed. This also occurs when C1q binds directly to the surface of the pathogen. Such binding leads to conformational changes in the C1q molecule, which leads to the activation of two C1r molecules. C1r is a serine protease. They then cleave C1s (another serine protease). The C1r²s² component now splits C4 and then C2, producing C4a, C4b, C2a, and C2b (historically, the larger fragment of C2 was called C2a but is now referred to as C2b). C4b and C2b bind to form the classical pathway C3-convertase (C4b2b complex), which promotes cleavage of C3 into C3a and C3b. C3b later joins with C4b2b to make C5 convertase (C4b2b3b complex).

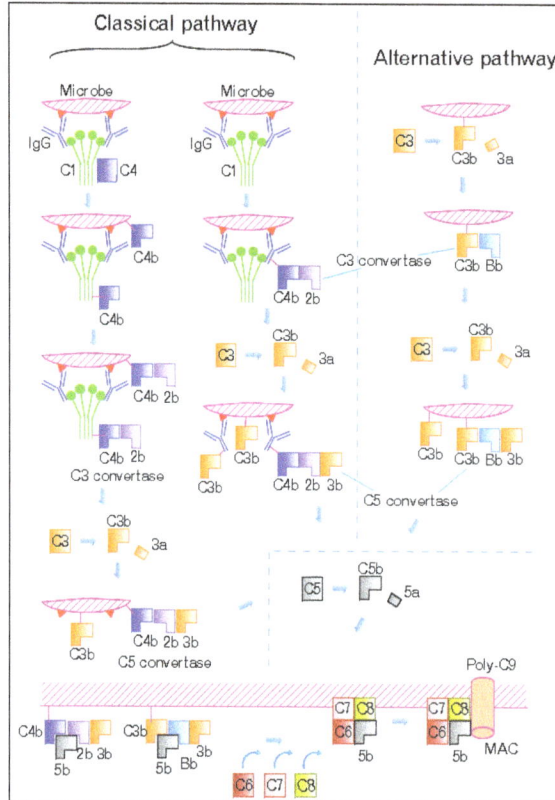

The classical and alternative complement pathways.

Alternative Pathway

The alternative pathway is continuously activated at a low level, analogous to a car engine at idle, as a result of spontaneous C3 hydrolysis due to the breakdown of the internal thioester bond (C3 is mildly unstable in aqueous environment). The alternative pathway does not rely on pathogen-binding antibodies like the other pathways. C3b that is generated from C3 by a C3 convertase enzyme complex in the fluid phase is rapidly inactivated by factor H and factor I, as is the C3b-like C3 that is the product of spontaneous cleavage of the internal thioester. In contrast, when the internal thioester of C3 reacts with a hydroxyl or amino group of a molecule on the surface of a cell or pathogen, the C3b that is now covalently bound to the surface is protected from factor H-mediated inactivation. The surface-bound C3b may now bind factor B to form C3bB. This complex in the presence of factor D will be cleaved into Ba and Bb. Bb will remain associated with C3b to form C3bBb, which is the alternative pathway C3 convertase.

The C3bBb complex is stabilized by binding oligomers of factor P (properdin). The stabilized C3 convertase, C3bBbP, then acts enzymatically to cleave much more C3, some of which becomes covalently attached to the same surface as C3b. This newly bound C3b recruits more B, D and P activity and greatly amplifies the complement activation. When complement is activated on a cell surface, the activation is limited by endogenous complement regulatory proteins, which include CD35, CD46, CD55 and CD59, depending on the cell. Pathogens, in general, don't have complement regulatory proteins (there are many exceptions, which reflect adaptation of microbial pathogens to vertebrate immune defenses). Thus, the alternative complement pathway is able to distinguish self from non-self on the basis of the surface expression of complement regulatory proteins. Host cells don't accumulate cell surface C3b (and the proteolytic fragment of C3b called iC3b) because this is prevented by the complement regulatory proteins, while foreign cells, pathogens and abnormal surfaces may be heavily decorated with C3b and iC3b. Accordingly, the alternative complement pathway is one element of innate immunity.

Once the alternative C3 convertase enzyme is formed on a pathogen or cell surface, it may bind covalently another C3b, to form C3bBbC3bP, the C5 convertase. This enzyme then cleaves C5 to C5a, a potent anaphylatoxin, and C5b. The C5b then recruits and assembles C6, C7, C8 and multiple C9 molecules to assemble the membrane attack complex. This creates a hole or pore in the membrane that can kill or damage the pathogen or cell.

Lectin Pathway

The lectin pathway is homologous to the classical pathway, but with the opsonin, mannose-binding lectin (MBL), and ficolins, instead of C1q. This pathway is activated by binding of MBL to mannose residues on the pathogen surface, which activates the MBL-associated serine proteases, MASP-1, and MASP-2 (very similar to C1r and C1s, respectively), which can then split C4 into C4a and C4b and C2 into C2a and C2b. C4b and C2b then bind together to form the classical C3-convertase, as in the classical pathway. Ficolins are homologous to MBL and function via MASP in a similar way. Several single-nucleotide polymorphisms have been described in M-ficolin in humans, with effect on ligand-binding ability and serum levels. Historically, the larger fragment of C2 was named C2a, but it is now referred to as C2b. In invertebrates without an adaptive immune system, ficolins are expanded and their binding specificities diversified to compensate for the lack of pathogen-specific recognition molecules.

Complement Protein Fragment Nomenclature

Immunology textbooks have used different naming assignments for the smaller and larger fragments of C2 as C2a and C2b. The preferred assignment appears to be that the smaller fragment be designated as C2a: as early as 1994, a well known textbook recommended that the larger fragment of C2 should be designated C2b. However, this was amplified in their 1999 4th edition, to say that: "It is also useful to be aware that the larger active fragment of C2 was originally designated C2a, and is still called that in some texts and research papers. Here, for consistency, we shall call all large fragments of complement b, so the larger fragment of C2 will be designated C2b. In the classical and lectin pathways the C3 convertase enzyme is formed from membrane-bound C4b with C2b."

The assignment is mixed in the latter literature, though. Some sources designate the larger and smaller fragments as C2a and C2b respectively while other sources apply the converse. However, due to the widely established convention, C2b here is the larger fragment, which, in the classical pathway, forms C4b2b (classically C4b2a). It may be noteworthy that, in a series of editions of Janeway's book, 1st to 7th, in the latest edition they withdraw the stance to indicate the larger fragment of C2 as C2b.

Viral Inhibition

Fixation of the MBL protein on viral surfaces has also been shown to enhance neutralization of viral pathogens.

Activation pathway	Classic	Alternative	Lectin
Activator	Ag–Ab Complex	spontaneous hydrolysis of C3	MBL-Mannose Complex
C3-convertase	C4b2b	C3bBb	C4b2b
C5-convertase	C4b2b3b	C3bC3bBb	C4b2b3b
MAC development	C5b+C6+C7+C8+C9		

Activation of Complements by Antigen-associated Antibody

In the classical pathway, C1 binds with its C1q subunits to Fc fragments (made of CH2 region) of IgG or IgM, which has formed a complex with antigens. C4b and C3b are also able to bind to antigen-associated IgG or IgM, to its Fc portion.

Such immunoglobulin-mediated binding of the complement may be interpreted as that the complement uses the ability of the immunoglobulin to detect and bind to non-self antigens as its guiding stick. The complement itself can bind non-self pathogens after detecting their pathogen-associated molecular patterns (PAMPs), however, utilizing specificity of the antibody, complements can detect non-self enemies much more specifically.

Some components have a variety of binding sites. In the classical pathway, C4 binds to Ig-associated C1q and C1r²s² enzyme cleaves C4 to C4b and 4a. C4b binds to C1q, antigen-associated Ig (specifically to its Fc portion), and even to the microbe surface. C3b binds to antigen-associated Ig and to the microbe surface. Ability of C3b to bind to antigen-associated Ig would work effectively against antigen-antibody complexes to make them soluble.

Regulation

The complement system has the potential to be extremely damaging to host tissues, meaning its activation must be tightly regulated. The complement system is regulated by complement control proteins, which are present at a higher concentration in the blood plasma than the complement proteins themselves. Some complement control proteins are present on the membranes of self-cells preventing them from being targeted by complement. One example is CD59, also known as protectin, which inhibits C9 polymerisation during the formation of the membrane attack complex. The classical pathway is inhibited by C1-inhibitor, which binds to C1 to prevent its activation.

C3-convertase can be inhibited by Decay accelerating factor (DAF), which is bound to erythrocyte plasma membranes via a GPI anchor.

Role in Disease

Complement Deficiency

It is thought that the complement system might play a role in many diseases with an immune component, such as Barraquer–Simons Syndrome, asthma, lupus erythematosus, glomerulonephritis, various forms of arthritis, autoimmune heart disease, multiple sclerosis, inflammatory bowel disease, paroxysmal nocturnal hemoglobinuria, atypical hemolytic uremic syndrome and ischemia-reperfusion injuries, and rejection of transplanted organs.

The complement system is also becoming increasingly implicated in diseases of the central nervous system such as Alzheimer's disease and other neurodegenerative conditions such as spinal cord injuries.

Deficiencies of the terminal pathway predispose to both autoimmune disease and infections (particularly Neisseria meningitidis, due to the role that the membrane attack complex ("MAC") plays in attacking Gram-negative bacteria).

Infections with *N. meningitidis* and *N. gonorrhoeae* are the only conditions known to be associated with deficiencies in the MAC components of complement. 40–50% of those with MAC deficiencies experience recurrent infections with *N. meningitidis*.

Deficiencies in Complement Regulators

Mutations in the complement regulators factor H and membrane cofactor protein have been associated with atypical hemolytic uremic syndrome. Moreover, a common single nucleotide polymorphism in factor H (Y402H) has been associated with the common eye disease age-related macular degeneration. Polymorphisms of complement component 3, complement factor B, and complement factor I, as well as deletion of complement factor H-related 3 and complement factor H-related 1 also affect a person's risk of developing age-related macular degeneration. Both of these disorders are currently thought to be due to aberrant complement activation on the surface of host cells.

Mutations in the C1 inhibitor gene can cause hereditary angioedema, a genetic condition resulting from reduced regulation of bradykinin by C1-INH.

Paroxysmal nocturnal hemoglobinuria is caused by complement breakdown of RBCs due to an inability to make GPI. Thus the RBCs are not protected by GPI anchored proteins such as DAF.

Diagnostic Tools

Diagnostic tools to measure complement activity include the total complement activity test.

The presence or absence of complement fixation upon a challenge can indicate whether particular antigens or antibodies are present in the blood. This is the principle of the complement fixation test.

Modulation by Infections

Recent research has suggested that the complement system is manipulated during HIV/AIDS, in a way that further damages the body.

Lymphatic System

The lymphatic system is part of the vascular system and an important part of the immune system, comprising a large network of lymphatic vessels that carry a clear fluid called lymph directionally towards the heart. The lymphatic system was first described in the seventeenth century independently by Olaus Rudbeck and Thomas Bartholin. Unlike the circulatory system, the lymphatic system is not a closed system. The human circulatory system processes an average of 20 litres of blood per day through capillary filtration, which removes plasma while leaving the blood cells. Roughly 17 litres of the filtered plasma is reabsorbed directly into the blood vessels, while the remaining three litres remain in the interstitial fluid. One of the main functions of the lymph system is to provide an accessory return route to the blood for the surplus three litres.

The other main function is that of defense in the immune system. Lymph is very similar to blood plasma: it contains lymphocytes. It also contains waste products and cellular debris together with bacteria and proteins. Associated organs composed of lymphoid tissue are the sites of lymphocyte production. Lymphocytes are concentrated in the lymph nodes. The spleen and the thymus are also lymphoid organs of the immune system. The tonsils are lymphoid organs that are also associated with the digestive system. Lymphoid tissues contain lymphocytes, and also contain other types of cells for support. The system also includes all the structures dedicated to the circulation and production of lymphocytes (the primary cellular component of lymph), which also includes the bone marrow, and the lymphoid tissue associated with the digestive system.

The blood does not come into direct contact with the parenchymal cells and tissues in the body (except in case of an injury causing rupture of one or more blood vessels), but constituents of the blood first exit the microvascular exchange blood vessels to become interstitial fluid, which comes into contact with the parenchymal cells of the body. Lymph is the fluid that is formed when interstitial fluid enters the initial lymphatic vessels of the lymphatic system. The lymph is then moved along the lymphatic vessel network by either intrinsic contractions of the lymphatic passages or by extrinsic compression of the lymphatic vessels via external tissue forces (e.g., the contractions of skeletal muscles), or by lymph hearts in some animals. The organization of lymph nodes and drainage follows the organization of the body into external and internal regions; therefore, the lymphatic drainage of the head, limbs, and body cavity walls follows an external route, and the lymphatic drainage of the thorax, abdomen, and pelvic cavities follows an internal route. Eventually, the lymph vessels empty into the lymphatic ducts, which drain into one of the two subclavian veins, near their junction with the internal jugular veins.

Structure

The lymphatic system consists of lymphatic organs, a conducting network of lymphatic vessels, and the circulating lymph.

The primary or central lymphoid organs generate lymphocytes from immature progenitor cells.

The thymus and the bone marrow constitute the primary lymphoid organs involved in the production and early clonal selection of lymphocyte tissues. Bone marrow is responsible for both the creation of T cells and the production and maturation of B cells. From the bone marrow, B cells immediately join the circulatory system and travel to secondary lymphoid organs in search of pathogens. T cells, on the other hand, travel from the bone marrow to the thymus, where they develop further. Mature T cells join B cells in search of pathogens. The other 95% of T cells begin a process of apoptosis, a form of programmed cell death.

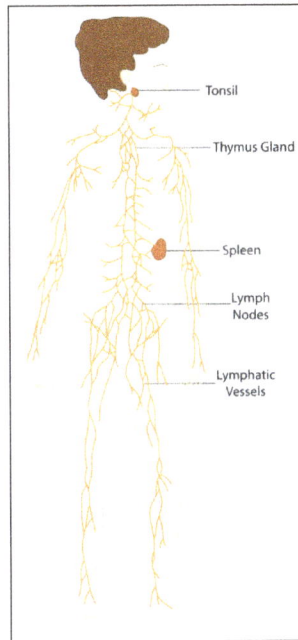

Lymphatic system

Secondary or peripheral lymphoid organs, which include lymph nodes and the spleen, maintain mature naive lymphocytes and initiate an adaptive immune response. The peripheral lymphoid organs are the sites of lymphocyte activation by antigens. Activation leads to clonal expansion and affinity maturation. Mature lymphocytes recirculate between the blood and the peripheral lymphoid organs until they encounter their specific antigen.

Secondary lymphoid tissue provides the environment for the foreign or altered native molecules (antigens) to interact with the lymphocytes. It is exemplified by the lymph nodes, and the lymphoid follicles in tonsils, Peyer's patches, spleen, adenoids, skin, etc. that are associated with the mucosa-associated lymphoid tissue (MALT).

In the gastrointestinal wall the appendix has mucosa resembling that of the colon, but here it is heavily infiltrated with lymphocytes.

Tertiary lymphoid organs (TLO) are abnormal lymph node–like structures that form in peripheral tissues at sites of chronic inflammation, such as chronic infection, transplanted organs undergoing graft rejection, some cancers, and autoimmune and autoimmune-related diseases. TLOs are regulated differently from the normal process whereby lymphoid tissues are formed during ontogeny, being dependent on cytokines and hematopoietic cells, but still drain interstitial fluid and transport lymphocytes in response to the same chemical messengers and gradients. TLOs typically contains far fewer lymphocytes, and assumes an immune role only when challenged with antigens that result in inflammation. It achieves this by importing the lymphocytes from blood and lymph.

Lymphoid Tissue

Thymus

The thymus is a primary lymphoid organ and the site of maturation for T cells, the lymphocytes of the adaptive immune system. The thymus increases in size from birth in response to postnatal antigen stimulation, then to puberty and regresses thereafter. The loss or lack of the thymus results in severe immunodeficiency and subsequent high susceptibility to infection. In most species, the thymus consists of lobules divided by septa which are made up of epithelium and is therefore an epithelial organ. T cells mature from thymocytes, proliferate and undergo selection process in the thymic cortex before entering the medulla to interact with epithelial cells.

The thymus provides an inductive environment for development of T cells from hematopoietic progenitor cells. In addition, thymic stromal cells allow for the selection of a functional and self-tolerant T cell repertoire. Therefore, one of the most important roles of the thymus is the induction of central tolerance.

The thymus is largest and most active during the neonatal and pre-adolescent periods. By the early teens, the thymus begins to atrophy and thymic stroma is mostly replaced by adipose tissue. Nevertheless, residual T lymphopoiesis continues throughout adult life.

Spleen

The main functions of the spleen are:

1. To produce immune cells to fight antigens.

2. To remove particulate matter and aged blood cells, mainly red blood cells.

3. To produce blood cells during fetal life.

The spleen synthesizes antibodies in its white pulp and removes antibody-coated bacteria and antibody-coated blood cells by way of blood and lymph node circulation. A study published in 2009 using mice found that the spleen contains, in its reserve, half of the body's monocytes within the red pulp. These monocytes, upon moving to injured tissue (such as the heart), turn into dendritic cells and macrophages while promoting tissue healing. The spleen is a center of activity of the mononuclear phagocyte system and can be considered analogous to a large lymph node, as its absence causes a predisposition to certain infections.

Like the thymus, the spleen has only efferent lymphatic vessels. Both the short gastric arteries and the splenic artery supply it with blood.

The germinal centers are supplied by arterioles called penicilliary radicles.

Up to the fifth month of prenatal development the spleen creates red blood cells. After birth the bone marrow is solely responsible for hematopoiesis. As a major lymphoid organ and a central player in the reticuloendothelial system, the spleen retains the ability to produce lymphocytes. The spleen stores red blood cells and lymphocytes. It can store enough blood cells to help in an emergency. Up to 25% of lymphocytes can be stored at any one time.

Lymph Nodes

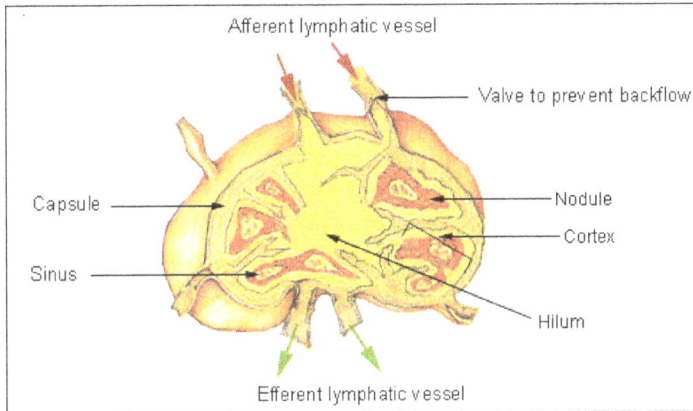

A lymph node showing afferent and efferent lymphatic vessels.

A lymph node is an organized collection of lymphoid tissue, through which the lymph passes on its way back to the blood. Lymph nodes are located at intervals along the lymphatic system. Several afferent lymph vessels bring in lymph, which percolates through the substance of the lymph node, and is then drained out by an efferent lymph vessel. There are between five and six hundred lymph nodes in the human body, many of which are grouped in clusters in different regions as in the underarm and abdominal areas. Lymph node clusters are commonly found at the base of limbs (groin, armpits) and in the neck, where lymph is collected from regions of the body likely to sustain pathogen contamination from injuries.

The substance of a lymph node consists of lymphoid follicles in an outer portion called the cortex. The inner portion of the node is called the medulla, which is surrounded by the cortex on all sides except for a portion known as the hilum. The hilum presents as a depression on the surface of the lymph node, causing the otherwise spherical lymph node to be bean-shaped or ovoid. The efferent lymph vessel directly emerges from the lymph node at the hilum. The arteries and veins supplying the lymph node with blood enter and exit through the hilum.

The region of the lymph node called the paracortex immediately surrounds the medulla. Unlike the cortex, which has mostly immature T cells, or thymocytes, the paracortex has a mixture of immature and mature T cells. Lymphocytes enter the lymph nodes through specialised high endothelial venules found in the paracortex.

A lymph follicle is a dense collection of lymphocytes, the number, size and configuration of which change in accordance with the functional state of the lymph node. For example, the follicles expand significantly when encountering a foreign antigen. The selection of B cells, or *B lymphocytes*, occurs in the germinal centre of the lymph nodes.

Lymph nodes are particularly numerous in the mediastinum in the chest, neck, pelvis, axilla, inguinal region, and in association with the blood vessels of the intestines.

Other Lymphoid Tissue

Lymphoid tissue associated with the lymphatic system is concerned with immune functions in defending the body against infections and the spread of tumours. It consists of connective tissue formed of reticular fibers, with various types of leukocytes, (white blood cells), mostly lymphocytes enmeshed in it, through which the lymph passes. Regions of the lymphoid tissue that are densely packed with lymphocytes are known as lymphoid follicles. Lymphoid tissue can either be structurally well organized as lymph nodes or may consist of loosely organized lymphoid follicles known as the mucosa-associated lymphoid tissue.

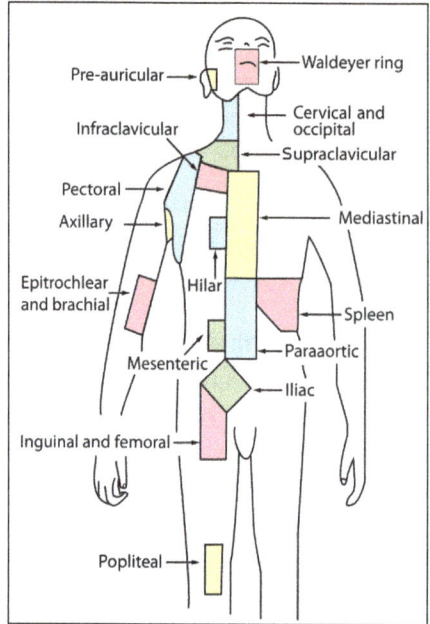

Regional lymph nodes.

The central nervous system also has lymphatic vessels, as discovered by the University of Virginia Researchers. The search for T-cell gateways into and out of the meninges uncovered functional meningeal lymphatic vessels lining the dural sinuses, anatomically integrated into the membrane surrounding the brain.

Lymphatic Vessels

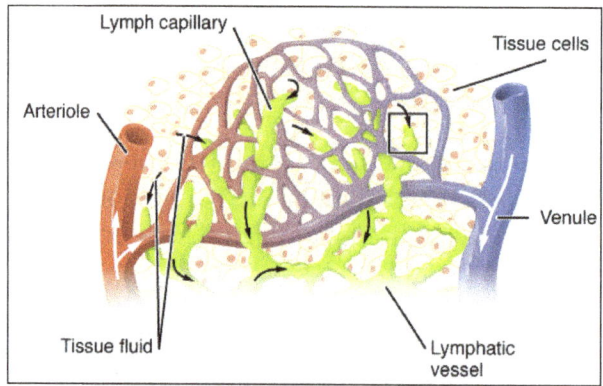

Lymph capillaries in the tissue spaces.

The lymphatic vessels, also called lymph vessels, conduct lymph between different parts of the body. They include the tubular vessels of the lymph capillaries, and the larger collecting vessels—the right lymphatic duct and the thoracic duct (the left lymphatic duct). The lymph capillaries are mainly responsible for the absorption of interstitial fluid from the tissues, while lymph vessels propel the absorbed fluid forward into the larger collecting ducts, where it ultimately returns to the bloodstream via one of the subclavian veins. These vessels are also called the lymphatic channels or simply lymphatics.

The lymphatics are responsible for maintaining the balance of the body fluids. Its network of capillaries and collecting lymphatic vessels work to efficiently drain and transport extravasated fluid, along with proteins and antigens, back to the circulatory system. Numerous intraluminal valves in the vessels ensure a unidirectional flow of lymph without reflux. Two valve systems are used to achieve this one directional flow—a primary and a secondary valve system. The capillaries are blind-ended, and the valves at the ends of capillaries use specialised junctions together with anchoring filaments to allow a unidirectional flow to the primary vessels. The collecting lymphatics, however, act to propel the lymph by the combined actions of the intraluminal valves and lymphatic muscle cells.

Development

Lymphatic tissues begin to develop by the end of the fifth week of embryonic development. Lymphatic vessels develop from lymph sacs that arise from developing veins, which are derived from mesoderm.

The first lymph sacs to appear are the paired jugular lymph sacs at the junction of the internal jugular and subclavian veins. From the jugular lymph sacs, lymphatic capillary plexuses spread to the thorax, upper limbs, neck and head. Some of the plexuses enlarge and form lymphatic vessels in their respective regions. Each jugular lymph sac retains at least one connection with its jugular vein, the left one developing into the superior portion of the thoracic duct.

The next lymph sac to appear is the unpaired retroperitoneal lymph sac at the root of the mesentery of the intestine. It develops from the primitive vena cava and mesonephric veins. Capillary plexuses and lymphatic vessels spread from the retroperitoneal lymph sac to the abdominal viscera and diaphragm. The sac establishes connections with the cisterna chyli but loses its connections with neighbouring veins.

The last of the lymph sacs, the paired posterior lymph sacs, develop from the iliac veins. The posterior lymph sacs produce capillary plexuses and lymphatic vessels of the abdominal wall, pelvic region, and lower limbs. The posterior lymph sacs join the cisterna chyli and lose their connections with adjacent veins.

With the exception of the anterior part of the sac from which the cisterna chyli develops, all lymph sacs become invaded by mesenchymal cells and are converted into groups of lymph nodes.

The spleen develops from mesenchymal cells between layers of the dorsal mesentery of the stomach. The thymus arises as an outgrowth of the third pharyngeal pouch.

Function

The lymphatic system has multiple interrelated functions:

- It is responsible for the removal of interstitial fluid from tissues.

- It absorbs and transports fatty acids and fats as chyle from the digestive system.

- It transports white blood cells to and from the lymph nodes into the bones.

- The lymph transports antigen-presenting cells, such as dendritic cells, to the lymph nodes where an immune response is stimulated.

Fat Absorption

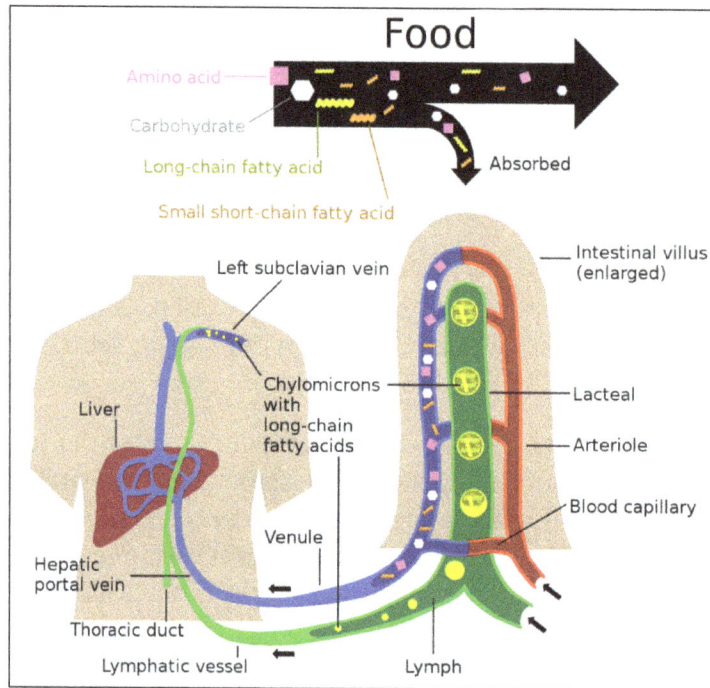

Nutrients in food are absorbed via intestinal vili (greatly enlargened in the picture) to blood and lymph. Long-chain fatty acids (and other lipids with similar fat solubility like some medicines) are absorbed to the lymph and move in it enveloped inside chylomicrons. They move via thoracic duct of the lymphatic system and finally enter the blood via the left subclavian vein thus bypassing the liver's first pass metabolism completely.

Lymph vessels called lacteals are at the beginning of the gastrointestinal tract, predominantly in the small intestine. While most other nutrients absorbed by the small intestine are passed on to the portal venous system to drain via the portal vein into the liver for processing, fats (lipids) are passed on to the lymphatic system to be transported to the blood circulation via the thoracic duct. (There are exceptions, for example medium-chain triglycerides are fatty acid esters of glycerol that passively diffuse from the GI tract to the portal system.) The enriched lymph originating in the lymphatics of the small intestine is called chyle. The nutrients that are released into the circulatory system are processed by the liver, having passed through the systemic circulation.

Immune Function

The lymphatic system plays a major role in the body's immune system, as the primary site for cells relating to adaptive immune system including T-cells and B-cells. Cells in the lymphatic system react to antigens presented or found by the cells directly or by other dendritic cells. When an antigen is recognized, an immunological cascade begins involving the activation and recruitment of more and more cells, the production of antibodies and cytokines and the recruitment of other immunological cells such as macrophages.

Clinical Significance

The study of lymphatic drainage of various organs is important in the diagnosis, prognosis, and treatment of cancer. The lymphatic system, because of its closeness to many tissues of the body, is responsible for carrying cancerous cells between the various parts of the body in a process called metastasis. The intervening lymph nodes can trap the cancer cells. If they are not successful in destroying the cancer cells the nodes may become sites of secondary tumours.

Enlarged Lymph Nodes

Lymphadenopathy refers to one or more enlarged lymph nodes. Small groups or individually enlarged lymph nodes are generally reactive in response to infection or inflammation. This is called local lymphadenopathy. When many lymph nodes in different areas of the body are involved, this is called generalised lymphadenopathy. Generalised lymphadenopathy may be caused by infections such as infectious mononucleosis, tuberculosis and HIV, connective tissue diseases such as SLE and rheumatoid arthritis, and cancers, including both cancers of tissue within lymph nodes, and metastasis of cancerous cells from other parts of the body, that have arrived via the lymphatic system.

Lymphedema

Lymphedema is the swelling caused by the accumulation of lymph, which may occur if the lymphatic system is damaged or has malformations. It usually affects limbs, though the face, neck and abdomen may also be affected. In an extreme state, called elephantiasis, the edema progresses to the extent that the skin becomes thick with an appearance similar to the skin on elephant limbs.

Causes are unknown in most cases, but sometimes there is a previous history of severe infection, usually caused by a parasitic disease, such as lymphatic filariasis.

Lymphangiomatosis is a disease involving multiple cysts or lesions formed from lymphatic vessels.

Lymphedema can also occur after surgical removal of lymph nodes in the armpit (causing the arm to swell due to poor lymphatic drainage) or groin (causing swelling of the leg). Conventional treatment is by manual lymphatic drainage and compression garments. Two drugs for the treatment of lymphedema are in clinical trials: Lymfactin and Ubenimex/Bestatin.

There is no evidence to suggest that the effects of manual lymphatic drainage are permanent.

Cancer

Cancer of the lymphatic system can be primary or secondary. Lymphoma refers to cancer that arises from lymphatic tissue. Lymphoid leukaemias and lymphomas are now considered to be tumours of the same type of cell lineage. They are called "leukaemia" when in the blood or marrow and "lymphoma" when in lymphatic tissue. They are grouped together under the name "lymphoid malignancy".

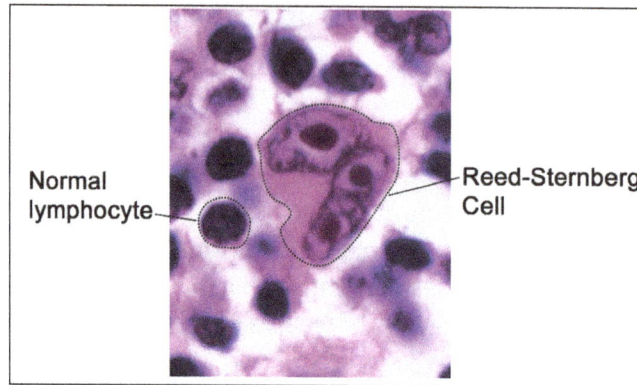

Reed–Sternberg cells.

Lymphoma is generally considered as either Hodgkin lymphoma or non-Hodgkin lymphoma. Hodgkin lymphoma is characterised by a particular type of cell, called a Reed–Sternberg cell, visible under microscope. It is associated with past infection with the Epstein-Barr Virus, and generally causes a painless "rubbery" lymphadenopathy. It is staged, using Ann Arbor staging. Chemotherapy generally involves the ABVD and may also involve radiotherapy. Non-Hodgkin lymphoma is a cancer characterised by increased proliferation of B-cells or T-cells, generally occurs in an older age group than Hodgkin lymphoma. It is treated according to whether it is *high-grade* or *low-grade*, and carries a poorer prognosis than Hodgkin lymphoma.

Lymphangiosarcoma is a malignant soft tissue tumour, whereas lymphangioma is a benign tumour occurring frequently in association with Turner syndrome. Lymphangioleiomyomatosis is a benign tumour of the smooth muscles of the lymphatics that occurs in the lungs.

Lymphoid leukaemia is another form of cancer where the host is devoid of different lymphatic cells.

Others are:

- Castleman's disease;
- Chylothorax;
- Kawasaki disease;
- Kikuchi disease;
- Lipedema;
- Lymphangitis;
- Lymphatic filariasis;
- Lymphocytic choriomeningitis;
- Solitary lymphatic nodule.

White Blood Cell

White blood cells (also called leukocytes or leucocytes and abbreviated as WBCs) are the cells of the immune system that are involved in protecting the body against both infectious disease and foreign invaders. All white blood cells are produced and derived from multipotent cells in the bone marrow known as hematopoietic stem cells. Leukocytes are found throughout the body, including the blood and lymphatic system.

All white blood cells have nuclei, which distinguishes them from the other blood cells, the anucleated red blood cells (RBCs) and platelets. Types of white blood cells can be classified in standard ways. Two pairs of broadest categories classify them either by structure (granulocytes or agranulocytes) or by cell lineage (myeloid cells or lymphoid cells). These broadest categories can be further divided into the five main types: neutrophils, eosinophils (acidophiles), basophils, lymphocytes, and monocytes. These types are distinguished by their physical and functional characteristics. Monocytes and neutrophils are phagocytic. Further subtypes can be classified; for example, among lymphocytes, there are B cells, T cells, and NK cells.

The number of leukocytes in the blood is often an indicator of disease, and thus the *white blood cell count* is an important subset of the complete blood count. The normal white cell count is usually between 4×10^9/L and 1.1×10^{10}/L. In the US, this is usually expressed as 4,000 to 11,000 white blood cells per microliter of blood. White blood cells make up approximately 1% of the total blood volume in a healthy adult, making them substantially less numerous than the red blood cells at 40% to 45%. However, this 1% of the blood makes a large difference to health, because immunity depends on it. An increase in the number of leukocytes over the upper limits is called leukocytosis. It is normal when it is part of healthy immune responses, which happen frequently. It is occasionally abnormal, when it is neoplastic or autoimmune in origin. A decrease below the lower limit is called leukopenia. This indicates a weakened immune system.

Types

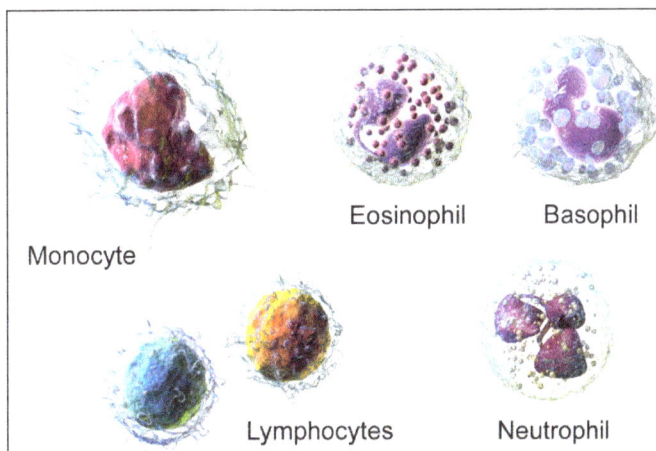

3D rendering of various types of white blood cells.

All white blood cells are nucleated, which distinguishes them from the anucleated red blood cells and platelets. Types of leukocytes can be classified in standard ways. Two pairs of broadest categories classify them either by structure (granulocytes or agranulocytes) or by cell lineage (myeloid cells or lymphoid cells). These broadest categories can be further divided into the five main types: Neutrophils, eosinophils, basophils, lymphocytes, and monocytes. These types are distinguished by their physical and functional characteristics. Monocytes and neutrophils are phagocytic. Further subtypes can be classified.

Granulocytes are distinguished from agranulocytes by their nucleus shape (lobed versus round, that is, polymorphonuclear versus mononuclear) and by their cytoplasm granules (present or absent, or more precisely, visible on light microscopy or not thus visible). The other dichotomy is by lineage: Myeloid cells (neutrophils, monocytes, eosinophils and basophils) are distinguished from lymphoid cells (lymphocytes) by hematopoietic lineage (cellular differentiation lineage). Lymphocytes can be further classified as T cells, B cells, and natural killer cells.

Type	Approx. % in adults	Diameter (μm)	Main targets	Nucleus	Granules	Lifetime
Neutrophil	62%	10–12	• Bacteria • Fungi	Multi-lobed	Fine, faintly pink (H&E stain)	6 hours–few days(days in spleen and other tissue)
Eosinophil	2.3%	10–12	• Larger parasites • Modulate allergic inflammatory responses	Bi-lobed	Full of pink-orange (H&E stain)	8–12 days (circulate for 4–5 hours)
Basophil	0.4%	12–15	• Release histamine for inflammatory responses	Bi-lobed or tri-lobed	Large blue	A few hours to a few days

Lymphocyte	30%	Small lymphocytes 7–8
		
		Large lymphocytes 12–15
			• B cells: releases antibodies and assists activation of T cells
			• T cells:
			  ◦ CD4+ Th (T helper) cells: activate and regulate T and B cells
			  ◦ CD8+ cytotoxic T cells: virus-infected and tumor cells.
			  ◦ γδ T cells: bridge between innate and adaptive immune responses; phagocytosis
			  ◦ Regulatory (suppressor) T cells: Returns the functioning of the immune system to normal operation after infection; prevents autoimmunity
			• Natural killer cells: virus-infected and tumor cells.
				Deeply staining, eccentric	NK-cells and cytotoxic (CD8+) T-cells	Years for memory cells, weeks for all else.

Monocyte	5.3%	15–30	• Monocytes migrate from the bloodstream to other tissues and differentiate into tissue resident macrophages, Kupffer cells in the liver.	Kidney shaped	None	Hours to days

Neutrophil

Neutrophils are the most abundant white blood cell, constituting 60-70% of the circulating leukocytes, and including two functionally unequal subpopulations: Neutrophil-killers and neutrophil-cagers. They defend against bacterial or fungal infection. They are usually first responders to microbial infection; their activity and death in large numbers form pus. They are commonly referred to as polymorphonuclear (PMN) leukocytes, although, in the technical sense, PMN refers to all granulocytes. They have a multi-lobed nucleus, which consists of three to five lobes connected by slender strands. This gives the neutrophils the appearance of having multiple nuclei, hence the name polymorphonuclear leukocyte. The cytoplasm may look transparent because of fine granules that are pale lilac when stained. Neutrophils are active in phagocytosing bacteria and are present in large amount in the pus of wounds. These cells are not able to renew their lysosomes (used in digesting microbes) and die after having phagocytosed a few pathogens. Neutrophils are the most common cell type seen in the early stages of acute inflammation. The average lifespan of inactivated human neutrophils in the circulation has been reported by different approaches to be between 5 and 135 hours.

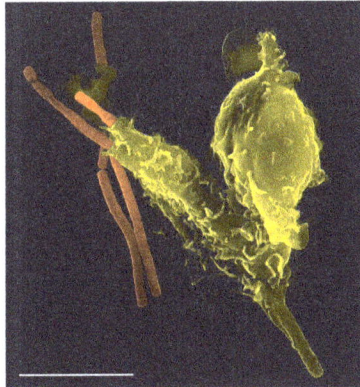

Neutrophil engulfing anthrax bacteria.

Eosinophil

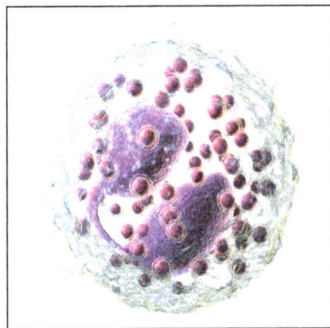

Eosinophils compose about 2-4% of the WBC total. This count fluctuates throughout the day, seasonally, and during menstruation. It rises in response to allergies, parasitic infections, collagen diseases, and disease of the spleen and central nervous system. They are rare in the blood, but numerous in the mucous membranes of the respiratory, digestive, and lower urinary tracts.

They primarily deal with parasitic infections. Eosinophils are also the predominant inflammatory cells in allergic reactions. The most important causes of eosinophilia include allergies such as asthma, hay fever, and hives; and also parasitic infections. They secrete chemicals that destroy these large parasites, such as hook worms and tapeworms, that are too big for any one WBC to phagocytize. In general, their nucleus is bi-lobed. The lobes are connected by a thin strand. The cytoplasm is full of granules that assume a characteristic pink-orange color with eosin staining.

Basophil

Basophils are chiefly responsible for allergic and antigen response by releasing the chemical histamine causing the dilation of blood vessels. Because they are the rarest of the white blood cells (less than 0.5% of the total count) and share physicochemical properties with other blood cells, they are difficult to study. They can be recognized by several coarse, dark violet granules, giving them a blue hue. The nucleus is bi- or tri-lobed, but it is hard to see because of the number of coarse granules that hide it.

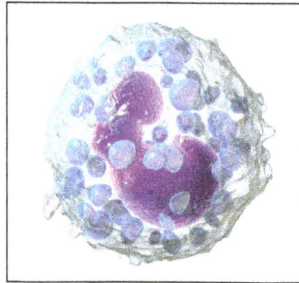

The movement of leukocytes in the blood. Phase-contrast microscopy.

They excrete two chemicals that aid in the body's defenses: histamine and heparin. Histamine is responsible for widening blood vessels and increasing the flow of blood to injured tissue. It also makes blood vessels more permeable so neutrophils and clotting proteins can get into connective tissue more easily. Heparin is an anticoagulant that inhibits blood clotting and promotes the movement of white blood cells into an area. Basophils can also release chemical signals that attract eosinophils and neutrophils to an infection site.

Lymphocyte

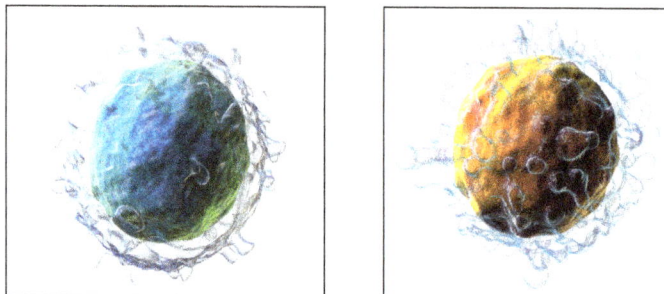

Lymphocytes are much more common in the lymphatic system than in blood. Lymphocytes are distinguished by having a deeply staining nucleus that may be eccentric in location, and a relatively small amount of cytoplasm. Lymphocytes include:

- B cells make antibodies that can bind to pathogens, block pathogen invasion, activate the complement system, and enhance pathogen destruction.

- T cells:

  ◦ CD4+ helper T cells: T cells displaying co-receptor CD4 are known as CD4+ T cells. These cells have T-cell receptors and CD4 molecules that, in combination, bind antigenic peptides presented on major histocompatibility complex (MHC) class II molecules on antigen-presenting cells. Helper T cells make cytokines and perform other functions that help coordinate the immune response. In HIV infection, these T cells are the main index to identify the individual's immune system integrity.

  ◦ CD8+ cytotoxic T cells: T cells displaying co-receptor CD8 are known as CD8+ T cells. These cells bind antigens presented on MHC I complex of virus-infected or tumour cells and kill them. Nearly all nucleated cells display MHC I.

  ◦ γδ T cells possess an alternative T cell receptor (different from the αβ TCR found on conventional CD4+ and CD8+ T cells). Found in tissue more commonly than in blood, γδ T cells share characteristics of helper T cells, cytotoxic T cells, and natural killer cells.

- Natural killer cells are able to kill cells of the body that do not display MHC class I molecules, or display stress markers such as MHC class I polypeptide-related sequence A (MIC-A). Decreased expression of MHC class I and up-regulation of MIC-A can happen when cells are infected by a virus or become cancerous.

Monocyte

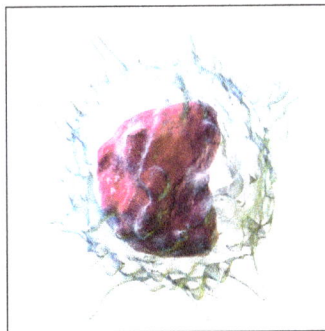

Monocytes, the largest type of WBCs, share the "vacuum cleaner" (phagocytosis) function of neutrophils, but are much longer lived as they have an extra role: they present pieces of pathogens to T cells so that the pathogens may be recognized again and killed. This causes an antibody response to be mounted. Monocytes eventually leave the bloodstream and become tissue macrophages, which remove dead cell debris as well as attack microorganisms. Neither dead cell debris nor attacking microorganisms can be dealt with effectively by the neutrophils. Unlike neutrophils, monocytes are able to replace their lysosomal contents and are thought to have a much longer active life. They have the kidney shaped nucleus and are typically agranulated. They also possess abundant cytoplasm.

Fixed Leucocytes

In figure, HSC=Hematopoietic stem cell, Progenitor=Progenitor cell, L-blast=Lymphoblast, Lymphocyte, Mo-blast=Monoblast, Monocyte, Myeloblast, Pro-M=Promyelocyte, Myelocyte, Meta-M=Metamyelocyte, Neutrophil, Eosinophil, Basophil, Pro-E=Proerythroblast, Baso-E=Basophilic erythroblast, poly-E=Polychromatic erythroblast, Ortho-E=Orthochromatic erythroblast, Erythrocyte, Promegakaryocyte, Megakaryocyte, Platelet.

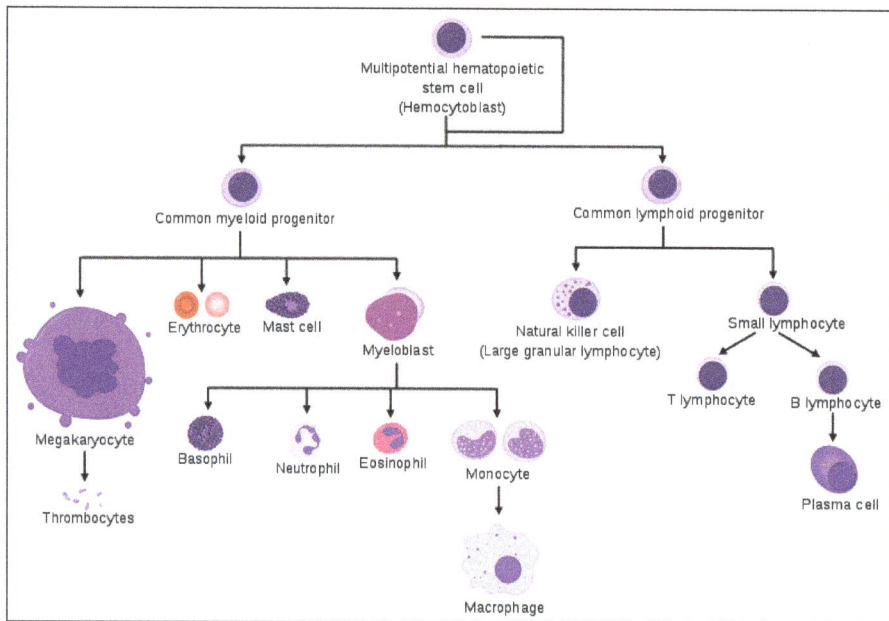

Some leucocytes migrate into the tissues of the body to take up a permanent residence at that location rather than remaining in the blood. Often these cells have specific names depending upon which tissue they settle in, such as fixed macrophages in the liver, which become known as Kupffer cells. These cells still serve a role in the immune system.

- Histiocytes;

- Dendritic cells (Although these will often migrate to local lymph nodes upon ingesting antigens);

- Mast cells;

- Microglia.

Disorders

The two commonly used categories of white blood cell disorders divide them quantitatively into those causing excessive numbers (proliferative disorders) and those causing insufficient numbers (leukopenias). Leukocytosis is usually healthy (e.g., fighting an infection), but it also may be dysfunctionally proliferative. WBC proliferative disorders can be classed as myeloproliferative and lymphoproliferative. Some are autoimmune, but many are neoplastic.

Another way to categorize disorders of white blood cells is qualitatively. There are various disorders in which the number of white blood cells is normal but the cells do not function normally.

Neoplasia of WBCs can be benign but is often malignant. Of the various tumors of the blood and lymph, cancers of WBCs can be broadly classified as leukemias and lymphomas, although those categories overlap and are often grouped as a pair.

Leucopenias

A range of disorders can cause decreases in white blood cells. This type of white blood cell decreased is usually the neutrophil. In this case the decrease may be called neutropenia or granulocytopenia. Less commonly, a decrease in lymphocytes (called lymphocytopenia or lymphopenia) may be seen.

Neutropenia

Neutropenia can be acquired or intrinsic. A decrease in levels of neutrophils on lab tests is due to either decreased production of neutrophils or increased removal from the blood.

- Medications - chemotherapy, sulfas or other antibiotics, phenothiazenes, benzodiazepines, antithyroids, anticonvulsants, quinine, quinidine, indomethacin, procainamide, thiazides,
- Radiation,
- Toxins - alcohol, benzenes,
- Intrinsic disorders - fanconi's, Kostmann's, cyclic neutropenia, Chédiak–Higashi,
- Immune dysfunction - disorders of collagen, AIDS, rheumatoid arthritis,
- Blood cell dysfunction - megaloblastic anemia, myelodysplasia, marrow failure, marrow replacement, acute leukemia,
- Any major infection,
- Miscellaneous - starvation, hypersplenism.

Symptoms of neutropenia are associated with the underlying cause of the decrease in neutrophils. For example, the most common cause of acquired neutropenia is drug-induced, so an individual may have symptoms of medication overdose or toxicity. Treatment is also aimed at the underlying cause of the neutropenia. One severe consequence of neutropenia is that it can increase the risk of infection.

Lymphocytopenia

Defined as total lymphocyte count below 1.0×10^9/L, the cells most commonly affected are CD4+ T cells. Like neutropenia, lymphocytopenia may be acquired or intrinsic and there are many causes.

- Inherited immune deficiency - severe combined immunodeficiency, common variable immune deficiency, ataxia-telangiectasia, Wiskott-Aldrich syndrome, immunodeficiency with short-limbed dwarfism, immunodeficiency with thymoma, purine nucleoside phosphorylase deficiency, genetic polymorphism.
- Blood cell dysfunction - aplastic anemia.
- Infectious diseases - viral (AIDS, SARS, West Nile encephalitis, hepatitis, herpes, measles, others), bacterial (TB, typhoid, pneumonia, rickettsiosis, ehrlichiosis, sepsis), parasitic (acute phase of malaria).

- Medications - chemotherapy (antilymphocyte globulin therapy, alemtuzumab, glucocorticoids).

- Radiation.

- Major surgery.

- Miscellaneous - ECMO, kidney or bone marrow transplant, hemodialysis, kidney failure, severe burn, celiac disease, severe acute pancreatitis, sarcoidosis, protein-losing enteropathy, strenuous exercise, carcinoma.

- Immune dysfunction - arthritis, systemic lupus erythematosus, Sjögren syndrome, myasthenia gravis, systemic vasculitis, Behcet-like syndrome, dermatomyositis, granulomatosis with polyangiitis.

- Nutritional/Dietary - alcohol abuse, zinc deficiency.

Like neutropenia, symptoms and treatment of lymphocytopenia are directed at the underlying cause of the change in cell counts.

Proliferative Disorders

An increase in the number of white blood cells in circulation is called leukocytosis. This increase is most commonly caused by inflammation. There are four major causes: increase of production in bone marrow, increased release from storage in bone marrow, decreased attachment to veins and arteries, decreased uptake by tissues. Leukocytosis may affect one or more cell lines and can be neutrophilic, eosinophilic, basophilic, monocytosis, or lymphocytosis.

Neutrophilia

Neutrophilia is an increase in the absolute neutrophil count in the peripheral circulation. Normal blood values vary by age. Neutrophilia can be caused by a direct problem with blood cells (primary disease). It can also occur as a consequence of an underlying disease (secondary). Most cases of neutrophilia are secondary to inflammation.

Primary Causes:

- Conditions with normally functioning neutrophils – hereditary neutrophilia, chronic idiopathic neutrophilia.

- Pelger–Huet anomaly.

- Down syndrome.

- Leukocyte adhesion deficiency.

- Familial cold urticaria.

- Leukemia (chronic myelogenous (CML)) and other myeloproliferative disorders.

- Surgical removal of spleen.

Secondary Causes:

- Infection.

- Chronic inflammation – especially juvenile rheumatoid arthritis, rheumatoid arthritis, Still's disease, Crohn's disease, ulcerative colitis, granulomatous infections (for example, tuberculosis), and chronic hepatitis.

- Cigarette smoking – occurs in 25–50% of chronic smokers and can last up to 5 years after quitting.

- Stress – exercise, surgery, general stress.

- Medication induced – corticosteroids (for example, prednisone, β-agonists, lithium).

- Cancer – either by growth factors secreted by the tumor or invasion of bone marrow by the cancer.

- Increased destruction of cells in peripheral circulation can stimulate bone marrow. This can occur in hemolytic anemia and idiopathic thrombocytopenic purpura.

Eosinophilia

A normal eosinophil count is considered to be less than 0.65×10^9/L. Eosinophil counts are higher in newborns and vary with age, time (lower in the morning and higher at night), exercise, environment, and exposure to allergens. Eosinophilia is never a normal lab finding. Efforts should always be made to discover the underlying cause, though the cause may not always be found.

Counting and Reference Ranges

The complete blood cell count is a blood panel that includes the overall WBC count and various subsets such as the absolute neutrophil count. Reference ranges for blood tests specify the typical counts in healthy people.

TLC- (Total leucocyte count): Normal TLC in an adult person is 6000-8000WBC/mm^3 of blood.

DLC- (Differential leucocyte count): Number/ (%) of different type of leucocyte in per cubic mm. of blood.

Phagocyte

Phagocytes are a type of white blood cell that use phagocytosis to engulf bacteria, foreign particles, and dying cells to protect the body. They bind to pathogens and internalise them in a phagosome, which acidifies and fuses with lysosomes in order to destroy the contents.

They are a key component of the innate immune system. There are three main groups of phagocytes: Monocytes and macrophages, granulocytes, and dendritic cells, all of which have a slightly different function in the body.

Monocytes

Monocytes are a type of phagocyte found in the bloodstream. They circulate around the body, and when a tissue is infected or inflamed they may leave the bloodstream and enter the tissue.

In the tissue they differentiate into macrophages, which form the major resident population of phagocytes in normal tissues. Monocytes are phagocytic but since most infections occur in tissues, it is the ability of monocytes to differentiate that is particularly key. If a particular set of signals are present, it is also possible for monocytes to differentiate into dendritic cells in the tissues.

Monocytes are the largest type of phagocyte, with a kidney bean shaped nucleus when seen under a microscope.

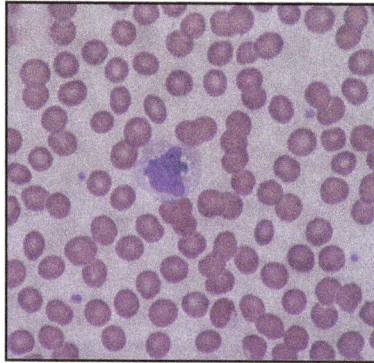

Figure: Electron micrograph showing a monocyte surrounded by red blood cells.

Macrophages

Macrophages are derived from monocytes and are found in the tissues. They have a major role as a first defence mechanism in phagocytosis of cellular debris, microbes and any other foreign substances.

They also help initiate the adaptive immune response by presenting antigens to T cells and secreting factors to induce inflammation and recruit other cells.

Macrophages may be termed differently depending on their location: microglia are present in the CNS and Kupffer cells are in the liver.

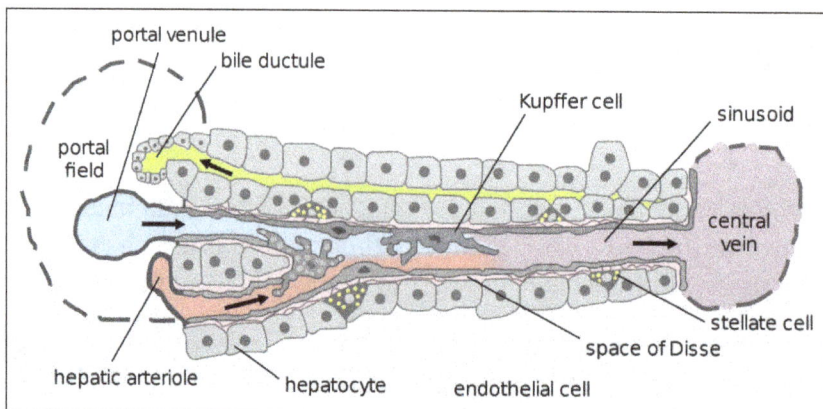

Diagram showing the location of Kupffer cells within the liver.

Dendritic Cells

The major function of dendritic cells is as a link between the innate and the adaptive immune systems. As immature dendritic cells they travel in the bloodstream and migrate through tissues and continually sample the pathogens they find via macropinocytosis.

Following phagocytosis, the cell becomes mature and migrates to a peripheral lymphoid organ such as a lymph node, the spleen, or gut-associated lymphoid tissue to present the antigen to a T cell. This then activates the T cell to initiate an adaptive immune response.

Dendritic cells can be recognised by the presence of multiple cytoplasmic projections from their surface, giving them a large surface area to volume ratio that aids close contact with multiple cells. These processes look similar to the dendrites of neurons, which gave dendritic cells their name.

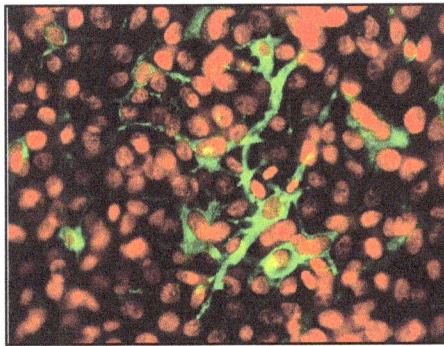

Dendritic cells (stained green) located in the corneal epithelium.

Granulocytes

Granulocytes are a group of cells with dense granules in their cytoplasm, and include neutrophils, eosinophils, and basophils.

Neutrophils are the most phagocytic of these cells: they are the most abundant white blood cell, and can be identified by their granular cytoplasm and lobulated nuclei (usually 2-5 lobules). They are formed from myeloid stem cells found within bone marrow.

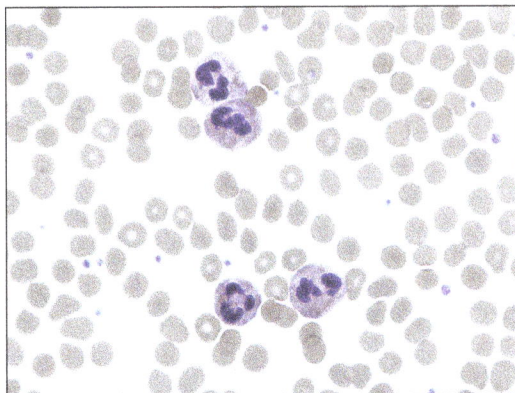

Electron micrograph showing neutrophils on a blood smear.

They are normally found within the bloodstream, but during the acute phase of infection they are among the first inflammatory cells to reach the site of infection. They are particularly specialised at killing intracellular pathogens due to cytoplasmic granules with toxic substances such as anti-microbial peptides, enzymes, and reactive oxygen species.

Neutrophils are short-lived cells and normally die following phagocytosis and use of their granules- dying or dead neutrophils are a major part of the pus seen with infection. Neutrophils are also important for inducing inflammation and recruiting inflammatory cells through release of cytokines and other inflammatory factors.

Innate Lymphoid Cell

Innate lymphoid cells (ILCs) are a group of innate immune cells that are derived from common lymphoid progenitor (CLP) and belong to the lymphoid lineage. These cells are defined by absence of antigen specific B or T cell receptor because of the lack of recombination activating gene (RAG). ILCs do not express myeloid or dendritic cell markers.

This relatively newly described group of cells has varying physiological functions; some functions are analogous to helper T cells, while the group also includes cytotoxic NK cells. Accordingly, they have an important role in protective immunity and the regulation of homeostasis and inflammation, so their dysregulation can lead to immune pathology such as allergy, bronchial asthma and autoimmune disease. In addition, they can regulate adipose function and metabolic homeostasis, in part by eliciting beiging.

Classification

ILCs can be divided based on the cytokines that they can produce, and the transcription factors that regulate their development and function. For each newly discovered branch of the ILC family, it will be important to determine whether a cell type represents a stable lineage or just a stage of differentiation or activation. The emerging body of data about the transcription factors and cytokine signals that differentiate ILCs contributes to the evolving classification system used to identify ILCs.

In 2013 a nomenclature and classification system was proposed that divides the known ILCs into three groups.

Group 1 ILCs

Group 1 ILCs constitutively express transcription factor T-bet and is able to produce Th1 cytokines (notably IFNγ and TNF) after stimulation with IL-12 or IL-18.

ILC1 cells comprise NK cells, CD127low CD103+ intraepithelial ILC1s and CD127high ILC1s.

- ILC1s are weakly cytotoxic cells closely related to Group 3 ILCs, from which they even appear to arise. ILC1s are analogous to T_h1 cells and share the common transcription factor of T-bet.

- Natural killer ('NK') cells are cytotoxic innate effector cells analogous to the cytotoxic T cells of the adaptive immune system. They are distributed throughout the blood, organs, and lymphoid tissue and make up around 15% of the peripheral blood lymphocytes. NK cells play a role in tumor surveillance and the rapid elimination of virus-infected cells. They do not require the missing "self" signal of MHC Class I and can recognize stressed cells in the absence of antibodies, allowing them to react much more quickly than the adaptive immune system. NK cells, discovered in 1975, are the prototypical innate lymphoid cell, and have been described as large granular lymphocytes that lack the T cell receptor.

Group 2 ILCs

Group 2 ILCs can produce type 2 cytokines (e.g. IL-4, IL-5, IL-9, IL-13).

ILC2s (also termed natural helper cells, nuocytes, or innate helper 2 cells) play the crucial role of secreting type 2 cytokines in response to helminth infection. They have also been implicated in the development of allergic lung inflammation. They express characteristic surface markers and receptors for chemokines, which are involved in distribution of lymphoid cells to specific organ sites. They require IL-7 for their development, which activates two transcription factors (both required by these cells)—RORα and GATA3. After stimulation with Th2 polarising cytokines (e.g. IL-25, IL-33, TSLP) ILC2s start to produce IL-5, IL-13, IL-9, IL-4. ILC2s are critical for primary responses to local Th2 antigens e.g. helminths and viruses and that is why ILC2s are abundant in tissues of skin, lungs, livers and gut.

In mice, ILC2s can regulate adipose function and metabolic homeostasis in part via production of enkephalin peptides that elicit beiging.

Group 3 ILCs

Group 3 ILCs are defined by their capacity to produce cytokines IL-17A and/or IL-22. They are the innate counterpart to T_h17 cells, and share the common transcription factor of RORγt. They comprise ILC3s and lymphoid tissue-inducer (LTi) cells:

- ILC3s are a lymphoid cell population that can produce IL-22 and expresses NKp46 (an NK cell activating receptor). Nevertheless, ILC3s differ from NK cells, as they are dependent on transcription factor RORγt, they lack cytotoxic effectors (perforin, granzymes and death receptors) and they do not produce IFNγ or TNF. They are found mainly in mucosal tissues and particularly in the intestinal tract.

- Lymphoid tissue inducer ('LTi') cells Lymphoid tissue inducer cells are a subset of innate lymphoid cells belonging to lymphoid lineage of hematopoetic origin. They are represented by embryonic lymphoid tissue inducer cells, which have the pivotal role in primary and secondary lymphoid tissue organization, and adult lymphoid tissue inducer cells, regulating adaptive immune response and maintaining secondary lymhoid tissue structure.

Characterization of LTi Cells

LTi are cells positive for IL7+CD45+CD4+ and negative for CD3 marker expressing LTαβ. Additionally, they express TNF-related activation-induced chemokine (TRANCE), Tumor Necrosis

Factor Superfamily Member 14 (TNFSF14, also known as LIGHT) and Tumor Necrosis Factor Alpha (TNFα), which are all ligands of the tumor necrosis factor (TNF) family. They also express chemokine receptors, such as C-X-C chemokine receptor type 5 (CXCR5), C-X-C chemokine receptor type 7 (CXCR7), and adhesion molecules Very Late Antigen-4 (VLA-4, also known as Integrin α4β1), Integrin α4β7 and Intercellular Adhesion Molecule 1 (ICAM-1). Furthermore, LTis are positive for CD25, CD44, CD90, CD117, CD122, CD132 markers.

Generation of LTi Cells

LTi cells are the very earliest hematopoietic cells colonizing lymphoid node anlagen, fetal spleen and intestine induced Peyer's patches and the nasal associated lymphoid tissue. They are derived from IL-7Rα+ fetal liver precursor cells. LTi cells induce the development of secondary lymphoid organ anlagen through interaction with LTβR being expressed by mesenchymal cells. The presence of the transcription factor Ikaros and the protein Id2 (member of the Id family) is a prerequisite for differentiation of progenitor cells into CD45+CD4+CD3- LTi cells. Another molecule required for the generation of LTi is the nuclear retinoic acid related-orphan receptor RORγt. TRANCE-R triggering leads to enhanced expression of LTαβ on LTi cells. Signaling via the IL-7R or via the TRANCE-R are important for intiatiot of surface LTαβ expression in LTi cells.

Development

CLPs, or common lymphoid precursors have the ability to differentiate into a number of different cell types including T cells, B cells, and ILCs, depending on the cellular signals present. With the exception of NK cells, all ILCs require IL-7 signaling for survival. Transcriptional repressor ID2 appears to antagonize B and T cell differentiation, yielding an ID2-dependent precursor that can further differentiate with lineage-specific transcription factors. There is evidence that the different branches of ILCs share a common precursor. Notch signaling may also be involved in the initial differentiation to a common ILC precursor. The development of ILCs is not completely understood. ILC3s may be necessary precursors to ILC1s.

Function

ILCs are a multifunctional group of cells. Their ability to rapidly secrete immunoregulatory cytokines allows them to contribute early on in immune responses to infection. They often reside at mucosal surfaces, where they are exposed to infectious agents in the environment.

Helminth Infection

ILC2 cells play a crucial role in the protection against helminthic infection. They are a major early source of IL-13, which can activate T cells and induce physiological responses that will help expel a parasite. These physiological responses include stimulating goblet cell mucus secretion and contraction of smooth muscle. In addition, they secrete signals that recruit and activate mast cells and eosinophils, and which stimulate B cell proliferation. They also secrete Amphiregulin, a member of the epidermal growth factor family, that stimulates tissue repair. This can function to enhance the barrier function of the epithelium and slow pathogen entry.

Enteric Pathogens

In the environment of intestinal tract, ILC3s have a crucial role in mediating the balance between symbiotic microbiota and the intestinal immune system. In response to inflammatory signals from the dendridic cells and gut epithelium, they produce IL-22 which increase the production of antimicrobial peptides and defensins. ILC3s also assist in immune responses to extracellular bacteria by maintaining the homeostasis of epithelia. Therefore, when malfunction appears, these cells may participate in the development of inflammatory bowel diseases (IBD).

Tumor Surveillance

Different groups of Innate lymphoid cells have ability to influence tumorigenesis in several ways.

ILC1 are the major population of ILC with anti-tumorigenic potential. The best explored ILC1 are NK cells. Their function is regulated by signals from stimulatory and inhibitory receptors. NK cells have ability to recognize missing MHC class I on tumor cell. In this way, they act in a complementary manner with the cytotoxic T cells that recognize and kill tumor cells which present a foreign antigen on MHC class I. NK cells express a number of cell surface activating NK cell receptors with specificity for stress induced ligands overexpressed on tumor cell. In humans, receptor NKG2D recognize ULBP1-6 and MICA, MICB and RAET1E, whereas in mice it binds RAE1 family molecules, H60 family molecules and MULT1 protein. Another family of activating NK cell receptors are NCRs (natural cytotoxicity receptors), DNAM1 (DNAX Accessory Molecule-1 CD266) and CD16 (mediate ADCC after binding of tumor specific antibody on tumor antigen).

ILC1 influence tumor microenvironment by production of several cytokines e.g. IFNg and TNFa which at the beginning of immune response polarize other immune cells into inflammatory phenotype, e.g. M1 macrophages. ILC1 also recruit DC and cytotoxic T cells. On the other hand, IFN g and TNF a play important role in induction of immunosuppressive phenotype of immune cells or MDSC, production of anti-inflammatory cytokines and formation of metastases.

Other ILC populations also influence tumor microenvironment.

ILC2 produce cytokines that promote anti-inflammatory immune response e.g. IL-13, IL-4, Amphiregulin. However, in some settings ILC2 produce IL-5 and promote cytotoxic response of eosinophils and antitumor response and metastasis suppression.

ILC3 are involved in inflammation-related tumorigenesis by production of IL-17, IL-22, IL-23 cytokines. This microenvironment leads to tumor development and progression and contribute for better survival of cancer cells.

Metabolism

Research identified ILC2s in adipose tissue as a factor in the development of obesity in mice. ILC2s are critical in energy homeostasis by producing methionine-enkephalin peptides in response to IL-33. This production promotes the emergence of beige adipocytes in white adipose tissue. The process of beiging leads to increased energy expenditure and decreased adiposity.

Pathology

Allergy and Asthma

ILC2s play a variety of roles in allergy. Primarily, they provide a source of the type 2 cytokines that orchestrate the allergic immune response. They produce a profile of signals in response to pro-allergenic cytokines IL-25 and IL-33 that is similar to those produced in response to helminthic infection. Their contribution to this signaling appears to be comparable to that of T cells. In response to allergen exposure in the lungs, ILC2s produce IL-13, a necessary cytokine in the pathogenesis of allergic reactions. This response appears to be independent of T and B cells. Further, allergic responses that resemble asthma-like symptoms have been induced in mice that lack T and B cells using IL-33. It has also been found that ILC2s are present in higher concentrations in tissues where allergic symptoms are present, such as in the nasal polyps of patients with chronic rhinosinusitis and the skin from patients with atopic dermatitis.

Autoimmune Disease

NK cells express many cell-surface receptors that can be activating, inhibitory, adhesion, cytokine, or chemotactic. The integration of information collected through these numerous inputs allows NK cells to maintain self-tolerance and recognize self-cell stress signals. If the nuanced, dynamic regulation of NK cell activation becomes unbalanced in favor of attacking self cells, autoimmune disease pathology. NK cell dysregulation has been implicated in a number of autoimmune disorders including multiple sclerosis, systemic lupus erythematosus, and type I diabetes mellitus.

Innate or Adaptive

Historically, the distinction between the innate and adaptive immune system focused on the innate system's nonspecific nature and lack of memory. As information has emerged about the functions of NK cells and other ILCs as effectors and orchestrators of the adaptive immune response, this distinction has become less clear. Some researchers suggest that the definition should focus more on the germline-coding of receptors in the innate immune system versus the rearranged receptors of the adaptive immune system.

Cytokine

Cytokines/immunocytokines, were initially used to separate the immunomodulatory proteins, also called immunotransmitters, from other growth factors that modulate proliferation and bioactivities of non-immune cells. Some cytokines are produced by a rather limited number of different cell types while others are produced by almost the entire spectrum of known cell types.

Recombinant cytokines are in clinical use, and continues attempts are made to develop hybrid molecules from cytokines. 1 must be aware of the fact that current knowledge is still limited. Cytokines are powerful two-edged weapons that can trigger a cascade of reactions, and may show activities that often go beyond the single highly specific property that it is hoped they possess. New factors are being discovered constantly and they extend our knowledge about the Cytokine network.

The understanding of the biological mechanisms governing cytokine actions are an important contribution to medical knowledge. The biochemistry and molecular biology of cytokine actions explain some well-known and sometimes also some of the more obscure clinical aspects of diseases. Knowledge that cytokines create regulatory hierarchies and provide independent and/or interrelated regulatory mechanisms that can confer distinct and interactive developmental functions lays a solid, albeit rather complicated foundation, for current and future clinical experiences.

The concept of "1 producer cell - 1 cytokine - 1 target cell" has been falsified for practically every cytokine investigated more closely. To classify these factors based on their producer or target cells is therefore also problematic.

Classifications based upon identical or shared biological activities of cytokines especially with broad definitions is also problematic for example: BCDF (B-cell differentiation factors), BCGF (B-cell growth factors), Motogenic cytokines, Chemotactic cytokines (Chemokines), CSF (colony stimulating factors), angiogenesis factors, or TRF (T-cell replacing factors). Designations such as HBGF group (heparin binding growth factors) take into account biochemical shared properties by a variety of cytokines which also problematic.

The term cytokine is used today as a generic name for a diverse group which includes proteins and peptides that act in nano-picomolar concentrations as humoral regulators and modulate the functional activities of individual cells and tissues. Cytokines also mediate interactions between cells and regulate processes taking place in the extracellular environment. Many growth factors and cytokines act as cellular survival factors by preventing programmed cell death.

Cytokines resemble hormones in their biological activity and systemic level, for example, inflammation, systemic inflammatory response syndrome, acute phase reaction, wound healing, and the neuroimmune network.

Cytokines act on a wider spectrum of target cells than hormones. The major feature distinguishing cytokines from hormones is the fact that cytokines are not produced by specialized cells organized in specialized glands. Cytokines are secreted proteins which means that their expression sites does not predict where they exert their biological function.

Several cytokines primary structure was found to be identical with enzymes. Cytokines do not possess enzymatic activities although there is a growing list of exceptions. Other cytokines require proteolytic activation.

Cytokines include Interleukins, Lymphokines, Monokines, Interferons (IFN), colony stimulating factors (CSF), Chemokines and a variety of other proteins.

Type-1 cytokines are cytokines produced by Th1 T-helper cells while Type-2 cytokines are those produced by Th2 T-helper cells. Type-1 cytokines include IL-2 (IL2), IFN-gamma (IFN-G), IL-12 (IL12) & TNF-beta (TNF-b), while Type 2 cytokines include IL-4 (IL4), IL-5 (IL5), IL-6 (IL6), IL-10(IL10), and IL-13 (IL13).

Comparison of cytokine sequences shows that primate cytokines (non-human) are closely related. An example: IL-1 alpha (IL1a), IL-1 beta (IL1b), IL-2 (IL2), IL-4 (IL4), IL-5 (IL5), IL-6 (IL6) , IL8 (IL-8), IL-10 (IL10), IL-12 (IL12), IL-15 (IL15), IFN-alpha (IFNA), IFN-gamma (IFN-G), and

TNF-alpha (TNFA) which share 93% to 99 % homology at the protein & nucleic acid level with the human sequences.

Cytokines can also be classified into family groups according to the types of secondary and tertiary structure. An example: IL-6 (IL6), IL-11 (IL11), CNTF (C-NTF), LIF, OSM (Oncostatin-M), EPO (Erythropoietin), G-CSF (GCSF), GH (Growth Hormone), PRL (Prolactin), IL-10 (IL10), IFN-alpha (IFN-A), IFN-beta (IFN-B) form long chain 4 helix bundles. IL-2 (IL2), IL-4 (IL4), IL-7 (IL7), IL-9 (IL9), IL-13 (IL13), IL-3 (IL3), IL-5 (IL5), GM-CSF (GMCSF), M-CSF (MCSF), SCF, IFN-gamma (IFNG) form short chain 4 helix bundles. Beta-trefoil structures are formed by IL1-alpha (IL1A), IL1-beta (IL1B), aFGF (FGF-acidic), bFGF (FGF-basic), INT-2 (INT2), KGF (FGF7). EGF, TGF-alpha (TGF-A), Betacellulin (BTC), SCDGF, Amphiregulin, HB-EGF, form EGF-like antiparallel beta-sheets.

Many cytokines are secreted by cells using secretory pathways and therefore are considered glycoproteins. Most genes encoding cytokines give rise to variety of cytokines by means of alternative splicing, yielding molecules with slightly different but biologically significant bioactivities. Usually the expression patterns of different forms of cytokines or of members of a cytokine family are overlapping only partially, suggesting a specific role for each factor.

Membrane-bound cytokines have been are associated with the extracellular matrix. The switching between soluble and membrane forms of cytokines is an important regulatory event. In some cases membrane forms of a cytokine have been found to be indispensable for normal development, with soluble forms being unable to entirely substitute for them.

Numerous cytokines are not stored inside cells though TGF-beta (TGF-b) and PDGF (P-DGF) are stored in platelets or TNF-alpha (TNF-A) and IL-8 (IL8) are found in human skin mast cells. Most of the cytokine's expression is regulated tightly at practically all levels. The factors are usually produced only by cells after cell activation in response to an induction signal. The production and secretion of cytokines and growth factors frequently is context dependent, i.e., their expression is influenced by individual signals received but also by the balance of signals received through one or more receptors (which themselves may be subject to inducible/repressible expression).

Cytokine's expression is regulated at the transcription level, translation level, and protein synthesis. The expression of cytokines also seems to be regulated differentially, depending on cell type and developmental age. Secretion or release from the producer cells is a regulated process. Once released, their behavior in the circulation may be regulated by soluble receptors and specific or unspecific binding proteins. Regulation also is at work at the receptor level on target cells and at the level of signaling pathways governing alterations in the behavior of responder cells.

Numerous cytokines are pleiotropic effectors showing multiple biological activities. Multiple cytokines have overlapping activities therefore a single cell frequently interacts with multiple cytokines with seemingly identical responses (cross-talk). A possible consequence of this functional overlap is the observation that 1 factor may frequently functionally replace another factor altogether or at least partially compensate for the lack of another factor. Since most cytokines have ubiquitous biological activities, their physiologic significance as normal regulators of physiology is often difficult to assess.

Gene function studies in experimental transgenic knock-out animals in which a cytokine gene has been functionally inactivated by gene targeting are very important in cytokine-research since, unlike in vitro studies, they provide information about the true in vivo functions of a given cytokine by highlighting the effects of their absence. In many instances these studies have shown that null mutations of particular cytokine genes do not have the effects in vivo expected from their activities in vitro.

Cytokines show stimulating or inhibitory activities and synergize or antagonize the actions of other factors. 1 sole Cytokine elicits reactions under certain circumstances that are the reverse of those shown under other circumstances. The type, the duration, and also the extent of cellular activities induced by a particular cytokine can be influenced considerably by the micro-environment of a cell, depending, for example, on the growth state of the cells (sparse or confluent), the type of neighboring cells, cytokine concentrations, the combination of other cytokines present at the same time, and even on the temporal sequence of several cytokines acting on the same cell. Under such circumstances combinatorial effects thus allow a single cytokine to transmit diverse signals to different subsets of cells.

Although some cytokines are known to share at least some biological effects, the observations that single cells usually show different patterns of gene expression in response to different cytokines can be taken as evidence for the existence of cytokine receptor-specific signal transduction pathways. Shared and different transcriptional activators that transduce a signal from a cytokine receptor to a transcription regulatory element of DNA are involved in these processes such as STAT proteins.

Basic FGF (bFGF) is a strong mitogen for fibroblasts at low concentrations and a chemoattractant at high concentrations. FGFb (FGF-b) has been shown also to be a biphasic regulator of human hepatoblastoma-derived HepG2 cells, depending upon the concentration. Interferon-gamma (IFN-gamma) can stimulate the proliferation of B-cells prestimulated with Anti-IgM, and inhibits the activities of the same cells induced by IL-4 (IL4). On the other hand, IL-4 (Interleukin-4) activates B-cells and promotes their proliferation while inhibiting the effects induced by IL2 in the same cells. The activity of at least two cytokines such as IL1-A (IL1A) and IL1-B (IL1B) is regulated by an endogenous receptor antagonist, the IL1 receptor anagonist (IL1TA). Cytokines, such as TNFA (TNF-A), IFN-gamma (IFN-G), IL-2 (IL2) & IL-4 (IL4), are inhibited by soluble receptors. Cytokines including IL-10 (IL10) and TGF-beta (TGF-B), inhibit other cytokines.

Early Cytokines preactivate cells so that they then can respond to late-acting cytokines. Cytokines induce the synthesis of novel gene products once they have bound to their corresponding. Several of the novel products are themselves cytokines. In addition, there are a variety of biological response modifiers that function as Anti-cytokines.

Cytokine mediators swiftly remote areas of a multicellular organism and multiple target cells can be degraded quickly, One can assume that cytokines play a pivotal role in all sorts of cell-to-cell communication processes although many of the mechanisms of their actions have not yet been elucidated in full detail.

Thorough examination of the physiological effects of the expression of cytokines in complex organisms has shown that these mediators are involved in all systemic reactions of an organism, including the important processes as regulation of immune responses, for example: BCDF(B-cell growth and differentiation factors), BCGF (B-cell growth factors) TRF (T-cell replacing factors), Isotype switching, inflammatory processes, hematopoiesis, and wound healing.

Embryogenesis and organ development inlvolves important mediators called Cytokines. Their activities in these processes may differ from those observed postnatally. Cytokines play a key role in neuroimmunological, neuroendocrinological, and neuroregulatory processes. Cytokines also regulate cell cycle, differentiation, migration, cell survival and cell death, and cell transformation. Viral infectious agents exploit the cytokine repertoire of organisms to evade immune responses of the host. Virus-encoded factors affect the activities of cytokines in at least four different ways: by inhibiting the synthesis and release of cytokines from infected cells; by interfering with the interaction between cytokines and their receptors; by inhibiting signal transmission pathways of cytokines; and by synthesizing virus-encoded cytokines that antagonize the effects of host cytokines mediating antiviral processes. Bacteria and micro-organisms also appear to produce substances with activities resembling those of cytokines and which they utilize to subvert host responses.

Cytokines are rarely related among eachother in their primary sequences. Some appear to have common 3 dimensional features and some of them can be grouped into families. An example is the TNF ligand superfamily members (with the exception of LT-alpha) are type 2 membrane glycoproteins (N-terminus inside) with homology to TNF in the extracellular domain (overall homologies, 20 %). The HBNF family includes members of the group of fibroblast growth factors. The chemokine group which contain diverse factors also have conserved sequence features. Analysis of crystal structures of several cytokines with very little sequence homology has revealed a common overall topology that is not deducible from sequence comparisons.

Cytokine biological activity of is mediated by specific membrane receptors, which are expressed on all cell types known. Cytokine expression is also subject to several regulatory although some receptors are expressed also constitutively.

Cytokine receptor proteins are multi-subunit structures that bind ligands and at the same time possess functions as signal transducers due to their intrinsic tyrosine kinase. Many receptors often share common signal transducing receptor components in the same family, which explains, at least in part, the functional redundancy of cytokines. Cross-communication between different signaling systems allows integration diversity of stimuli, which a cell can be subjected to under varying physiological situations. This and the ubiquitous cellular distribution of certain cytokine receptors have hampered attempts to define critical responsive cell populations and the physiologically important cell-specific functions of cytokines in vivo. Numerous receptors are associated with special signal transducing proteins in the interior of the cell. Receptors bind more than 1 cytokine. Cytokine receptors shown to be converted into soluble binding proteins that regulate ligand access to the cell by specific proteolytic cleavage of receptor ectodomains.

Specific activities of cytokines have been the basis for current concepts of therapeutical intervention, in particular of the treatment of hematopoietic malfunctions and tumor therapy. Applications involve the support of chemo- and radiotherapy, bone marrow transplantation, and general immunostimulation.

References

- Immune-system, Conditions And Treatments, health: betterhealth.vic.gov.au, Retrieved 13 May, 2019

- Alberts B, Johnson A, Lewis J, Raff M, Roberts K, Walters P (2002). Molecular Biology of the Cell (4th ed.). New York and London: Garland Science. ISBN 0-8153-3218-1

- "Lymph - Definition and More from the Free Merriam-Webster Dictionary". Www.merriam-webster.com. Retrieved 2010-05-29

- Cytokines: prospecbio.com, Retrieved 8 January, 2019

- International Human Genome Sequencing Consortium (October 2004). "Finishing the euchromatic sequence of the human genome". Nature. 431 (7011): 931–45. Doi:10.1038/nature03001. PMID 15496913

- Abbas AK, Lichtman AH, Pillai S (2010). Cellular and Molecular Immunology (6th ed.). Elsevier. Pp. 272–288. ISBN 978-1-4160-3123-9

- Phagocytes, cells-immune-system, immune-system: teachmephysiology.com, Retrieved 21 May, 2019

- Complement Deficiencies Workup: Laboratory Studies, Imaging Studies, Other Tests". Emedicine.medscape.com. Retrieved 2018-04-26

Immune System Receptors $\quad\boxed{3}$

- **Immune Receptor**

- **Co-receptor**

- **Cytokine Receptor**

- **TNF Receptor Superfamily**

- **Chemokine Receptor**

- **Killer-cell Immunoglobulin-like Receptor**

- **Leukocyte Immunoglobulin-like Receptors**

Receptors that bind to a substance and cause a response in the immune system are termed as immune system receptors. Some of these receptors are cytokine receptors, killer-cell immunoglobulin-like receptors, leukocyte immunoglobulin-like receptors and chemokine receptors. This chapter discusses in detail these receptors of the immune system.

Immune Receptor

Before any immune mechanism can go into action, there must be a recognition that something exists for it to act against. Normally this means foreign material such as a virus, bacterium or other infectious organism. This recognition is carried out by a series of recognition molecules or receptors. Some of these circulate freely in blood or body fluids, others are fixed to the membranes of various cells or reside inside the cell cytoplasm. In every case, some constituent of the foreign material must interact with the recognition molecule like a key fitting into the right lock. This initial act of recognition opens the door that leads eventually to a full immune response.

These receptors are quite different in the innate and the adaptive immune system. The innate system possesses a limited number, known as pattern-recognition receptors (PRRs), which have been selected during evolution to recognize structures common to groups of disease causing organisms such as the lipopolysaccharide (LPS) in some bacterial cell walls. These PRRs act as the 'early warning' system of immunity, triggering a rapid inflammatory response which precedes and is essential for a subsequent adaptive response. In contrast, the adaptive system has thousands of millions of different receptors on its B and T lymphocytes, each one exquisitely sensitive to one individual molecular structure. The responses triggered by these receptors offer more effective protection against infection, but are usually much slower to develop. Linking the two systems are the families of major histocompatibility complex (MHC) molecules, specialized for 'serving up' foreign molecules to T lymphocytes. Another set of 'linking' receptors are those by which molecules such as antibody and complement become bound to cells, where they can themselves act as receptors.

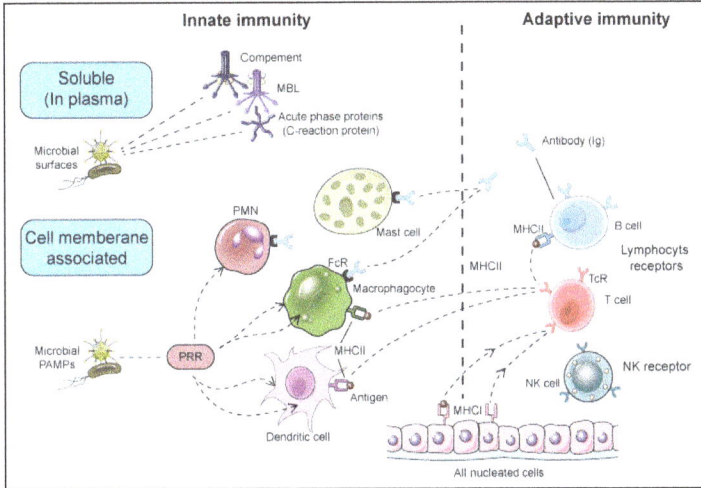

The immune recognition and receptors in innate and adaptive immunity.

The innate immune system recognizes molecular structures that are produced by microbial pathogens. The microbial substances that stimulate innate immunity are often shared by classes of microbes and are called pathogen-associated molecular patterns (PAMPs). Different types of microbes express different PAMPs. These structures include: nucleic acids that are unique to microbes, such as double stranded RNA found in replicating viruses and unmethylated CpG DNA sequences found in bacteria; features of proteins that are found in microbes, such as initiation by N-formylmethionine, which is typical of bacterial proteins; and complex lipids and carbohydrates that are synthesized by microbes but not by mammalian cells, such as lipopolysaccharide (LPS) in gram-negative bacteria, lipoteichoic acid in gram-positive bacteria, and oligosaccharides with terminal mannose residues found in microbial but not in mammalian glycoproteins. Whereas the innate immune system has evolved to recognize only a limited number of molecules that are unique to microbes, the adaptive immune system is capable of recognizing many more diverse foreign substances whether or not they are products of microbes.

Table: Examples of PAMPs.

Pathogen-Associated Molecular Patterns		Microbe Type
Nucleic acids	ssRNA	Virus
	dsRNA	Virus
	CpG	Virus, bacteria
Proteins	Pilin	Bacteria
	Flagellin	Bacteria
Cell wall lipids	LPS	Gram-negative bacteria
	Lipoteichoic acid	Gram-positive bacteria
Carbohydrates	Mannan	Fungi, bacteria
	Glucans	Fungi

The innate immune system uses several types of cellular receptors, present in different locations in cells, and soluble molecules in the blood and mucosal secretions to recognize PAMPs. Cell-associated recognition molecules of the innate immune system are expressed by phagocytes (primarily macrophages and neutrophils), dendritic cells, epithelial cells that form the barrier interface between the body and the external environment, and many other types of cells that occupy tissues and organs. These cellular receptors for pathogens and damage-associated molecules are often called pattern recognition receptors. They are expressed on the surface, in phagocytic vesicles, and in the cytosol of various cell types, all of which are locations where microbes may be present.

Table: Pattern Recognition Molecules of the Innate Immune System.

Pattern Recognition Receptors	Location	Specific Examples	PAMP/DAMP Ligands
Cell-Associated			
Toll-like receptors (TLRs)	Plasma membrane and endosomal membranes of dendritic cells, phagocytes, B cells, endothelial cells, and many other cell types	TLRs 1-9	Various microbial molecules including bacterial LPS and peptidoglycans, viral nucleic acids
NOD-like receptors (NLRs)	Cytosol of phagocytes, epithelial cells, and other cells	NOD1/2 NLRP family (inflammasomes)	Bacterial cell wall peptidoglycans Intracellular crystals (urate, silica); changes in cytosolic ATP and ion concentrations; lysosomal damage
RIG-like receptors (RLRs)	Cytosol of phagocytes and other cells	RIG-1, MDA-5	Viral RNA
Cytosolic DNA sensors (CDSs)	Cytosolic DNA sensors (CDSs)	AIM2; STING-associated CDSs	Bacterial and viral DNA
C-type lectin–like receptors (CLRs)	C-type lectin–like receptors (CLRs)	Mannose receptor Dectin	Microbial surface carbohydrates with terminal mannose and fructose Glucans present in fungal cell walls
Scavenger receptors	Plasma membranes of phagocytes	CD36	Microbial diacylglycerides
N-Formyl met-leu-phe receptors	Plasma membranes of phagocytes	FPR and FPRL1	Peptides containing N-formylmethionyl residues
Soluble			
Pentraxins	Plasma	C-reactive protein	Microbial phosphorylcholine and phosphatidylethanolamine
Collectins	Plasma	Mannose-binding lectin	Carbohydrates with terminal mannose and fructose
	Alveoli	Surfactant proteins SP-A and SP-D	Various microbial structures
Ficolins	Plasma	Ficolin	N-Acetylglucosamine and lipoteichoic acid components of the cell walls of gram-positive bacteria
Complement	Plasma	Various complement proteins	Microbial surfaces

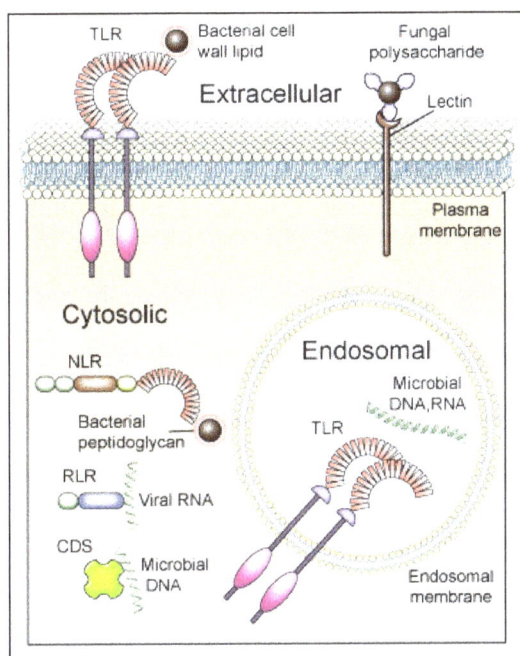

Cellular locations of pattern recognition receptors of the innate immune system.

Cell-associated PRR

Toll-Like Receptors: Toll-like receptors (TLRs) are an evolutionarily conserved family of pattern recognition receptors expressed on many cell types that recognize products of a wide variety of microbes as well as molecules expressed or released by stressed and dying cells. The TLRs are type I integral membrane glycoproteins that contain leucine-rich repeats flanked by characteristic cysteine-rich motifs in their extracellular regions, which are involved in ligand binding, and a Toll/IL-1 receptor (TIR) homology domain in their cytoplasmic tails, which is essential for signaling. TIR domains are also found in the cytoplasmic tails of the receptors for the cytokines IL-1 and IL-18, and similar signaling pathways are engaged by TLRs, IL-1, and IL-18.

Cytosolic Receptors

NOD-Like Receptors: NOD-like receptors (NLRs) are a family of more than 20 different cytosolic proteins, some of which recognize PAMPs and recruit other proteins to form signaling complexes that promote inflammation. This family of proteins is named after NOD (nucleotide oligomerization domain–containing protein). Typical NLR proteins contain at least three different domains with distinct structures and functions. These include a leucine-rich repeat domain that senses the presence of ligand, similar to the leucine-rich repeats of TLRs; a NACHT (neuronal apoptosis inhibitory protein [NAIP], CIITA, HET-E, and TP1) domain, which allows NLRs to bind to one another and form oligomers; and an effector domain, which recruits other proteins to form signaling complexes. The NLRP subfamily of NOD-like receptors respond to cytosolic PAMPs by forming signaling complexes called inflammasomes, which generate active forms of the inflammatory cytokines IL-1 and IL-18.

RIG-Like Receptors: RIG-like receptors (RLRs) are cytosolic sensors of viral RNA that respond to viral nucleic acids by inducing the production of the antiviral type I interferons. RLRs can recognize double-stranded RNA and RNA-DNA heteroduplexes, which include the genomes of RNA viruses and RNA transcripts of RNA and DNA viruses. The two best characterized RLRs are RIG-I (retinoic acid–inducible gene I) and MDA5 (melanoma differentiation-associated gene 5). Both of these proteins contain two N-terminal caspase recruitment domains that interact with other signaling proteins, an RNA-helicase domain, and a C-terminal domain, the latter two being involved in RNA recognition.

Co-receptor

A co-receptor is a cell surface receptor that binds a signalling molecule in addition to a primary receptor in order to facilitate ligand recognition and initiate biological processes, such as entry of a pathogen into a host cell.

Properties

The term co-receptor is prominent in literature regarding signal transduction, the process by which external stimuli regulate internal cellular functioning. The key to optimal cellular functioning is maintained by possessing specific machinery that can carry out tasks efficiently and effectively. Specifically, the process through which intermolecular reactions forward and amplify extracellular signals across the cell surface has developed to occur by two mechanisms. First, cell surface receptors can directly transduce signals by possessing both serine and threonine or simply serine in the cytoplasmic domain. They can also transmit signals through adaptor molecules through their cytoplasmic domain which bind to signalling motifs. Secondly, certain surface receptors lacking a cytoplasmic domain can transduce signals through ligand binding. Once the surface receptor binds the ligand it forms a complex with a corresponding surface receptor to regulate signalling. These categories of cell surface receptors are prominently referred to as co-receptors. Co-receptors are also referred to as accessory receptors, especially in the fields of biomedical research and immunology.

Co-receptors are proteins that maintain a three-dimensional structure. The large extracellular domains make up approximately 76–100% of the receptor. The motifs that make up the large extracellular domains participate in ligand binding and complex formation. The motifs can include glycosaminoglycans, EGF repeats, cysteine residues or ZP-1 domains. The variety of motifs leads to co-receptors being able to interact with two to nine different ligands, which themselves can also interact with a number of different co-receptors. Most co-receptors lack a cytoplasmic domain and tend to be GPI-anchored, though a few receptors have been identified which contain short cytoplasmic domains that lack intrinsic kinase activity.

Localization and Function

Depending on the type of ligand a co-receptor binds, its location and function can vary. Various ligands include interleukins, neurotrophic factors, fibroblast growth factors, transforming growth factors, vascular endothelial growth factors and epidermal growth factors. Co-receptors prominent in embryonic tissue have an essential role in morphogen gradient formation or tissue differentiation. Co-receptors localized in endothelial cells function to enhance cell proliferation and cell migration. With such variety in regards to location, co-receptors can participate in many different cellular activities. Co-receptors have been identified as participants in cell signalling cascades, embryonic development, cell adhesion regulation, gradient formation, tissue proliferation and migration.

Classical Examples

CD Family

The CD family of co-receptors are a well-studied group of extracellular receptors found in immunological cells. The CD receptor family typically act as co-receptors, illustrated by the classic example of CD4 acting as a co-receptor to the T cell receptor (TCR) to bind major histocompatibility complex II (MHC-II). This binding is particularly well-studied in T-cells where it serves to activate T-cells that are in their resting (or dormant) phase and to cause active cycling T-cells to undergo programmed cell death. Boehme *et al.* demonstrated this interesting dual outcome by blocking the binding of CD4 to MHC-II which prevented the programmed cell death reaction that active T-cells typically display. The CD4 receptor is composed of four concatamerized Ig-like domains and is anchored to the cell membrane by a single transmembrane domain. CD family receptors are typically monomers or dimers, though they are all primarily extracellular proteins. The CD4 receptor in particular interacts with murine MHC-II following the "ball-on-stick" model, where the Phe-43 ball fits into the conserved hydrophobic $\alpha2$ and $\beta2$ domain residues. During binding with MHC-II, CD4 maintains independent structure and does not form any bonds with the TCR receptor.

The members of the CD family of co-receptors have a wide range of function. As well as being involved in forming a complex with MHC-II with TCR to control T-cell fate, the CD4 receptor is infamously the primary receptor that HIV envelope glycoprotein GP120 binds to. In comparison, CD28 acts as a 'co-coreceptor' for the MHC-II binding with TCR and CD4. CD28 increases the Il-2 secretion from the T-cells if it is involved in the initial activation; however, CD28 blockage has no effect on programmed cell death after the T-cell has been activated.

CCR Family of Receptors

The CCR family of receptors are a group of g-protein coupled receptors (GPCRs) that normally operate as chemokine receptors. They are primarily found on immunological cells, especially T-cells. CCR receptors are also expressed on neuronal cells, such as dendrites and microglia. Perhaps the most famous and well-studied of the CCR family is CCR5 (and its near-homologue CXCR4) which acts as the primary co-receptor for HIV viral infection. The HIV envelope glycoprotein GP120 binds to CD4 as its primary receptor, CCR5 then forms a complex with CD4 and HIV, allowing viral entry into the cell. CCR5 is not the only member of the CCR family that allows for HIV infection. Due to the commonality of structures found throughout the family, CCR2b, CCR3, and CCR8 can be utilized by some HIV strains as co-receptors to facilitate infection. CXCR4 is very similar to CCR5 in structure. While only some HIV strains can utilize CCR2b, CCR3 and CCR8, all HIV strains can infect through CCR5 and CXCR4.

CCR5 is known to have an affinity for macrophage inflammatory protein (MIP) and is thought to play a role in inflammatory immunological responses. The primary role of this receptor is less understood than its role in HIV infection, as inflammation responses remain a poorly understood facet of the immune system. CCR5's affinity for MIP makes it of great interest for practical applications such as tissue engineering, where attempts are being made to control host inflammatory and immunological responses at a cellular signalling level. The affinity for MIP has been utilized in-vitro to prevent HIV infection through ligand competition; however, these entry-inhibitors have failed in-vivo due to the highly adaptive nature of HIV and toxicity concerns.

Clinical Significance

Because of their importance in cell signaling and regulation, co-receptors have been implicated in a number of diseases and disorders. Co-receptor knockout mice are often unable to develop and such knockouts generally result in embryonic or perinatal lethality. In immunology in particular, the term "co-receptor" often describes a secondary receptor used by a pathogen to gain access to the cell, or a receptor that works alongside T cell receptors such as CD4, CD8, or CD28 to bind antigens or regulate T cell activity in some way.

Inherited Co-receptor Autosomal Disorders

Many co-receptor-related disorders occur due to mutations in the receptor's coding gene. LRP5 (low-density lipoprotein receptor-related protein 5) acts as a co-receptor for the Wnt-family of glycoproteins which regulate bone mass. Malfunctions in this co-receptor lead to lower bone density and strength which contribute to osteoporosis.

Loss of function mutations in LRP5 have been implicated in Osteoporosis-pseudoglioma syndrome, Familial exudative vitreoretinopathy, and a specific missense mutation in the first β-propeller region of LRP5 can lead to abnormally high bone density or osteopetrosis. Mutations in LRP1 have also been found in cases of Familial Alzheimer's disease

Loss of function mutations in the Cryptic co-receptor can lead to random organ positioning due to developmental left-right orientation defects.

Gigantism is believed to be caused, in some cases, by a loss of function of the Glypican 3 co-receptor.

Cancer

Carcinoembryonic antigen cell adhesion molecule-1 (Caecam1) is an immunoglobulin-like co-receptor that aids in cell adhesion in epithelial, endothelial and hematopoietic cells, and plays a vital role during vascularization and angiogenesis by binding vascular endothelial growth factor (VEGF).

Angiogenesis is important in embryonic development but it is also a fundamental process of tumor growth. Deletion of the gene in Caecam1-/- mice results in a reduction of the abnormal vascularization seen in cancer and lowered nitric oxide production, suggesting a therapeutic possibility through targeting of this gene. The neuropilin co-receptor family mediates binding of VEGF in conjunction with the VEGFR1/VEGFR2 and Plexin signaling receptors, and therefore also plays a role in tumor vascular development.

CD109 acts as a negative regulator of the tumor growth factor β (TGF-β) receptor. Upon binding TGF-β, the receptor is internalized via endocytosis through CD109's action which lowers signal transmission into the cell. In this case, the co-receptor is functioning in a critical regulatory manner to reduce signals that instruct the cell to grow and migrate – the hallmarks of cancer. In conjunction, the LRP co-receptor family also mediates binding of TGF-β with a variety of membrane receptors.

Interleukins 1, 2, and 5 all rely on interleukin co-receptors to bind to the primary interleukin receptors.

Syndecans 1 and 4 have been implicated in a variety of cancer types including cervical, breast, lung, and colon cancer, and abnormal expression levels have been associated with poorer prognosis.

HIV

In order to infect a cell, the envelope glycoprotein GP120 of the HIV virus interacts with CD4 (acting as the primary receptor) and a co-receptor: either CCR5 or CXCR4. This binding results in membrane fusion and the subsequent intracellular signaling that facilitates viral invasion. In approximately half of all HIV cases, the viruses using the CCR5 co-receptor seem to favor immediate infection and transmission while those using the CXCR4 receptor do not present until later in the immunologically suppressed stage of the disease. The virus will often switch from using CCR5 to CXCR4 during the course of the infection, which serves as an indicator for the progression of the disease. Recent evidence suggests that some forms of HIV also use the large integrin a4b7 receptor to facilitate increased binding efficiency in mucosal tissues.

Hepatitis C

The Hepatitis C virus requires the CD81 co-receptor for infection. Studies suggest that the tight junction protein Claudin-1 (CLDN1) may also play a part in HCV entry. Claudin family abnormalities are also common in hepatocellular carcinoma, which can result from HPV infection.

Blockade as a Treatment for Autoimmunity

It is possible to perform a CD4 co-receptor blockade, using antibodies, in order to lower T cell activation and counteract autoimmune disorders. This blockade appears to elicit a "dominant" effect, that is to say, once blocked, the T cells do not regain their ability to become active. This effect then spreads to native T cells which then switch to a CD4+CD25+GITR+FoxP3+ T regulatory phenotype.

Currently, the two most prominent areas of co-receptor research are investigations regarding HIV and cancer. HIV research is highly focused on the adaption of HIV strains to a variety of host co-receptors. Cancer research is mostly focused on enhancing the immune response to tumor cells, while some research also involves investigating the receptors expressed by the cancerous cells themselves.

HIV-based Co-receptor

Most HIV-based co-receptor research focuses on the CCR5 co-receptor. The majority of HIV strains use the CCR5 receptor. HIV-2 strains can also use the CXCR4 receptor though the CCR5 receptor is the more predominantly targeted of the two. Both the CCR5 and the CXCR4 co-receptors are seven-trans-membrane (7TM) G protein-coupled receptors. Different strains of HIV work on different co-receptors, although the virus can switch to utilizing other co-receptors. For example,

R5X4 receptors can become the dominant HIV co-receptor target in main strains. HIV-1 and HIV-2 can both use the CCR8 co-receptor. The crossover of co-receptor targets for different strains and the ability for the strains to switch from their dominant co-receptor can impede clinical treatment of HIV. Treatments such as WR321 mAb can inhibit some strains of CCR5 HIV-1, preventing cell infection. The mAb causes the release of HIV-1-inhibitory b-chemokines, preventing other cells from becoming infected.

Cancer

Cancer-based research into co-receptors includes the investigation of growth factor activated co-receptors, such as Transforming Growth Factor (TGF-β) co-receptors. Expression of the co-receptor endoglin, which is expressed on the surface of tumor cells, is correlated with cell plasticity and the development of tumors. Another co-receptor of TGF-β is CD8. Although the exact mechanism is still unknown, CD8 co-receptors have been shown to enhance T-cell activation and TGF-β-mediated immune suppression. TGF-β has been shown to influence the plasticity of cells through integrin and focal adhesion kinase. The co-receptors of tumor cells and their interaction with T-cells provide important considerations for tumor immunotherapy. Recent research into co-receptors for p75, such as the sortilin co-receptor, has implicated sortillin in connection to neurotrophins, a type of nerve growth factor. The p75 receptor and co-receptors have been found to influence the aggressiveness of tumors, specifically via the ability of neurotrophins to rescue cells from certain forms of cell death. Sortilin, the p75 co-receptor, has been found in natural killer cells, but with only low levels of neurotrophin receptor. The sortilin co-receptor is believed to work with a neurotrophin homologue that can also cause neurotrophin to alter the immune response.

Cytokine Receptor

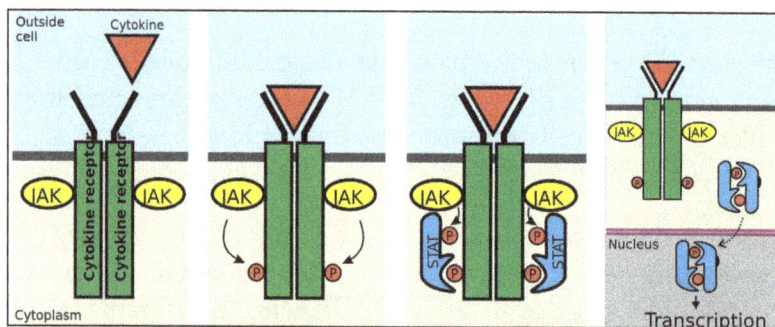

Key steps of the JAK-STAT pathway for type 1 and 2 cytokine receptors.

Cytokine receptors are receptors that bind to cytokines.

In recent years, the cytokine receptors have come to demand the attention of more investigators than cytokines themselves, partly because of their remarkable characteristics, and partly because a deficiency of cytokine receptors has now been directly linked to certain debilitating immunodeficiency states. In this regard, and also because the redundancy and pleiotropy of cytokines are a consequence of their homologous receptors, many authorities are now of the opinion that a classification of cytokine receptors would be more clinically and experimentally useful.

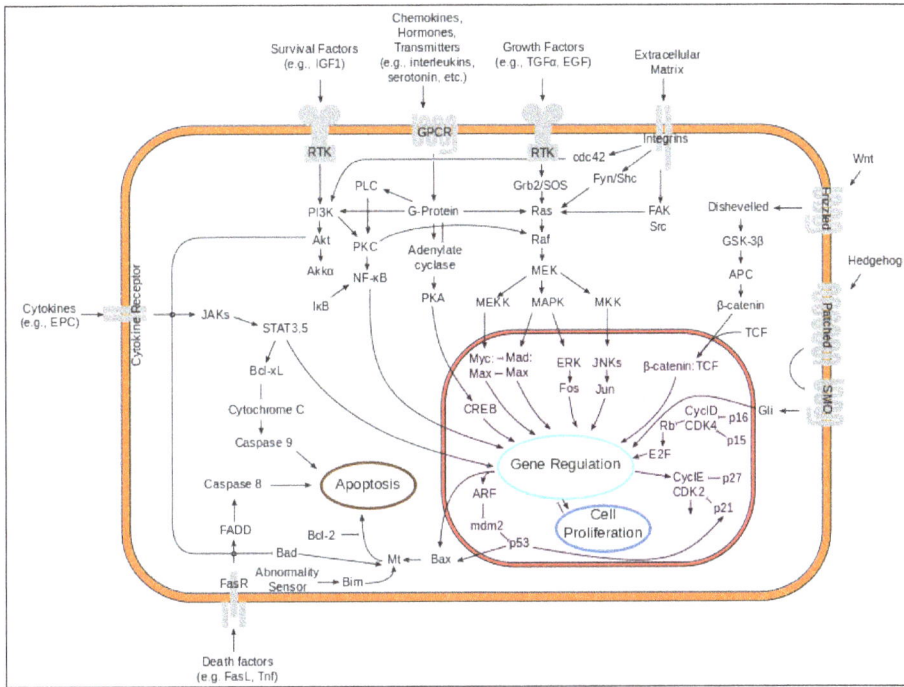

Signal transduction. (Cytokine receptor at center left.).

Classification

A classification of cytokine receptors based on their three-dimensional structure has been attempted. (Such a classification, though seemingly cumbersome, provides several unique perspectives for attractive pharmacotherapeutic targets).

- Type I cytokine receptors, whose members have certain conserved motifs in their extracellular amino-acid domain. The IL-2 receptor belongs to this chain, whose γ-chain (common to several other cytokines) deficiency is directly responsible for the x-linked form of Severe Combined Immunodeficiency (X-SCID).

- Type II cytokine receptors, whose members are receptors mainly for interferons.

- Immunoglobulin (Ig) superfamily, which are ubiquitously present throughout several cells and tissues of the vertebrate body.

- Tumor necrosis factor receptor family, whose members share a cysteine-rich common extracellular binding domain, and includes several other non-cytokine ligands like receptors, CD40, CD27 and CD30, besides the ligands on which the family is named (TNF).

- Chemokine receptors, two of which acting as binding proteins for HIV (CXCR4 and CCR5). They are G protein coupled receptors.

- TGF-beta receptor family, which are Serine/threonine kinase receptors. Includes the TGF beta receptors.

Solubility

Cytokine receptors may be both membrane-bound and soluble. Soluble cytokine receptors are extremely common regulators of cytokine function. Soluble cytokine receptors typically consist of the extracellular portions of membrane-bound receptors.

TNF Receptor Superfamily

The tumor necrosis factor receptor superfamily (TNFRSF) is a protein superfamily of cytokine receptors characterized by the ability to bind tumor necrosis factors (TNFs) via an extracellular cysteine-rich domain. With the exception of nerve growth factor (NGF), all TNFs are homologous to the archetypal TNF-alpha. In their active form, the majority of TNF receptors form trimeric complexes in the plasma membrane. Accordingly, most TNF receptors contain transmembrane domains (TMDs), although some can be cleaved into soluble forms (e.g. TNFR1), and some lack a TMD entirely (e.g. DcR3). In addition, most TNF receptors require specific adaptor protein such as TRADD, TRAF, RIP and FADD for downstream signalling. TNF receptors are primarily involved in apoptosis and inflammation, but they can also take part in other signal transduction pathways, such as proliferation, survival, and differentiation. TNF receptors are expressed in a wide variety of tissues in mammals, especially in leukocytes.

The term death receptor refers to those members of the TNF receptor superfamily that contain a death domain, such as TNFR1, Fas receptor, DR4 and DR5. They were named after the fact that they seemed to play an important role in apoptosis (programmed cell death), although they are now known to play other roles as well.

In the strict sense, the term TNF receptor is often used to refer to the archetypal members of the superfamily, namely TNFR1 and TNFR2, which recognize TNF-alpha.

Members

There are 27 family members, numerically classified as TNFRSF#, where # denotes the member number, sometimes followed a letter.

Type	Protein (member)#	Synonyms	Gene	Ligand(s)
1	Tumor necrosis factor receptor 1 (1A)	CD120a	TNFRSF1A	TNF-alpha (cachectin)
	Tumor necrosis factor receptor 2 (1B)	CD120b	TNFRSF1B	
3	Lymphotoxin beta receptor (3)	CD18	LTBR	Lymphotoxin beta (TNF-C)
4	OX40 (4)	CD134	TNFRSF4	OX40L
5	CD40 (5)	Bp50	CD40	CD154
6	Fas receptor (6)	Apo-1, CD95	FAS	FasL
	Decoy receptor 3 (6B)	TR6, M68	TNFRSF6B	FasL, LIGHT, TL1A
7	CD27 (7)	S152, Tp55	CD27	CD70, Siva
8	CD30 (8)	Ki-1	TNFRSF8	CD153
9	4-1BB (9)	CD137	TNFRSF9	4-1BB ligand

10	Death receptor 4 (10A)	TRAILR1, Apo-2, CD261	TNFRSF10A	TRAIL
	Death receptor 5 (10B)	TRAILR2, CD262	TNFRSF10B	
	Decoy receptor 1 (10C)	TRAILR3, LIT, TRID, CD263	TNFRSF10C	
	Decoy receptor 2 (10D)	TRAILR4, TRUNDD, CD264	TNFRSF10D	
11	RANK (11A)	CD265	TNFRSF11A	RANKL
	Osteoprotegerin (11B)	OCIF, TR1	TNFRSF11B	
12	TWEAK receptor (12A)	Fn14, CD266	TNFRSF12A	TWEAK
13	TACI (13B)	IGAD2, CD267	TNFRSF13B	APRIL, BAFF, CAMLG
	BAFF receptor (13C)	CD268	TNFRSF13C	BAFF
14	Herpesvirus entry mediator (14)	ATAR, TR2, CD270	TNFRSF14	LIGHT
16	Nerve growth factor receptor (16)	p75NTR, CD271	NGFR	NGF, BDNF, NT-3, NT-4
17	B-cell maturation antigen (17)	TNFRSF13A, CD269	TNFRSF17	BAFF
18	Glucocorticoid-induced TN-FR-related (18)	AITR, CD357	TNFRSF18	GITR ligand
19	TROY (19)	TAJ, TRADE	TNFRSF19	unknown
21	Death receptor 6 (21)	CD358	TNFRSF21	
25	Death receptor 3 (25)	Apo-3, TRAMP, LARD, WS-1	TNFRSF25	TL1A
27	Ectodysplasin A2 receptor (27)	XEDAR	EDA2R	EDA-A2

Chemokine Receptor

Chemokine receptors (nomenclature as agreed by the NC-IUPHAR Subcommittee on Chemokine Receptors comprise a large subfamily of 7TM proteins that bind one or more chemokines, a large family of small cytokines typically possessing chemotactic activity for leukocytes. Additional hematopoietic and non-hematopoietic roles have been identified for many chemokines in the areas of embryonic development, immune cell proliferation, activation and death, viral infection, and as antibiotics, among others. Chemokine receptors can be divided by function into two main groups: G protein-coupled chemokine receptors, which mediate leukocyte trafficking, and "Atypical chemokine receptors", which may signal through non-G protein-coupled mechanisms and act as chemokine scavengers to downregulate inflammation or shape chemokine gradients.

Chemokines in turn can be divided by structure into four subclasses by the number and arrangement of conserved cysteines. CC (also known as β-chemokines; n= 28), CXC (also known as α-chemokines; n= 17) and CX3C (n= 1) chemokines all have four conserved cysteines, with zero, one and three amino acids separating the first two cysteines respectively. C chemokines (n= 2) have only the second and fourth cysteines found in other chemokines. Chemokines can also be classified by function into homeostatic and inflammatory subgroups. Most chemokine receptors are able to bind multiple high-affinity chemokine ligands, but the ligands for a given receptor are almost always restricted to the same structural subclass. Most chemokines bind to more than one receptor subtype. Receptors for inflammatory chemokines are typically highly promiscuous with regard to ligand specificity, and may lack a selective endogenous ligand. G protein-coupled chemokine receptors are named acccording to the class of chemokines bound, whereas ACKR is the root acronym for atypical chemokine receptors. There can be substantial cross-species differences in the sequences of both chemokines and chemokine receptors, and in the pharmacology and biology of chemokine receptors. Endogenous and microbial non-chemokine ligands have also been identified for chemokine receptors. Many chemokine receptors function as HIV co-receptors, but CCR5 is the only one demonstrated to play an essential role in HIV/AIDS pathogenesis.

Killer-cell Immunoglobulin-like Receptor

Killer-cell immunoglobulin-like receptors (KIRs), are a family of type I transmembrane glycoproteins expressed on the plasma membrane of natural killer (NK) cells and a minority of T cells. They regulate the killing function of these cells by interacting with major histocompatibility (MHC) class I molecules, which are expressed on all nucleated cell types. KIR receptors can distinguish between major histocompatibility (MHC) class I allelic variants, which allows them to detect virally infected cells or transformed cells. Most KIRs are inhibitory, meaning that their recognition of MHC molecules suppresses the cytotoxic activity of their NK cell. Only a limited number of KIRs are activating, meaning that their recognition of MHC molecules activates the cytotoxic activity of their cell. Initial expression of KIRs on NK cells is stochastic, but there is an educational process that NK cells undergo as they mature that alters the expression of KIRs to maximize the balance between effective defense and self-tolerance. As a result of KIR's role in killing unhealthy self-cells and not killing healthy self-cells, KIRs are involved in protection against and propensity to viral infection, autoimmune disease, and cancer. KIR molecules are highly polymorphic, meaning that their gene sequences differ greatly between individuals, and polygenic so that it is extremely rare for two unrelated individuals to possess the same KIR genotype.

Function

Role in Natural Killer Cells

Natural killer (NK) cells are a type of lymphocyte cell involved in the innate immune system's response to viral infection and tumor transformation of host cells. Like T cells, NK cells have many qualities characteristic of the adaptive immune system, including the production of "memory" cells that persist following encounter with antigens and the ability to create a secondary recall response. Unlike T cells, NK cell receptors are germline encoded, and therefore do not require somatic gene rearrangements. Because NK cells target self cells, they have an intricate mechanism by which they differentiate self and non-self cells in order to minimize the destruction of healthy cells and maximize the destruction of unhealthy cells.

Natural killer cell cytolysis of target cells and cytokine production is controlled by a balance of inhibitory and activating signals, which are facilitated by NK cell receptors. NK cell inhibitory receptors are part of either the immunoglobulin-like (IgSF) superfamily or the C-type lectin-like receptor (CTLR) superfamily. Members of the IgSF family include the human killer cell immunoglobulin-like receptor (KIR) and the Immunoglobulin-like transcripts (ILT). CTLR inhibitory receptors include the CD94/NKG2A and the murine Ly49, which is probably analogous to the human KIR.

Role in T Cells

KIR and CD94 (CTLR) receptors are expressed by 5% of peripheral blood T cells.

Nomenclature and Classification

KIR receptors are named based on the number of their extracellular Ig-like domains (2D or 3D) and by the length of their cytoplasmic tail (long (L), short (S), or pseudogene (P)). The number following the L, S, or P in the case of a pseudogene, differentiates KIR receptors with the same number of extracellular domains and length of cytoplasmic tail. Finally, the asterisk after this nomenclature indicates allelic variants.

Single substitutions, insertions, or deletions in the genetic material that encodes KIR receptors changes the site of termination for the gene, causing the cytoplasmic tail to be long or short, depending on the site of the stop codon. These single nucleotide alterations in the nucleotide sequence fundamentally alter KIR function. With the exception of KIR2DL4, which has both activating and inhibitory capabilities, KIR receptors with long cytoplasmic tails are inhibitory and those with short tails are activating.

Receptor Types

Inhibitory Receptors

Inhibitory receptors recognize self-MHC class I molecules on target self cells, causing the activation of signaling pathways that stop the cytolytic function of NK cells. Self-MHC class I molecules are always expressed under normal circumstance. According to the missing-self hypothesis, inhibitory KIR receptors recognize the downregulation of MHC class I molecules in virally-infected or transformed self cells, leading these receptors to stop sending the inhibition signal, which then leads to the lysis of these unhealthy cells. Because natural killer cells target virally infected host cells and tumor cells, inhibitory KIR receptors are important in facilitating self-tolerance.

KIR inhibitory receptors signal through their immunoreceptor tyrosine-based inhibitory motif (ITIM) in their cytoplasmic domain. When inhibitory KIR receptors bind to a ligand, their ITIMs are tyrosine phosphorylated and protein tyrosine phosphatases, including SHP-1, are recruited. Inhibition occurs early in the activation signaling pathway, likely through the interference of the pathway by these phosphatases.

Activating Receptors

Activating receptors recognize ligands that indicate host cell aberration, including induced-self antigens (which are markers of infected self cells and include MICA, MICB, and ULBP, all of which are related to MHC class 1 molecules), altered-self antigens (MHC class I antigens laden with foreign peptide), and/or non-self (pathogen encoded molecules). The binding of activating KIR receptors to these molecules causes the activation of signaling pathways that cause NK cells to lyse virally infected or transformed cells.

Activating receptors do not have the immunoreceptor tyrosine-base inhibition motif (ITIM) characteristic of inhibitory receptors, and instead contain a positively charged lysine or arginine residue in their transmembrane domain (with the exception of KIR2B4) that helps to bind DAP12, an adaptor molecule containing a negatively charged residue as well as immunoreceptor tyrosine-based activation motifs (ITAM). Activating KIR receptors include KIR2DS, KIR2DL, and KIR3DS.

Much less is known about activating receptors compared to inhibitory receptors. A significant proportion of the human population lacks activating KIR receptors on the surface of their NK cells as a result of truncated variants of KIR2DS4 and 2DL4, which are not expressed on the cell surface, in individuals who are heterozygous for the KIR group A haplotype. This suggests that a lack of activating KIR receptors is not incredibly detrimental, likely because there are other families of activating NK cell surface receptors that bind MHC class I molecules that are probably expressed in individuals with this phenotype. Because little is known about the function of activating KIR receptors, however, it is possible that there is an important function of activating KIR receptors of which we are not yet aware.

Activating receptors have lower affinity for their ligands than do inhibitory receptors. Although the purpose of this difference in affinity is unknown, it is possible that the cytolysis of target cells occurs preferentially under conditions in which the expression of stimulating MHC class I molecules on target cells is high, which may occur during viral infection. This difference, which is also present in Ly49, the murine homolog to KIR, tips the balance towards self-tolerance.

Expression

Activating and inhibitory KIR receptors are expressed on NK cells in patchy, variegated combinations, leading to distinct NK cells. The IgSF and CTLR superfamily inhibitory receptors expressed on the surface of NK cells are each expressed on a subset of NK cells in such a way that not all classes of inhibitory NK cell receptors are expressed on each NK cell, but there is some overlap. This creates unique repertoires of NK cells, increasing the specificity with which NK cells recognize virally-infected and transformed self-cells. Expression of KIR receptors is determined primarily by genetic factors, but recent studies have found that epigenetic mechanisms also play a role in KIR receptor expression. Activating and inhibitory KIR receptors that recognize the same class I MHC molecule are mostly not expressed by the same NK cell. This pattern of expression is beneficial in that target cells that lack inhibitory MHC molecules but express activating MHC molecules are extremely sensitive to cytolysis.

Although initial expression of inhibitory and activating receptors on NK cells appears to be stochastic, there is an education process based on MHC class I alleles expressed by the host that determines the final repertoire of NK receptor expression. This process of education is not well understood. Different receptor genes are expressed primarily independently of other receptor genes, which substantiates the idea that initial expression of receptors is stochastic. Receptors are not expressed entirely independently of each other, however, which supports the idea that there is an education process that reduces the amount of randomness associated with receptor expression. Further, once an NK receptor gene is activated in a cell, its expression is maintained for many cell generations. It appears that some proportion of NK cells are developmentally immature and therefore lack inhibitory receptors, making them hyporesponsive to target cells. In the human fetal liver, KIR and CD49 receptors are already expressed by NK cells, indicating that at least some KIR receptors are present in fetal NK cells, although more studies are needed to substantiate this idea. Although the induction of NK receptor expression is not fully understood, one study found that human progenitor cells cultured in vitro with cytokines developed into NK cells, and many of these cells expressed CD94/NKG2A receptors, a CTLR receptor. Moreover, there was little to no KIR receptor expression in these cells, so additional signals are clearly required for KIR induction.

The balance between effective defense and self-tolerance is important to the functioning of NK cells. It is thought that NK cell self-tolerance is regulated by the educational process of receptor expression described above, although the exact mechanism is not known. The "at least one" hypothesis is an attractive, though not yet fully substantiated, hypothesis that tries to explain the way in which self-tolerance is regulated in the education process. This hypothesis posits that the NK cell repertoire is regulated so that at least one inhibitory receptor (either of the IgSF or CTLR superfamily) is present on every NK cell, which would ensure self-tolerance. Effective defense requires an opposing pattern of receptor expression. The co-expression of many MHC-specific receptors by NK cells is disfavored, likely because cells that co-express receptors are less able to attack virally infected or transformed cells that have down-regulated or lost one MHC molecule compared to NK cells that co-express receptors to a lesser degree. Minimization of co-expression, therefore, is important for mounting an effective defense by maximizing the sensitivity of response.

Structure

Gene Structure

The KIR gene cluster has approximately 150 kb and is located in the leukocyte receptor complex (LRC) on human chromosome 19q13.4. KIR genes have 9 exons, which are strongly correlated with KIR receptor protein domains (leader, D0, D1, and D2, stem, transmembrane, and cytosolic domains). Furthermore, the promoter regions of the KIR genes share greater than 90% sequence identity, which indicates that there is similar transcriptional regulation of KIR genes.

The human killer cell immunoglobulin-like receptors superfamily (which share 35-50% sequence identity and the same fold as KIR) includes immunoglobulin-like transcripts (ILT, also known as leukocyte immunoglobulin-like receptors (LIRs)), leukocyte-associated Ig-like receptors (LAIR), paired Ig-like receptors (PIR), and gp49. Moreover, it has been reported that between 12 and 17 KIR receptors have been identified. There was a single ancestral gene from which all extant KIR receptor genes arose via duplications, recombinations, and mutations, and all KIR receptors share more than 90% sequence identity.

Genes

- Two domains, long cytoplasmic tail: KIR2DL1, KIR2DL2, KIR2DL3, KIR2DL4, KIR2DL5A, KIR2DL5B,

- Two domains, short cytoplasmic tail: KIR2DS1, KIR2DS2, KIR2DS3, KIR2DS4, KIR2DS5,

- Three domains, long cytoplasmic tail: KIR3DL1, KIR3DL2, KIR3DL3,

- Three domains, short cytoplasmic tail: KIR3DS1.

Protein Structure

NK cell receptors bind directly to the MHC class I molecules on the surface of target cells. Human killer cell immunoglobulin-like receptors recognize the α1 and α2 domains of class I human leukocyte antigens (HLA-A, -B, and −C), which are the human versions of MHCs. Position 44 in the D1 domain of KIR receptors and position 80 in HLA-C are important for the specificity of KIR-HLA binding.

Diversity

Allelic Diversity

All but two KIR genes (KIR2DP1 and KIR3DL3) have multiple alleles, with KIR3DL2 and KIR3DL1 having the most variations (12 and 11, respectively). In total, as of 2012 there were 614 known KIR nucleotide sequences encoding 321 distinct KIR proteins. Further, inhibitory receptors are more polymorphic than activating receptors. The great majority (69%) of substitutions in the KIR DNA sequence are nonsynonymous, and 31% are synonymous. The ratio of nonsynonymous to synonymous substitutions (dN/dS) is greater than one for every KIR and every KIR domain, indicating that positive selection is occurring. Further, the 5` exons, which encode the leader peptide and the Ig-like domains, have a larger proportion of nonsynonymous substitutions than do the 3` exons, which encode the stem, transmembrane region, and the cytoplasmic tail. This indicates that stronger selection is occurring on the 5` exons, which encodes the extracellular part of the KIR that binds to the MHC. There is, therefore, evidence of strong selection on the KIR ligand binding sites, which is consistent with the high specificity of the KIR ligand binding site, as well as the rapid evolution of class I MHC molecules and viruses.

Genotype and Haplotype Diversity

Human genomes differ in their amount of KIR genes, in their proportion of inhibitory versus activating genes, and in their allelic variations of each gene. As a result of these polygenic and polymorphic variations, less than 2% of unrelated individuals have the same KIR genotype, and ethnic populations have broadly different KIR genotype frequencies. This incredible diversity likely reflects the pressure from rapidly evolving viruses. 30 distinct haplotypes have been classified, all of which can be broadly characterized by group A and group B haplotypes. The Group A haplotype has a fixed set of genes, which are KIR3DL3, 2L3, 2DP1, 2DL1, 3DP1, 2DL4, 3DL1, 2DS4, and 3DL2. Group B haplotypes encompass all other haplotypes, and therefore have a variable set of genes, including several genes absent from group A, including KIR2DS1, 2DS2, 2DS3, 2DS5, 2DL2, 2DL5, and 3DS1. Because group B has both gene and allelic diversity (compared to just allelic diversity in group A), group B is even more diverse than group A. Four KIR genes (2DL4, 3DL2, 3DL3, AND 3DP1) are present in nearly all KIR haplotypes and as a result are known as framework genes. Inheritance of maternal and paternal haplotypes results in further diversity of individual KIR genotype.

Group A only has one activating KIR receptor, whereas Group B contains many activating KIR receptors, and as a result group B haplotype carriers have a stronger response to virally infected and transformed cells. As a result of the huge migrations peoples indigenous to India, Australia, and the Americas made from Africa, activating KIR receptors became advantageous to these populations, and as a result these populations acquired activating KIR receptors.

A study of the genotypes of 989 individuals representing eight distinct populations found 111 distinct KIR genotypes. Individuals with the most frequent genotype, which comprised 27% of the individuals studied, are homozygous for the group A haplotype. The remaining 110 KIR genotypes found in this study are either group A and group B heterozygotes or group B homozygotes (who are indistinguishable from heterozygotes by genotype alone). 41% (46) of the genotypes identified were found in only one individual, and 90% of individuals had the same 40 genotypes. Clearly, there is extensive diversity in human KIR genotypes, which allows for rapid evolution in response to rapidly evolving viruses.

Role in Disease

Genotypes that are inhibitory KIR receptor dominant are likely susceptible to infection and reproductive disorders but protective against autoimmune diseases, whereas activating KIR receptor dominant genotypes are likely susceptible to autoimmunity but protective against viral infection and cancer. The relationship between inhibitory vs stimulatory KIR genotype dominance, however, is more complicated than this because diseases are so diverse and have so many different causes, and immune activation or de-activation may not be protective or harmful at every stage of disease. KIR2DS2 or 2DS1, which are activating receptors, are strongly correlated with most autoimmune diseases, which is logical because activating receptors induce signaling pathways that lead to cytolysis of target cells. Another activating receptor, KIR3DS1, is protective to hepatitis-C virus infection, is associated with slowing down of AIDs progression, and is associated with cervical cancer, which is associated with a distinct strain of HPV. It is likely that KIR3DS1 is associated with cervical cancer despite its stimulatory nature because cervical tumors generally associate with localized inflammation.

As a Drug Target

1-7F9 is a human monoclonal antibody that binds to KIR2DL1/2L3. Very similar Lirilumab is intended for the treatment of cancers e.g. leukemia.

Leukocyte Immunoglobulin-like Receptors

MHC class I (MHC-I) polymorphisms are associated with the outcome of some viral infections and autoimmune diseases. MHC-I proteins present antigenic peptides and are recognized by receptors on natural killer cells and cytotoxic T lymphocytes, thus enabling the immune system to detect self-antigens and eliminate targets lacking self or expressing foreign antigens. Recognition of MHC-I, however, extends beyond receptors on cytotoxic leukocytes. Members of the leukocyte Ig-like receptor (LILR) family are expressed on monocytic cells and can recognize both classical and non-classical MHC-I alleles. Despite their relatively broad specificity when compared to the T cell receptor or killer Ig-like receptors, variations in the strength of LILR binding between different MHC-I alleles have recently been shown to correlate with control of HIV infection. We suggest that LILR recognition may mediate MHC-I disease association in a manner that does not depend on a binary discrimination of self/non-self by cytotoxic cells. Instead, the effects of LILR activity following engagement by MHC-I may represent a "degrees of self" model, whereby strength of binding to different alleles determines the degree of influence exerted by these receptors on immune cell functions. LILRs are expressed by myelomonocytic cells and lymphocytes, extending their influence across antigen-presenting cell subsets including dendritic cells, macrophages, and B cells. They have been identified as important players in the response to infection, inflammatory diseases, and cancer, with recent literature to indicate that MHC-I recognition by these receptors and consequent allelic effects could extend an influence beyond the immune system.

MHC class I (MHC-I) proteins are characterized by a high level of polymorphism, with thousands of allelic variants identified to date. Such extensive variation indicates powerful selection pressure to maintain a wide range of alleles. Disease associations for individual MHC-I alleles are well-documented. The most striking is that of HLA-B27, which is present in >90% of the patients with ankylosing spondylitis. MHC-I polymorphisms have also been shown to be associated with the outcome of viral infections, including the control of HIV infection, clearance of HCV infection, and protection from dengue hemorrhagic fever following secondary infection with this virus.

Proposed mechanisms to explain classical MHC-I disease associations have focused on the functional role(s) of these proteins. The best characterized of these roles is MHC presentation of short antigenic peptides for recognition by the T cell receptor (TCR) on cytotoxic T cells (CTL). Thus, many studies have examined the nature of the peptides presented by disease-associated alleles and of T cell responses restricted by these alleles. For example, a number of studies have examined the peptide specificities of HLA-B27 subtypes. In the context of HIV infection, a dominant HLA-B27 restricted viral peptide is thought to play a key role in the association of this allele with control of infection. Immune escape from the response against the dominant peptide results in a decrease in HIV-1 replication.

In humans, classical MHC-I are also recognized by members of the killer Ig-like receptor (KIR) family, which are encoded in the leukocyte receptor complex (LRC) on chromosome 19. KIR demonstrate allele (and in some cases, peptide) specificity, albeit at a lower level of precision for individual peptide/MHC complexes than that shown by classical TCR. KIR are expressed on natural killer (NK) cells and T cells where they inhibit the ability of these cytotoxic cells to lyse target cells that express self MHC-I alleles. As knowledge regarding their biology and MHC specificities has grown, KIR has been studied alongside MHC-I in conditions such as spondyloarthropathy, HIV, and HCV infections. There is considerable variation in KIR haplotypes such that any individual may not carry the relevant MHC ligand for every KIR receptor that they express and vice versa. A number of studies suggest that particular combinations of KIR and HLA alleles, believed to result in functional receptor/ligand interactions, are associated with protection from progression to AIDS following HIV infection.

A lesser-studied family of proteins encoded within the LRC is also capable of recognizing MHC class I. These leukocyte Ig-like receptors (LILR) do not appear to be involved in the cytolytic removal of targets bearing non-self MHC-I protein complexes. Instead, they are predominantly expressed on cells of the myelomonocytic lineage, and some of them show a broad specificity encompassing both classical and non-classical MHC-I. The observation that LILR vary in the strength of their binding to individual MHC-I alleles, however, raised the possibility that these innate immune receptors may contribute in some manner toward MHC-I disease associations. In support of this theory, a recent study of a large cohort of HIV-1 infected patients demonstrated that the overall binding strength of LILRB2 for the MHC-I haplotypes expressed by these individuals was positively associated with the level of viremia.

Leukocyte Ig-like Receptors

The various members of the LILR family are broadly categorized as inhibitory (LILRB) or activating (LILRA), according to the presence or absence of tyrosine-based signaling motifs in their cytoplasmic tail. In some cases, putative activating receptors have been shown to elicit inhibitory effects and vice versa for inhibitory receptors. Receptor engagement results in intracellular phosphorylation of the tyrosine-based motifs within the receptors themselves (LILRB) or on associated adaptor molecules (LILRA). Downstream signaling events can be mediated by phosphatases such as SHP-1, SHP-2, and SHIP and vary according to the receptor and/or cellular context. For example, SHP-2 may mediate production of IL-6 via the NF-kB pathway following LILRB2 engagement on dendritic cells or inhibition of the mTOR pathway following LILRB1 engagement on T lymphocytes.

There are multiple similarities between KIR and LILR in terms of Ig domain-based structure, gene location within the LRC, and ability to recognize MHC-I. Unlike their NK receptor counterparts, however, LILR orthologs (known as PIR) are found in rodents, where they demonstrate similar ligand binding, expression, and functional profiles. This may indicate a higher degree of evolutionary conservation for LILR than for KIR, with bovine orthologs also identified and similar proteins documented in chickens and fish. Within the murine system, there is a single inhibitory receptor, PIR-B, and multiple activating receptors (PIR-A). PIRs are involved in the regulation of lymphocyte, antigen-presenting cell, and granulocyte functions, and their study has enabled the identification of functions for both these receptors and their human counterparts, such as the regulation of synaptic plasticity and platelet activation by PIR-B and LILRB2.

Figure shows the known expression profiles of LILR on leukocyte subsets according to current literature. The known expression profiles for LILR are not exhaustive; expression of individual members of the family has been documented for macrophages, B-cells, NK cells, and other non-immune cells. These receptors are, therefore, likely to have far-reaching effects on a range of immunological functions. Immune cells, which have yet to be characterized in full for LILR expression, include invariant NK (iNKT), gamma delta (γδ), regulatory (Treg) and T helper 17 (Th17) T-cells, B-cell subsets, as well as the various APC subsets and granulocytes.

		Activating Receptor						Inhibitory Receptors				
		LILRA1	LILRA2	LILRA3	LILRA4	LILRA5	LILRA6	LILRB1	LILRB2	LILRB3	LILRB4	LILRB5
Expression	Macrophage			Secreted								
	Monocyte			Secreted		CD14+			CD14+		CD14+	
	mDC											
	pDC											
	moDC											
	Basophils											
	Eosinophils											
	T cell										Activated	
	B cell											
	NK cell											
	Oesteoclasts											
	Breast carcinoma											
	Placental stroma											
	Endothelial cells											
	Placental											
	Vascular smooth muscle										HIV+	
	Tissue-like memory B cells											
	Mast cell granules											intra-cell
	Human hematopoietic stem cells											

LILR expression profile, according to literature. Blue shaded squares indicate expression according to the literature; annotation within boxes indicates expression specifics (for example, observed during HIV infection or for a particular cell phenotype). Green denotes Group 1 LILR and red, Group 2 LILR.

Leukocyte Ig-like receptor activity can result in the upregulation or downregulation of both innate and adaptive functions with a range of effects on different cell types. For example, LILR and PIR have been shown to inhibit TLR-mediated functions of antigen-presenting cells such as inflammatory cytokine secretion. Inhibitory LILR have been shown to inhibit the upregulation of co-stimulatory proteins on antigen-presenting cells, thus favoring regulatory T cell responses. On lymphocytes, inhibitory LILR have been shown to inhibit T and B cell receptor signaling and downregulate antibody and cytokine production. Activating LILR have been shown to mediate monocyte activation and secretion of inflammatory cytokines and on basophils to trigger release of histamine.

MHC Recognition by LILR

Following the initial identification of LILRB1 as a receptor for self and viral MHC-I , structural studies predicted that several other members of the family would also recognize MHC-I. Members of the family were allocated into two groups on this basis, with Group 1 containing receptors predicted to bind MHC-I and Group 2 containing receptors that were not predicted to bind MHC-I. It was confirmed subsequently that the Group 1 members LILRA1, LILRA2, LILRA3, LILRB1, and LILRB2 can engage MHC-I. Members of the LILR family vary in their MHC-I binding preferences. LILRB2 demonstrates the broadest specificity, with the ability to recognize all classical and non-classical self MHC-I alleles and forms tested to date. Although LILRB2 binds to both the α3 and β2m regions of the MHC-I antigen-presenting structure, the major portion of its binding site lies within the highly conserved α3 domain. The degree of interaction between this receptor and the α3 domain is sufficient to allow LILRB2 to bind open conformers of MHC-I, which lack β2m. In contrast, the major LILRB1 binding site lies within β2m, thus this receptor can only associate with β2m-associated MHC-I. Recognition of open MHC-I conformers has also been observed for LILRA1 and LILRA3, which were shown in one study to have stronger binding to open confomers than to β2m-associated MHC-I. These findings indicate that alternatively folded forms of MHC-I may play a functional role in the immune response. It is also important to note that the members of the LILR family may interact in cis with MHC-I on the cell surface, as been demonstrated for PIR-B and LILRB1.

Despite their broad specificity, LILRB1 and LILRB2 show variation in their strength of binding to different MHC-I alleles. Binding occurs predominantly through the D1-D2 domains of the receptor, but it has been suggested that secondary binding sites in the D3 and D4 domains may contribute to allelic variations in the strength of LILR binding. The potential importance of such variations was first highlighted by the observation that MHC-I complexes differing by only one amino acid in the bound peptide showed different affinities for LILRB2, which corresponded with the extent of LILRB2-mediated modulation of antigen-presenting cell phenotype. A subsequent comparison of binding strength for different MHC-I alleles to LILRB1 and LILRB2 identified distinct preferences. LILRB1 has a lower affinity for some HLA-A alleles; those with Ala193 and Val194 have shown lower binding ability. Ser207 and Gln253 alleles also show weaker binding to LILRB1 and are in linkage disequilibrium with Ala193 and Val194. LILRB2 has been shown to bind most strongly to HLA-A and weakly to HLA-B alleles but with greater variability for these alleles than LILRB1. Its binding is weakest to a subset of alleles including HLA-B27 and HLA-B 5701. Some of these outliers were MHC-I alleles with known disease associations, leading to the suggestion that LILR recognition of MHC-I might influence susceptibility to, and outcome of, some viral infections or autoimmune diseases.

LILR, MHC and Infection

Viral infection may be regarded as the primary pathology in which MHC-I recognition is essential to achieve a successful immune response. MHC-I proteins present fragments of intracellular proteins to T cells in order to enable the lysis of infected cells, and the peptide binding specificity of particular MHC-I alleles may thus influence the course of disease. There is evidence to suggest that LILR expression is induced in response to infection and can be regarded as an indicator of an effective adaptive immune response. Studies are now beginning to highlight the relevance of LILR in particular infections and the influence of MHC-I recognition in the process.

Distinct LILR expression profiles were found to be associated with dendritic cell dysfunction during acute HIV-1 infection and with "elite" control of infection. As there are well-characterized associations for different MHC-I alleles with either HIV viral control or progression to AIDS and given that LILR have been implicated in its disease pathology, this viral infection represented a suitable model for testing the hypothesis that LILR may mediate MHC-I disease associations. Support for this theory was provided by studies, which demonstrated that MHC-I alleles and complexes associated with disease progression were preferential ligands for the inhibitory receptor LILRB2, whereas those associated with delayed onset of AIDS showed weaker binding to the receptor. It could therefore be hypothesized that weaker affinity for LILRB2 would result in a lack of inhibition of dendritic cell functions, resulting in a more effective anti-HIV immune response. One study sought to examine the MHC-I haplotype of HIV-1 patient cohorts in combination with the strength of their LILR binding in order to assess whether LILR recognition might influence the course of disease. An association with LILRB2, but not LILRB1, binding strength was observed, indicating that the strength of MHC-I recognition correlates with control of viral load. This study provided the first strong evidence that, despite the broad specificity of LILR, the strength of their binding preference for different MHC-I alleles could represent a novel mechanism for an MHC-I association during infection.

Binding of MHC-I by "Activating" members of the LILR family may also be relevant in HIV-1 infection. LILRA1 and LILRA3 preferentially bind HLA-C open conformers, and HLA-C variants have been associated with different outcomes of HIV infection. One particular polymorphism, −35C/T, lies 35 kb upstream of the HLA-C locus. The −35C allele corresponds with increased HLA-C expression, which in turn is associated with delayed onset of AIDS. HLA-C proteins are more stable in open conformer form than their HLA-A and -B counterparts and are upregulated following immune cell activation. It is, therefore, possible that LILRA1 or LILRA3 recognition of HLA-C might provide a further mechanism for MHC-I disease associations during HIV infection.

Leukocyte Ig-like receptor binding preferences for MHC-I alleles may influence the outcome of other viral infections. Expression of HLA-B27 is associated with spontaneous clearance of hepatitis C virus infection, and by analogy with HIV-1, it could be hypothesized that the low binding preference of LILRB2 for this allele might influence disease outcome. Another viral infection where LILR may be responsible for MHC-I-associated protective effects is dengue. Large case-control studies have identified MHC-I alleles with protective effects in dengue infection. Antibody opsonized dengue has recently been shown to co-ligate the inhibitory receptor LILRB1 when engaged by FcγR, leading to inhibition of FcγR signaling and indicating that LILRB1 may play a role in antibody-dependent dengue. Infection with DENV is highly inflammatory and results in a large influx of activated B-cells.

Autoimmunity

Individual LILR have been implicated in autoimmunity, and their preferences for MHC-I alleles may be relevant in these conditions. Of the receptors known to recognize MHC-I, LILRA3 has been found to be associated with a number of inflammatory conditions. Expressed only in a soluble form, LILRA3 possesses no known signaling capacity of its own but can bind ligands of cell-associated LILR. Some individuals do not express LILRA3 due to a large 6.7 kbp sequence deletion. The prevalence of this deletion polymorphism is population-dependent and ranges from 6 to 84%, with a particularly high relevance in the Japanese population, where a number of non-functional spliced isoforms have also been identified. The deletion has been associated with increased susceptibility and early onset of multiple sclerosis (MS) symptoms in a number of studies, although conflicting data have been observed in other populations.

LILRA3 deficiency may also be a risk factor for Sjögrens syndrome (SS), with increased prevalence of null allele homozygous individuals in certain populations, while the functional allele is a suggested risk factor in others. More recent studies have linked LILRA3 to rheumatoid arthritis (RA). In contrast to MS, increased serum level of functional LILRA3 is a proposed genetic risk factor for RA, with serum levels correlating directly with disease severity. Of further note is the prominent expression of LILRA2, A5, B2, and B3 in synovial tissues of RA patients, and the reduction of LILRA2, LILRB2, and LILRB3 in patients responsive to disease-modifying antirheumatic drugs (DMARDs). Functional LILRA3 has also been suggested as a risk factor for systemic lupus erythematosus (SLE) following a genotyping study in Han Chinese populations, which also found higher levels of LILRA3 mRNA in SLE patients.

Other Ligands and Functions of LILR

Direct recognition of dengue virus by LILRB1 highlights the relevance of future studies to characterize the full range of ligands for these receptors and compare their relative binding strengths. As described above, LILRB2 is known to be the most promiscuous receptor in the family in terms of its broad specificity for classical and non-classical MHC-I in folded and unfolded forms. LILRB2 has also been shown to bind a range of non-MHC ligands including angiopoietin-like proteins and NOGO, a myelin component. More recently, LILRA3 has also been shown to bind NOGO. These findings extend the relevance of LILR beyond immune responses to situations such as neurodegeneration, neural plasticity, angiogenesis, and other, as yet, unidentified scenarios where MHC-I may compete with other ligands for receptor binding. In the future, comparative binding assays may indicate how MHC-I allelic preferences might influence the ability of LILR to bind alternative ligands. Such investigations could cast light on previous observations regarding the relevance of MHC-I in neural plasticity and regeneration and associations with non-immune conditions such as Alzheimer's disease.

References

- Immune-recognition-and-receptors: creative-diagnostics.com, Retrieved 14 July, 2019

- Gomperts, BD.; Kramer, IM. Tatham, PER. (2002). Signal transduction. Academic Press. ISBN 0-12-289631-9 ISBN

- Kirkbridge, K.C., Ray, B.N., Blobe, G.C. (2005). "Cell-surface co-receptors: emerging roles in signaling and human disease". Trends Biochem. Sci. 30 (11): 611–21. Doi:10.1016/j.tibs.2005.09.003. PMID 16185874

- Brooks, Andrew J.; Dehkhoda, Farhad; Kragelund, Birthe B. (2017). "Cytokine Receptors". Principles of Endocrinology and Hormone Action. Springer International Publishing. Pp. 1–29. Doi:10.1007/978-3-319-27318-1_8-2. ISBN 9783319273181

- Locksley RM, Killeen N, Lenardo MJ (2001). "The TNF and TNF receptor superfamilies: integrating mammalian biology". Cell. 104 (4): 487–501. Doi:10.1016/S0092-8674(01)00237-9. PMID 11239407

- Family Display Forward, GRAC: guidetopharmacology.org, Retrieved 31 March, 2019

- Uhrberg M (January 2005). "The KIR gene family: life in the fast lane of evolution". European Journal of Immunology. 35 (1): 10–5. Doi:10.1002/eji.200425743. PMID 15580655

Concepts of Immunology 4

Some of the fundamental concepts of immunology are immune tolerance, antigen presentation, intrinsic immunity, immunoglobulin class switching, immune repertoire and immunological synapse. This chapter has been carefully written to provide an easy understanding of these key concepts of immunology.

Immune Tolerance

Tolerance is the prevention of an immune response against a particular antigen. For instance, the immune system is generally tolerant of self-antigens, so it does not usually attack the body's own cells, tissues, and organs. However, when tolerance is lost, disorders like autoimmune disease or food allergy may occur. Tolerance is maintained in a number of ways:

- When adaptive immune cells mature, there are several checkpoints in place to eliminate autoreactive cells. If a B cell produces antibodies that strongly recognize host cells, or if a T cell strongly recognizes self-antigen, they are deleted.

- Nevertheless, there are autoreactive immune cells present in healthy individuals. Autoreactive immune cells are kept in a non-reactive, or anergic, state. Even though they recognize the body's own cells, they do not have the ability to react and cannot cause host damage.

- Regulatory immune cells circulate throughout the body to maintain tolerance. Besides limiting autoreactive cells, regulatory cells are important for turning an immune response off after the problem is resolved. They can act as drains, depleting areas of essential nutrients that surrounding immune cells need for activation or survival.

- Some locations in the body are called immunologically privileged sites. These areas, like the eye and brain, do not typically elicit strong immune responses. Part of this is because of physical barriers, like the blood-brain barrier, that limit the degree to which immune cells may enter. These areas also may express higher levels of suppressive cytokines to prevent a robust immune response.

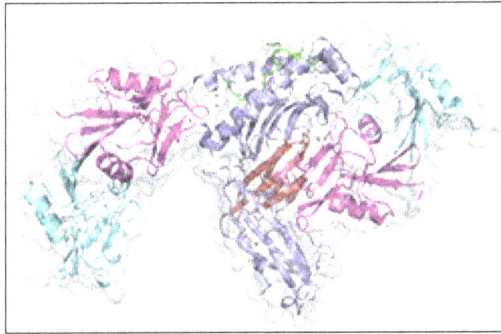

Inhibitory NK cell receptor (purple and light blue) binds to MHC-I
(blue and red), an interaction that prevents immune responses against self.

Fetomaternal tolerance is the prevention of a maternal immune response against a developing fetus. Major histocompatibility complex (MHC) proteins help the immune system distinguish between host and foreign cells. MHC also is called human leukocyte antigen (HLA). By expressing paternal MHC or HLA proteins and paternal antigens, a fetus can potentially trigger the mother's immune system. However, there are several barriers that may prevent this from occurring. The placenta reduces the exposure of the fetus to maternal immune cells, the proteins expressed on the outer layer of the placenta may limit immune recognition, and regulatory cells and suppressive signals may play a role.

Transplantation of a donor tissue or organ requires appropriate MHC or HLA matching to limit the risk of rejection. Because MHC or HLA matching is rarely complete, transplant recipients must continuously take immunosuppressive drugs, which can cause complications like higher susceptibility to infection and some cancers. Researchers are developing more targeted ways to induce tolerance to transplanted tissues and organs while leaving protective immune responses intact.

Immunity

In biology, immunity is the balanced state of multicellular organisms having adequate biological defenses to fight infection, disease, or other unwanted biological invasion, while having adequate tolerance to avoid allergy, and autoimmune diseases.

Innate and Adaptive

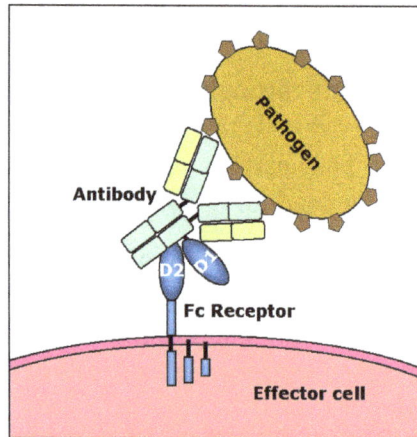

Scheme of a Fc receptor.

Immunity is the capability of multicellular organisms to resist harmful microorganisms from entering it. Immunity involves both specific and nonspecific components. The nonspecific components act as barriers or eliminators of a wide range of pathogens irrespective of their antigenic make-up. Other components of the immune system adapt themselves to each new disease encountered and can generate pathogen-specific immunity.

An immune system may contain innate and adaptive components. The innate system in mammalians, for example, is composed of primitive bone marrow cells that are programmed to recognise foreign substances and react. The adaptive system is composed of more advanced lymphatic cells that are programmed to recognise self-substances and don't react. The reaction to foreign substances is etymologically described as inflammation, meaning to set on fire. The non-reaction to self-substances is described as immunity, meaning to exempt or as immunotolerance. These two components of the immune system create a dynamic biological environment where "health" can be seen as a physical state where the self is immunologically spared, and what is foreign is inflammatorily and immunologically eliminated. "Disease" can arise when what is foreign cannot be eliminated or what is self is not spared.

Innate immunity, also called native immunity, exists by virtue of an organisms constitution, that is its genetic make-up, without an external stimulation or a previous infection. It is divided into two types: (a) Non-Specific innate immunity, a degree of resistance to all infections in general. (b) Specific innate immunity, a resistance to a particular kind of microorganism only. As a result, some races, particular individuals or breeds in agriculture do not suffer from certain infectious diseases.

Adaptive immunity can be sub-divided depending on how the immunity was introduced in 'naturally acquired' through chance contact with a disease-causing agent, whereas 'artificially acquired immunity' develops through deliberate actions such as vaccination. Both naturally and artificially acquired immunity can be further subdivided depending on whether the host built up immunity itself by antigen as 'active immunity' and lasts long-term, sometimes lifelong. 'Passive immunity' is acquired through transfer (injection or infusion) of antibodies or activated T-cells from an immune host; it is short lived—usually lasting only a few months. The diagram summarizes these divisions of immunity.

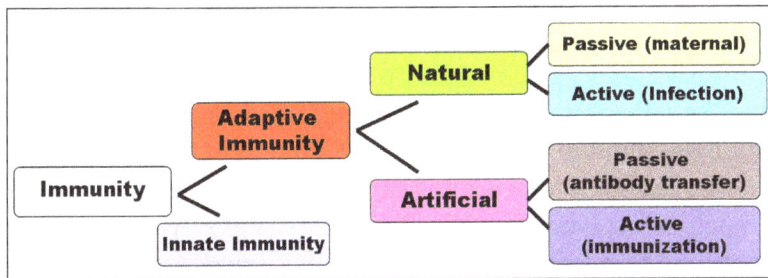

Adaptive immunity can also be divided by the type of immune mediators involved; humoral immunity is the aspect of immunity that is mediated by secreted antibodies, whereas cell mediated immunity involves T-lymphocytes alone. Humoral immunity is called active when the organism generates its antibodies, and passive when antibodies are transferred between individuals or species. Similarly, cell-mediated immunity is active when the organisms' T-cells are stimulated, and passive when T cells come from another organism.

Passive

Passive immunity is the transfer of active immunity, in the form of readymade antibodies, from one individual to another. Passive immunity can occur naturally, when maternal antibodies are transferred to the foetus through the placenta, and can also be induced artificially, when high levels of human (or horse) antibodies specific for a pathogen or toxin are transferred to non-immune individuals. Passive immunization is used when there is a high risk of infection and insufficient time for the body to develop its own immune response, or to reduce the symptoms of ongoing or immunosuppressive diseases. Passive immunity provides immediate protection, but the body does not develop memory, therefore the patient is at risk of being infected by the same pathogen later.

Naturally Acquired Passive Immunity

Maternal passive immunity is a type of naturally acquired passive immunity, and refers to antibody-mediated immunity conveyed to a fetus by its mother during pregnancy. Maternal antibodies (MatAb) are passed through the placenta to the fetus by an FcRn receptor on placental cells. This occurs around the third month of gestation. IgG is the only antibody isotype that can pass through the placenta. Passive immunity is also provided through the transfer of IgA antibodies found in breast milk that are transferred to the gut of the infant, protecting against bacterial infections, until the newborn can synthesize its antibodies. Colostrum present in mothers milk is an example of passive immunity.

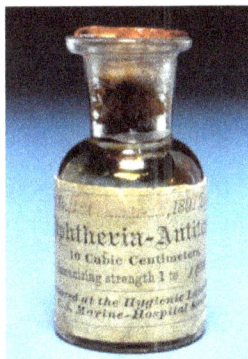

One of the first bottles of diphtheria antitoxin produced.

Artificially Acquired Passive Immunity

Artificially acquired passive immunity is a short-term immunization induced by the transfer of antibodies, which can be administered in several forms; as human or animal blood plasma, as pooled human immunoglobulin for intravenous (IVIG) or intramuscular (IG) use, and in the form of monoclonal antibodies (MAb). Passive transfer is used prophylactically in the case of immuno-deficiency diseases, such as hypogammaglobulinemia. It is also used in the treatment of several types of acute infection, and to treat poisoning. Immunity derived from passive immunization lasts for only a short period of time, and there is also a potential risk for hypersensitivity reactions, and serum sickness, especially from gamma globulin of non-human origin.

The artificial induction of passive immunity has been used for over a century to treat infectious disease, and before the advent of antibiotics, was often the only specific treatment for certain in-fections. Immunoglobulin therapy continued to be a first line therapy in the treatment of severe respiratory diseases until the 1930s, even after sulfonamide lot antibiotics were introduced.

Transfer of Activated T-cells

Passive or "adoptive transfer" of cell-mediated immunity, is conferred by the transfer of "sensitized" or activated T-cells from one individual into another. It is rarely used in humans because it requires histocompatible (matched) donors, which are often difficult to find. In unmatched donors this type of transfer carries severe risks of graft versus host disease. It has, however, been used to treat certain diseases including some types of cancer and immunodeficiency. This type of transfer differs from a bone marrow transplant, in which (undifferentiated) hematopoietic stem cells are transferred.

Active

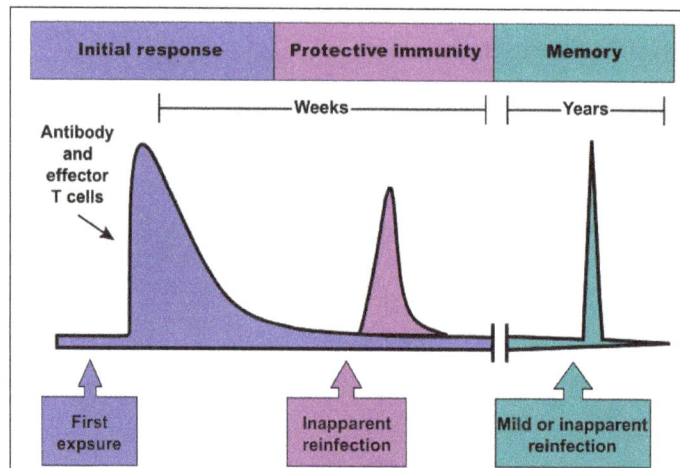

The time course of an immune response.

Due to the formation of immunological memory, reinfection at later time points leads to a rapid increase in antibody production and effector T cell activity. These later infections can be mild or even unapparent.

When B cells and T cells are activated by a pathogen, memory B-cells and T- cells develop, and the primary immune response results. Throughout the lifetime of an animal, these memory cells will "remember" each specific pathogen encountered, and can mount a strong secondary response if the pathogen is detected again. The primary and secondary responses were first described in 1921 by English immunologist Alexander Glenny although the mechanism involved was not discovered until later. This type of immunity is both active and adaptive because the body's immune system prepares itself for future challenges. Active immunity often involves both the cell-mediated and humoral aspects of immunity as well as input from the innate immune system.

Naturally Acquired Active Immunity

Naturally acquired active immunity occurs when a person is exposed to a live pathogen and develops a primary immune response, which leads to immunological memory. This type of immunity is "natural" because deliberate exposure does not induce it. Many disorders of immune system function can affect the formation of active immunity such as immunodeficiency (both acquired and congenital forms) and immunosuppression.

Artificially Acquired Active Immunity

Artificially acquired active immunity can be induced by a vaccine, a substance that contains antigen. A vaccine stimulates a primary response against the antigen without causing symptoms of the disease. Richard Dunning coined the term vaccination, a colleague of Edward Jenner, and adapted by Louis Pasteur for his pioneering work in vaccination. The method Pasteur used entailed treating the infectious agents for those diseases, so they lost the ability to cause serious disease. Pasteur adopted the name vaccine as a generic term in honor of Jenner's discovery, which Pasteur's work built upon.

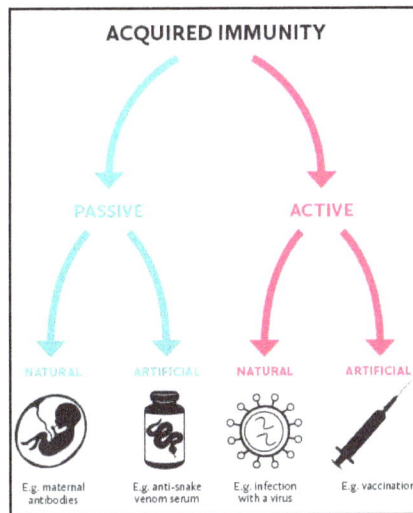

In 1807, Bavaria became the first group to require that their military recruits be vaccinated against smallpox, as the spread of smallpox was linked to combat. Subsequently, the practice of vaccination would increase with the spread of war.

There are four types of traditional vaccines:

- Inactivated vaccines are composed of micro-organisms that have been killed with chemicals and/or heat and are no longer infectious. Examples are vaccines against flu, cholera, plague, and hepatitis A. Most vaccines of this type are likely to require booster shots.

- Live, attenuated vaccines are composed of micro-organisms that have been cultivated under conditions which disable their ability to induce disease. These responses are more durable and do not generally require booster shots. Examples include yellow fever, measles, rubella, and mumps.

- Toxoids are inactivated toxic compounds from micro-organisms in cases where these (rather than the micro-organism itself) cause illness, used prior to an encounter with the toxin of the micro-organism. Examples of toxoid-based vaccines include tetanus and diphtheria.

- Subunit vaccines are composed of small fragments of disease-causing organisms. A characteristic example is the subunit vaccine against Hepatitis B virus.

Most vaccines are given by hypodermic or intramuscular injection as they are not absorbed reliably through the gut. Live attenuated polio and some typhoid and cholera vaccines are given orally in order to produce immunity based in the bowel.

Autoimmunity

Autoimmunity is the system of immune responses of an organism against its own healthy cells and tissues. Any disease that results from such an aberrant immune response is termed an "autoimmune disease". Prominent examples include celiac disease, diabetes mellitus type 1, sarcoidosis, systemic lupus erythematosus (SLE), Sjögren's syndrome, eosinophilic granulomatosis with polyangiitis, Hashimoto's thyroiditis, Graves' disease, idiopathic thrombocytopenic purpura, Addison's disease, rheumatoid arthritis (RA), ankylosing spondylitis, polymyositis (PM), dermatomyositis (DM) and multiple sclerosis (MS). Autoimmune diseases are very often treated with steroids.

In the later 19th century it was believed that the immune system was unable to react against the body's own tissues. Paul Ehrlich, at the turn of the 20th century, proposed the concept of *horror autotoxicus*. Ehrlich later adjusted his theory to recognize the possibility of autoimmune tissue attacks, but believed certain innate protection mechanisms would prevent the autoimmune response from becoming pathological.

In 1904 this theory was challenged by the discovery of a substance in the serum of patients with paroxysmal cold hemoglobinuria that reacted with red blood cells. During the following decades, a number of conditions could be linked to autoimmune responses. However, the authoritative status of Ehrlich's postulate hampered the understanding of these findings. Immunology became a biochemical rather than a clinical discipline. By the 1950s the modern understanding of autoantibodies and autoimmune diseases started to spread.

More recently it has become accepted that autoimmune responses are an integral part of vertebrate immune systems (sometimes termed "natural autoimmunity"). Autoimmunity should not be confused with alloimmunity.

Low-level Autoimmunity

While a high level of autoimmunity is unhealthy, a low level of autoimmunity may actually be beneficial. Taking the experience of a beneficial factor in autoimmunity further, one might hypothesize with intent to prove that autoimmunity is always a self-defense mechanism of the mammal system to survive. The system does not randomly lose the ability to distinguish between self and non-self, the attack on cells may be the consequence of cycling metabolic processes necessary to keep the blood chemistry in homeostasis.

Second, autoimmunity may have a role in allowing a rapid immune response in the early stages of an infection when the availability of foreign antigens limits the response (i.e., when there are few pathogens present). In their study, Stefanova et al. injected an anti-MHC Class II antibody into mice expressing a single type of MHC Class II molecule (H-2^b) to temporarily prevent CD4+ T cell-MHC interaction. Naive CD4+ T cells (those that have not encountered any antigens before) recovered from these mice 36 hours post-anti-MHC administration showed decreased responsiveness to the antigen pigeon cytochrome C peptide, as determined by Zap-70 phosphorylation, proliferation, and Interleukin-2 production. Thus Stefanova et al. demonstrated that self-MHC recognition (which, if too strong may contribute to autoimmune disease) maintains the responsiveness of CD4+ T cells when foreign antigens are absent.

Immunological Tolerance

Pioneering work by Noel Rose and Ernst Witebsky in New York, and Roitt and Doniach at University College London provided clear evidence that, at least in terms of antibody-producing B cells (B lymphocytes), diseases such as rheumatoid arthritis and thyrotoxicosis are associated with loss of immunological tolerance, which is the ability of an individual to ignore "self", while reacting to "non-self". This breakage leads to the immune system's mounting an effective and specific immune response against self determinants. The exact genesis of immunological tolerance is still elusive, but several theories have been proposed since the mid-twentieth century to explain its origin.

Three hypotheses have gained widespread attention among immunologists:

- Clonal Deletion theory, proposed by Burnet, according to which self-reactive lymphoid cells are destroyed during the development of the immune system in an individual. For their work Frank M. Burnet and Peter B. Medawar were awarded the 1960 Nobel Prize in Physiology or Medicine "for discovery of acquired immunological tolerance".

- Clonal Anergy theory, proposed by Nossal, in which self-reactive T- or B-cells become inactivated in the normal individual and cannot amplify the immune response.

- Idiotype Network theory, proposed by Jerne, wherein a network of antibodies capable of neutralizing self-reactive antibodies exists naturally within the body.

In addition, two other theories are under intense investigation:

- Clonal Ignorance theory, according to which autoreactive T cells that are not represented in the thymus will mature and migrate to the periphery, where they will not encounter the appropriate antigen because it is inaccessible tissues. Consequently, auto-reactive B cells, that escape deletion, cannot find the antigen or the specific helper T cell.

- Suppressor population or Regulatory T cell theory, wherein regulatory T-lymphocytes (commonly CD4+FoxP3$^+$ cells, among others) function to prevent, downregulate, or limit autoaggressive immune responses in the immune system.

Tolerance can also be differentiated into "Central" and "Peripheral" tolerance, on whether or not the above-stated checking mechanisms operate in the central lymphoid organs (Thymus and Bone Marrow) or the peripheral lymphoid organs (lymph node, spleen, etc., where self-reactive B-cells may be destroyed). It must be emphasised that these theories are not mutually exclusive, and evidence has been mounting suggesting that all of these mechanisms may actively contribute to vertebrate immunological tolerance.

A puzzling feature of the documented loss of tolerance seen in spontaneous human autoimmunity is that it is almost entirely restricted to the autoantibody responses produced by B lymphocytes. Loss of tolerance by T cells has been extremely hard to demonstrate, and where there is evidence for an abnormal T cell response it is usually not to the antigen recognised by autoantibodies. Thus, in rheumatoid arthritis there are autoantibodies to IgG Fc but apparently no corresponding T cell response. In systemic lupus there are autoantibodies to DNA, which cannot evoke a T cell response, and limited evidence for T cell responses implicates nucleoprotein antigens. In Celiac disease there are autoantibodies to tissue transglutaminase but the T cell response is to the foreign protein gliadin. This disparity has led to the idea that human autoimmune disease is in most cases (with probable exceptions including type I diabetes) based on a loss of B cell tolerance which makes use of normal T cell responses to foreign antigens in a variety of aberrant ways.

Immunodeficiency and Autoimmunity

There are a large number of immunodeficiency syndromes that present clinical and laboratory characteristics of autoimmunity. The decreased ability of the immune system to clear infections in these patients may be responsible for causing autoimmunity through perpetual immune system activation.

One example is common variable immunodeficiency (CVID) where multiple autoimmune diseases are seen, e.g.: inflammatory bowel disease, autoimmune thrombocytopenia and autoimmune thyroid disease.

Familial hemophagocytic lymphohistiocytosis, an autosomal recessive primary immunodeficiency, is another example. Pancytopenia, rashes, swollen lymph nodes and enlargement of the liver and spleen are commonly seen in such individuals. Presence of multiple uncleared viral infections due to lack of perforin are thought to be responsible.

In addition to chronic and/or recurrent infections many autoimmune diseases including arthritis, autoimmune hemolytic anemia, scleroderma and type 1 diabetes mellitus are also seen in X-linked agammaglobulinemia (XLA). Recurrent bacterial and fungal infections and chronic inflammation of the gut and lungs are seen in chronic granulomatous disease (CGD) as well. CGD is a caused by decreased production of nicotinamide adenine dinucleotide phosphate (NADPH) oxidase by neutrophils. Hypomorphic RAG mutations are seen in patients with midline granulomatous disease; an autoimmune disorder that is commonly seen in patients with granulomatosis with polyangiitis and NK/T cell lymphomas.

Wiskott-Aldrich syndrome (WAS) patients also present with eczema, autoimmune manifestations, recurrent bacterial infections and lymphoma.

In autoimmune polyendocrinopathy-candidiasis-ectodermal dystrophy (APECED) also autoimmunity and infections coexist: Organ-specific autoimmune manifestations (e.g. hypoparathyroidism and adrenocortical failure) and chronic mucocutaneous candidiasis.

Finally, IgA deficiency is also sometimes associated with the development of autoimmune and atopic phenomena.

Genetic Factors

Certain individuals are genetically susceptible to developing autoimmune diseases. This susceptibility is associated with multiple genes plus other risk factors. Genetically predisposed individuals do not always develop autoimmune diseases.

Three main sets of genes are suspected in many autoimmune diseases. These genes are related to:

- Immunoglobulins;
- T-cell receptors;
- The major histocompatibility complexes (MHC).

The first two, which are involved in the recognition of antigens, are inherently variable and susceptible to recombination. These variations enable the immune system to respond to a very wide variety of invaders, but may also give rise to lymphocytes capable of self-reactivity.

- HLA DR2 is strongly positively correlated with Systemic Lupus Erythematosus, narcolepsy and multiple sclerosis, and negatively correlated with DM Type 1;
- HLA DR3 is correlated strongly with Sjögren's syndrome, myasthenia gravis, SLE, and DM Type 1;
- HLA DR4 is correlated with the genesis of rheumatoid arthritis, Type 1 diabetes mellitus, and pemphigus vulgaris.

Fewer correlations exist with MHC class I molecules. The most notable and consistent is the association between HLA B27 and spondyloarthropathies like ankylosing spondylitis and reactive arthritis. Correlations may exist between polymorphisms within class II MHC promoters and autoimmune disease.

The contributions of genes outside the MHC complex remain the subject of research, in animal models of disease (Linda Wicker's extensive genetic studies of diabetes in the NOD mouse), and in patients (Brian Kotzin's linkage analysis of susceptibility to SLE).

Recently, PTPN22 has been associated with multiple autoimmune diseases including Type I diabetes, rheumatoid arthritis, systemic lupus erythematosus, Hashimoto's thyroiditis, Graves' disease, Addison's disease, Myasthenia Gravis, vitiligo, systemic sclerosis juvenile idiopathic arthritis, and psoriatic arthritis.

Sex

There is some evidence that a person's sex may also have some role in the development of autoimmunity; that is, most autoimmune diseases are sex-related. A few autoimmune diseases that men are just as or more likely to develop as women include: ankylosing spondylitis, type 1 diabetes mellitus, granulomatosis with polyangiitis, Crohn's disease, Primary sclerosing cholangitis and psoriasis.

Ratio of female/male incidence of autoimmune diseases	
Hashimoto's thyroiditis	10:1
Graves' disease	7:1
Multiple sclerosis (MS)	2:1
Myasthenia gravis	2:1
Systemic lupus erythematosus (SLE)	9:1
Rheumatoid arthritis	5:2
Primary sclerosing cholangitis	1:2

The reasons for the sex role in autoimmunity vary. Women appear to generally mount larger inflammatory responses than men when their immune systems are triggered, increasing the risk of autoimmunity. Involvement of sex steroids is indicated by that many autoimmune diseases tend to fluctuate in accordance with hormonal changes, for example: during pregnancy, in the menstrual cycle, or when using oral contraception. A history of pregnancy also appears to leave a persistent increased risk for autoimmune disease. It has been suggested that the slight, direct exchange of cells between mothers and their children during pregnancy may induce autoimmunity. This would tip the gender balance in the direction of the female.

Another theory suggests the female high tendency to get autoimmunity is due to an imbalanced X chromosome inactivation. The X-inactivation skew theory, proposed by Princeton University's Jeff Stewart, has recently been confirmed experimentally in scleroderma and autoimmune thyroiditis. Other complex X-linked genetic susceptibility mechanisms are proposed and under investigation.

Environmental Factors

An interesting inverse relationship exists between infectious diseases and autoimmune diseases. In areas where multiple infectious diseases are endemic, autoimmune diseases are quite rarely seen. The reverse, to some extent, seems to hold true. The hygiene hypothesis attributes these correlations to the immune manipulating strategies of pathogens. While such an observation has been variously termed as spurious and ineffective, according to some studies, parasite infection is associated with reduced activity of autoimmune disease.

The putative mechanism is that the parasite attenuates the host immune response in order to protect itself. This may provide a serendipitous benefit to a host that also suffers from autoimmune disease. The details of parasite immune modulation are not yet known, but may include secretion of anti-inflammatory agents or interference with the host immune signaling.

A paradoxical observation has been the strong association of certain microbial organisms with autoimmune diseases. For example, *Klebsiella pneumoniae* and coxsackievirus B have been strongly correlated with ankylosing spondylitis and diabetes mellitus type 1, respectively. This has been explained by the tendency of the infecting organism to produce super-antigens that are capable of polyclonal activation of B-lymphocytes, and production of large amounts of antibodies of varying specificities, some of which may be self-reactive.

Certain chemical agents and drugs can also be associated with the genesis of autoimmune conditions, or conditions that simulate autoimmune diseases. The most striking of these is the drug-induced lupus erythematosus. Usually, withdrawal of the offending drug cures the symptoms in a patient.

Cigarette smoking is now established as a major risk factor for both incidence and severity of rheumatoid arthritis. This may relate to abnormal citrullination of proteins, since the effects of smoking correlate with the presence of antibodies to citrullinated peptides.

Pathogenesis of Autoimmunity

Several mechanisms are thought to be operative in the pathogenesis of autoimmune diseases, against a backdrop of genetic predisposition and environmental modulation. A summary of some of the important mechanisms have been described:

- T-Cell Bypass – A normal immune system requires the activation of B-cells by T-cells before the former can undergo differentiation into plasma B-cells and subsequently produce antibodies in large quantities. This requirement of a T-cell can be bypassed in rare instances, such as infection by organisms producing super-antigens, which are capable of initiating polyclonal activation of B-cells, or even of T-cells, by directly binding to the β-subunit of T-cell receptors in a non-specific fashion.

- T-Cell-B-Cell discordance – A normal immune response is assumed to involve B and T cell responses to the same antigen, even if we know that B cells and T cells recognise very different things: conformations on the surface of a molecule for B cells and pre-processed peptide fragments of proteins for T cells. However, there is nothing as far as we know that requires this. All that is required is that a B cell recognising antigen X endocytoses and processes a protein Y (normally =X) and presents it to a T cell. Roosnek and Lanzavecchia showed that B cells recognising IgGFc could get help from any T cell responding to an antigen co-endocytosed with IgG by the B cell as part of an immune complex. In coeliac disease it seems likely that B cells recognising tissue transglutamine are helped by T cells recognising gliadin.

- Aberrant B cell receptor-mediated feedback – A feature of human autoimmune disease is that it is largely restricted to a small group of antigens, several of which have known signaling roles in the immune response (DNA, C1q, IgGFc, Ro, Con. A receptor, Peanut agglutinin receptor(PNAR)). This fact gave rise to the idea that spontaneous autoimmunity may result when the binding of antibody to certain antigens leads to aberrant signals being fed back to parent B cells through membrane bound ligands. These ligands include B cell receptor (for antigen), IgG Fc receptors, CD21, which binds complement C3d, Toll-like receptors 9 and 7 (which can bind DNA and nucleoproteins) and PNAR. More indirect aberrant activation of B cells can also be envisaged with autoantibodies to acetyl choline receptor (on thymic myoid cells) and hormone and hormone binding proteins. Together with the concept of T-cell-B-cell discordance this idea forms the basis of the hypothesis of self-perpetuating autoreactive B cells. Autoreactive B cells in spontaneous autoimmunity are seen as surviving because of subversion both of the T cell help pathway and of the feedback signal through B cell receptor, thereby overcoming the negative signals responsible for B cell self-tolerance without necessarily requiring loss of T cell self-tolerance.

- Molecular Mimicry – An exogenous antigen may share structural similarities with certain host antigens; thus, any antibody produced against this antigen (which mimics the self-antigens) can also, in theory, bind to the host antigens, and amplify the immune response. The idea of molecular mimicry arose in the context of Rheumatic Fever, which follows infection with Group A beta-haemolytic streptococci. Although rheumatic fever has been attributed to molecular mimicry for half a century no antigen has been formally identified (if anything too many have been proposed). Moreover, the complex tissue distribution of the disease (heart, joint, skin, basal ganglia) argues against a cardiac specific antigen. It remains entirely possible that the disease is due to e.g. an unusual interaction between immune complexes, complement components and endothelium.

- Idiotype Cross-Reaction – Idiotypes are antigenic epitopes found in the antigen-binding portion (Fab) of the immunoglobulin molecule. Plotz and Oldstone presented evidence that autoimmunity can arise as a result of a cross-reaction between the idiotype on an antiviral antibody and a host cell receptor for the virus in question. In this case, the host-cell receptor is envisioned as an internal image of the virus, and the anti-idiotype antibodies can react with the host cells.

- Cytokine Dysregulation – Cytokines have been recently divided into two groups according to the population of cells whose functions they promote: Helper T-cells type 1 or type 2. The second category of cytokines, which include IL-4, IL-10 and TGF-β (to name a few), seem to have a role in prevention of exaggeration of pro-inflammatory immune responses.

- Dendritic cell apoptosis – Immune system cells called dendritic cells present antigens to active lymphocytes. Dendritic cells that are defective in apoptosis can lead to inappropriate systemic lymphocyte activation and consequent decline in self-tolerance.

- Epitope spreading or epitope drift – When the immune reaction changes from targeting the primary epitope to also targeting other epitopes. In contrast to molecular mimicry, the other epitopes need not be structurally similar to the primary one.

- Epitope modification or Cryptic epitope exposure – This mechanism of autoimmune disease is unique in that it does not result from a defect in the hematopoietic system. Instead, disease results from the exposure of cryptic N-glycan (polysaccharide) linkages common to lower eukaryotes and prokaryotes on the glycoproteins of mammalian non-hematopoietic cells and organs. This exposure of phylogenically primitive glycans activates one or more mammalian innate immune cell receptors to induce a chronic sterile inflammatory state. In the presence of chronic and inflammatory cell damage, the adaptive immune system is recruited and self–tolerance is lost with increased autoantibody production. In this form of the disease, the absence of lymphocytes can accelerate organ damage, and intravenous IgG administration can be therapeutic. Although this route to autoimmune disease may underlie various degenerative disease states, no diagnostics for this disease mechanism exist at present, and thus its role in human autoimmunity is currently unknown.

The roles of specialized immunoregulatory cell types, such as regulatory T cells, NKT cells, γδ T-cells in the pathogenesis of autoimmune disease are under investigation.

Classification

Autoimmune diseases can be broadly divided into systemic and organ-specific or localised autoimmune disorders, depending on the principal clinico-pathologic features of each disease.

- Systemic autoimmune diseases include coeliac disease, lupus erythematosus, Sjögren's syndrome, sarcoidosis, scleroderma, rheumatoid arthritis, cryoglobulinemic vasculitis, and dermatomyositis. These conditions tend to be associated with autoantibodies to antigens which are not tissue specific. Thus although polymyositis is more or less tissue specific in presentation, it may be included in this group because the autoantigens are often ubiquitous t-RNA synthetases.

- Local syndromes which affect a specific organ or tissue:

  ◦ Endocrinologic: Diabetes mellitus type 1, Hashimoto's thyroiditis, Addison's disease.

  ◦ Gastrointestinal: Crohn's disease, pernicious anaemia.

  ◦ Dermatologic: Pemphigus vulgaris, vitiligo.

  ◦ Haematologic: Autoimmune haemolytic anaemia, idiopathic thrombocytopenic purpura.

  ◦ Neurological: Multiple sclerosis, myasthenia gravis, autoimmune encephalitis, gluten ataxia.

Using the traditional "organ specific" and "non-organ specific" classification scheme, many diseases have been lumped together under the autoimmune disease umbrella. However, many chronic inflammatory human disorders lack the telltale associations of B and T cell driven immunopathology. In the last decade it has been firmly established that tissue "inflammation against self" does not necessarily rely on abnormal T and B cell responses.

This has led to the recent proposal that the spectrum of autoimmunity should be viewed along an "immunological disease continuum," with classical autoimmune diseases at one extreme and diseases driven by the innate immune system at the other extreme. Within this scheme, the full spectrum of autoimmunity can be included. Many common human autoimmune diseases can be seen to have a substantial innate immune mediated immunopathology using this new scheme. This new classification scheme has implications for understanding disease mechanisms and for therapy development.

Diagnosis

Diagnosis of autoimmune disorders largely rests on accurate history and physical examination of the patient, and high index of suspicion against a backdrop of certain abnormalities in routine laboratory tests (example, elevated C-reactive protein). In several systemic disorders, serological assays which can detect specific autoantibodies can be employed. Localised disorders are best diagnosed by immunofluorescence of biopsy specimens. Autoantibodies are used to diagnose many autoimmune diseases. The levels of autoantibodies are measured to determine the progress of the disease.

Treatments

Treatments for autoimmune disease have traditionally been immunosuppressive, anti-inflammatory, or palliative. Managing inflammation is critical in autoimmune diseases. Non-immunological therapies, such as hormone replacement in Hashimoto's thyroiditis or Type 1 diabetes mellitus treat outcomes of the autoaggressive response, thus these are palliative treatments. Dietary manipulation limits the severity of celiac disease. Steroidal or NSAID treatment limits inflammatory symptoms of many diseases. IVIG is used for CIDP and GBS. Specific immuno-modulatory therapies, such as the TNFα antagonists (e.g. etanercept), the B cell depleting agent rituximab, the anti-IL-6 receptor tocilizumab and the costimulation blocker abatacept have been shown to be useful in treating RA. Some of these immunotherapies may be associated with increased risk of adverse effects, such as susceptibility to infection.

Helminthic therapy is an experimental approach that involves inoculation of the patient with specific parasitic intestinal nematodes (helminths). There are currently two closely related treatments available, inoculation with either Necator americanus, commonly known as hookworms, or Trichuris Suis Ova, commonly known as Pig Whipworm Eggs.

T cell vaccination is also being explored as a possible future therapy for autoimmune disorders.

Nutrition and Autoimmunity

Vitamin D/Sunlight:

- Because most human cells and tissues have receptors for vitamin D, including T and B cells, adequate levels of vitamin D can aid in the regulation of the immune system. Vitamin D plays a role in immune function by acting on T cells and natural killer cells. Research has demonstrated an association between low serum vitamin D and autoimmune diseases, including multiple sclerosis, type 1 diabetes, and Systemic Lupus Erythematosus (commonly referred to simply as lupus). However, since photosensitivity occurs in lupus, patients are advised to avoid sunlight which may be responsible for vitamin D deficiency seen in this disease. Polymorphisms in the vitamin D receptor gene are commonly found in people with autoimmune diseases, giving one potential mechanism for vitamin D's role in autoimmunity. There is mixed evidence on the effect of vitamin D supplementation in type 1 diabetes, lupus, and multiple sclerosis.

Omega-3 Fatty Acids:

- Studies have shown that adequate consumption of omega-3 fatty acids counteracts the effects of arachidonic acids, which contribute to symptoms of autoimmune diseases. Human and animal trials suggest that omega-3 is an effective treatment modality for many cases of Rheumatoid Arthritis, Inflammatory Bowel Disease, Asthma, and Psoriasis.

- While major depression is not necessarily an autoimmune disease, some of its physiological symptoms are inflammatory and autoimmune in nature. Omega-3 may inhibit production of interferon gamma and other cytokines which cause the physiological symptoms of depression. This may be due to the fact that an imbalance in omega-3 and omega-6 fatty acids, which have opposing effects, is instrumental in the etiology of major depression.

Probiotics/Microflora:

- Various types of bacteria and microflora present in fermented dairy products, especially Lactobacillus casei, have been shown to both stimulate immune response to tumors in mice and to regulate immune function, delaying or preventing the onset of nonobese diabetes.

This is particularly true of the Shirota strain of L. casei (LcS). The LcS strain is mainly found in yogurt and similar products in Europe and Japan, and rarely elsewhere.

Antioxidants:

- It has been theorized that free radicals contribute to the onset of type-1 diabetes in infants and young children, and therefore that the risk could be reduced by high intake of antioxidant substances during pregnancy. However, a study conducted in a hospital in Finland from 1997-2002 concluded that there was no statistically significant correlation between antioxidant intake and diabetes risk. This study involved monitoring of food intake through questionnaires, and estimated antioxidant intake on this basis, rather than by exact measurements or use of supplements.

Alloimmunity

Alloimmunity (sometimes called isoimmunity) is an immune response to nonself antigens from members of the same species, which are called alloantigens or isoantigens. Two major types of alloantigens are blood group antigens and histocompatibility antigens. In alloimmunity, the body creates antibodies against the alloantigens, attacking transfused blood, allotransplanted tissue, and even the fetus in some cases. Alloimmune (isoimmune) response results in graft rejection, which is manifested as deterioration or complete loss of graft function. In contrast, autoimmunity is an immune response to the self's own antigens. (The *allo-* prefix means "other", whereas the *auto-* prefix means "self".) Alloimmunization (isoimmunization) is the process of becoming alloimmune, that is, developing the relevant antibodies for the first time.

Alloimmunity is caused by the difference between products of highly polymorphic genes, primarily genes of the major histocompatibility complex, of the donor and graft recipient. These products are recognized by T-lymphocytes and other mononuclear leukocytes which infiltrate the graft and damage it.

Types of Rejection

Transfusion Reaction

A failure of cross-matching can allow donor blood of an incompatible blood group to be transfused, resulting in a transfusion reaction.

Hemolytic Disease of the Fetus and Newborn

Hemolytic disease of the fetus and newborn is similar to a transfusion reaction in that the mother's antibodies cannot tolerate the fetus's antigens, which happens when the immune tolerance of pregnancy is impaired. In many instances the maternal immune system attacks the fetal blood cells, resulting in fetal anemia. HDN ranges from mild to severe. Severe cases require intrauterine transfusions or early delivery to survive, while mild cases may only require phototherapy at birth.

Acute Rejection

Acute rejection is caused by antigen-specific Th1 and cytotoxic T-lymphocytes. They recognize transplanted tissue because of expression of alloantigens. A transplant is rejected during first several days or weeks after transplantation.

Hyperacute and Accelerated Rejection

Hyperacute and accelerated rejection is antibody-mediated immune response to the allograft. Recipient's blood already contains circulating antibodies before the transplantation – either IgM or antibodies incurred by previous immunization (e.g. by repeated blood transfusion). In case of hyperacute rejection, antibodies activate complement; moreover, the reaction can be enhanced by neutrophils. This type of rejection is very fast, the graft is rejected in a few minutes or hours after the transplantation. Accelerated rejection leads to phagocyte and NK cell activation (not of the complement) through their Fc receptors that bind Fc parts of antibodies. Graft rejection occurs within 3 to 5 days. This type of rejection is a typical response to xenotransplants.

Chronic Rejection

Chronic rejection is not yet fully understood, but it is known that it is associated with alloantibody and cytokine production. Endothelium of the blood vessels is being damaged, therefore the graft is not sufficiently supplied with blood and is replaced with fibrous tissue (fibrosis). It takes two months at least to reject the graft in this way.

Mechanisms of Rejection

CD4+ and CD8+ T-lymphocytes along with other mononuclear leukocytes (their exact function regarding the topic is not known) participate in the rejection. B-lymphocytes, NK cells and cytokines also play a role in it.

- Cellular rejection – CD4+ and CD8+ T-lymphocytes, NK cells.

- Humoral rejection – B-lymphocytes.

- Cytokines.

B-lymphocytes

Humoral (antibody-mediated) type of rejection is caused by recipient's B-lymphocytes which produce alloantibodies against donor MHC class I and II molecules. These alloantibodies can activate the complement – this leads to target cell lysis. Alternatively, donor cells are coated with alloantibodies that initiate phagocytosis through Fc receptors of mononuclear leukocytes. Mechanism of humoral rejection is relevant for hyperacute, accelerated and chronic rejection. Alloimmunity can be also regulated by neonatal B cells.

Cytokines

Cytokine microenvironment where CD4+ T-lymphocytes recognize alloantigens significantly influences polarization of the immune response.

- CD4+ T-lymphocytes differentiate into Th1 helper cells in the presence of IL-12 (which is usually secreted by mature dendritic cells). Th1 cells produce proinflammatory cytokine IFN-γ and destroy the allograft tissue.

- If there is IL-4, CD4+ T-lymphocytes become Th2 cells secreting IL-4 and IL-5. Then allograft tolerance is mostly observed.

- TGF-β induces expression of Foxp3 gene in the absence of proinflammatory cytokines and thus differentiation of CD4+ T-lymphocytes into regulatory T cells (Treg). Regulatory T cells produce anti-inflammatory cytokines IL-10 and TGF-β which ensures the allograft tolerance.

- However, in the presence of IL-6 or IL-21 along with TGF-β, CD4+ T-lymphocytes acquire tissue-destructive Th17 phenotype and secrete IL-17.

NK Cells

NK cells can also directly target the transplanted tissue. It depends on the balance of activating and inhibitory NK cell receptors and on their ligands expressed by the graft. Receptors of KIR (Killer-cell immunoglobulin-like receptor) family bind concrete MHC class I molecules. If the graft has these ligands on its surface, NK cell cannot be activated (KIR receptors provide inhibitory signal). So if these ligands are missing, there is no inhibitory signal and NK cell becomes activated. It recognizes target cells by "missing-self strategy" and induces their apoptosis by enzymes perforin and granzymes released from its cytotoxic granules. Alloreactive NK cells also secrete proinflammatory cytokines IFN-γ and TNF-α to increase expression of MHC molecules and costimulatory receptors on the surface of APCs (antigen-presenting cells). This promotes APC maturation which leads to amplification of T-cell alloreactivity by means of direct and also indirect pathway of alloantigen recognition. NK cells are able to kill Foxp3+ regulatory T-lymphocytes as well and shift the immune response from graft tolerance toward its rejection. Besides the ability of NK cells to influence APC maturation and T cell development, they can probably reduce or even prevent alloimmune response to transplanted tissue – either by killing the Donor APCs or by anti-inflammatory cytokine IL-10 and TGF-β secretion. However it is important to note that NK cell sub-populations differ in alloreactivity rate and in their immuno-modulatory potential. Concerning immunosuppressive drugs, the effects on NK cells are milder in comparison to T cells.

T-lymphocytes

Alloantigen Recognition

Alloantigen on APC surface can be recognized by recipient's T-lymphocytes through two different pathways:

- Direct allorecognition – Occurs when donor's APCs are presenting graft antigens. Recipient's T-lymphocytes can identify either MHC molecules alone or complex MHC molecule-foreign peptide as alloantigens. Specific T-cell receptors (TCR) of CD8+ T-lymphocytes recognize these peptides when form the complex with MHC class I molecules and TCR of CD4+ T-lymphocytes recognize a complex with MHC class II molecules.

- Indirect allorecognition – Recipient's APCs infiltrate transplanted tissue, then they process and present, as any other foreign peptides, donor's MHC glycoproteins by MHC class II molecules. Mechanism of indirect allorecognition and therefore the involvement of CD4+ T-lymphocytes is the main cause of graft rejection. That is why the compatibility between donor and recipient MHC class II molecules is the most important factor concerning transplantation.

Activation of T-lymphocytes

T-lymphocytes are fully activated under two conditions:

- T-lymphocytes must recognize complex MHC-alloantigen presented by APC through direct or indirect allorecognition pathway.

- T-lymphocytes must receive costimulatory signal. There are costimulatory molecules on T-cell surface and APCs express their ligands (e.g. molecule CD28, which is on the surface of all naïve CD4+ and CD8+ T-lymphocytes, can bind ligands CD80 and CD86). Receptor-ligand engagement triggers T-cell signaling resulting in IL-2 production, clonal expansion and therefore development of effector and memory T-lymphocytes. In contrast, there are also such receptors on T-lymphocytes that cause inhibition of T-cell activation (for instance CD152/CTLA-4 receptor which binds CD80 and CD86 as well). If T-lymphocyte does not receive costimulatory signal, its activation fails and it becomes anergic.

Alloimmune response can be enhanced by proinflammatory cytokines and by CD4+ T-lymphocytes that are responsible for APC maturation and IL-2 production. IL-2 is crucial for memory CD8+ T cell development. These cells may represent a serious problem after the transplantation. As the effect of being exposed to various infections in the past, antigen-specific T-lymphocytes have developed in patient's body. Part of them is kept in organism as memory cells and these cells could be a reason for "cross-reactivity" – immune response against unrelated but similar graft alloantigens. This immune response is called secondary and is faster, more efficient and more robust.

Graft Tolerance

Transplanted tissue is accepted by immunocompetent recipient if it is functional in the absence of immunosuppressive drugs and without histologic signs of rejection. Host can accept another graft from the same donor but reject graft from different donor. Graft acceptance depends on the balance of proinflammatory Th1, Th17 lymphocytes and anti-inflammatory regulatory T cells. This is influenced by cytokine microenvironment, as mentioned before, where CD4+ T-lymphocytes are activated and also by inflammation level (because pathogens invading organism activate the immune system to various degrees and causing proinflammatory cytokine secretion, therefore they support the rejection). Immunosuppressive drugs are used to suppress the immune response, but the effect is not specific. Therefore, organism can be affected by the infection much more easily. The goal of the future therapies is to suppress the alloimmune response specifically to prevent these risks. The tolerance could be achieved by elimination of most or all alloreactive T cells and by influencing alloreactive effector-regulatory T-lymphocytes ratio in favor of regulatory cells which could inhibit alloreactive effector cells. Another method would be based on costimulatory signal blockade during alloreactive T-lymphocytes activation.

Intrinsic Immunity

Intrinsic immunity refers to a set of recently discovered cellular-based anti-viral defense mechanisms, notably genetically encoded proteins which specifically target eukaryotic retroviruses. Unlike adaptive and innate immunity effectors, intrinsic immune proteins are usually expressed at a constant level, allowing a viral infection to be halted quickly.

Eukaryotic organisms have been exposed to viral infections for millions of years. The development of the innate and adaptive immune system reflects the evolutionary importance of fighting infection. Some viruses, however, have proven to be so deadly or refractory to conventional immune mechanisms that specific, genetically encoded cellular defense mechanisms have evolved to combat them. Intrinsic immunity comprises cellular proteins which are always active and have evolved to block infection by specific viruses or viral taxa.

The recognition of intrinsic immunity as a potent anti-viral defense mechanism is a recent discovery and is not yet discussed in most immunology courses or texts. Though the extent of protection intrinsic immunity affords is still unknown, it is possible that intrinsic immunity may eventually be considered a third branch of the traditionally bipartite immune system.

Relationship to the Immune System

Intrinsic Immunity combines aspects of the two traditional branches of the immune system - adaptive and innate immunity – but is mechanistically distinct. Innate cellular immunity recognizes viral infection using toll-like receptors (TLRs), or pattern recognition receptors, which sense Pathogen-associated molecular patterns (PAMPs), triggering the expression of nonspecific antiviral proteins. Intrinsic immune proteins, however, are specific both in virus recognition and their mechanism of viral attenuation. Like innate immunity, however, the intrinsic immune system does not respond differently upon repeat infection by the same pathogen. Also, like adaptive immunity, intrinsic immunity is specifically tailored to a single type or class of pathogens, notably retroviruses.

Unlike adaptive and innate immunity, which must sense the infection to be turned on (and can take weeks to become effective in the case of adaptive immunity) intrinsic immune proteins are constitutively expressed and ready to shut down infection immediately following viral entry. This is particularly important in retroviral infections since viral integration into the host genome occurs quickly after entry and reverse transcription and is largely irreversible.

Because the production of intrinsic immune mediating proteins cannot be increased during infection, these defenses can become saturated and ineffective if a cell is infected with a high level of virus.

Activities of Canonical Intrinsic Immune Proteins

- TRIM5α (Tripartite interaction motif five, splice variant α) is one of the most studied intrinsic immune proteins due to its connection with human immunodeficiency virus (HIV) and simian immunodeficiency virus (SIV). This constitutively expressed protein recognizes the capsid proteins of entering retroviruses and prevents viral uncoating and reverse transcription through an unknown mechanism. The rhesus monkey TRIM5α variant is able to recognize and prevent HIV infection, whereas the human TRIM5α protein can prevent SIV infection. This variation helps explain why HIV and SIV infect humans and monkeys respectively, and probably reflects a previous epidemic of what we now call HIV among ancestors of current rhesus monkey populations.

- APOBEC3G (Apolipoprotein editing complex 3G) is another intrinsic immune protein which interferes with HIV infection. APOBEC3G is a cytidine deaminase against single stranded DNA which introduces transversion mutations into the HIV genome during reverse transcription by randomly changing cytidine basepairs into uracil. Though this will not necessarily stop viral integration, the resulting progeny viral genomes are too riddled with mutations to be viable. APOBEC3G expression is disrupted by the HIV vif protein which induces its degradation through the ubiquitin/proteasome system. Vif actually exploits our intrinsic immunity, titrating the degree of APOBEC3G polyubiquitination in order to augment the genetic variability already present in HIV-1 (owing to its mutation-happy reverse transcriptase). Vif therefore acts via APOBEC3G to increase the likelihood of the generation of escape mutants in HIV-1 pathogenesis. If an HIVΔvif deletion mutant is created it will be able to infect a cell, but will produce non-viable progeny virus due to the action of APOBEC3G.

Other intrinsic immune proteins have been discovered which block Murine leukemia virus (MLV), Herpes simplex virus (HSV), and Human Cytomegalovirus (HCMV). In many cases, such as that of APOBEC3G above, viruses have evolved mechanisms for disrupting the actions of these proteins. Another example is the cellular protein Daxx, which silences viral promoters, but is degraded by an active HCMV protein early in infection.

Antibody

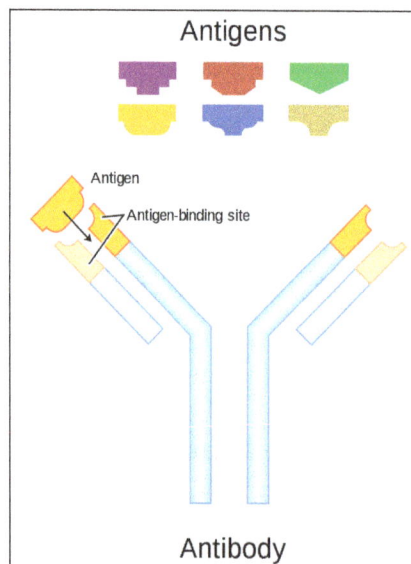

Each antibody binds to a specific antigen; an interaction similar to a lock and key.

An antibody (Ab), also known as an immunoglobulin (Ig), is a large, Y-shaped protein produced mainly by plasma cells that is used by the immune system to neutralize pathogens such as pathogenic bacteria and viruses. The antibody recognizes a unique molecule of the pathogen, called an antigen, via the fragment antigen-binding (Fab) variable region. Each tip of the "Y" of an antibody contains a paratope (analogous to a lock) that is specific for one particular epitope (similarly, analogous to a key) on an antigen, allowing these two structures to bind together with precision. Using this binding mechanism, an antibody can *tag* a microbe or an infected cell for attack by other parts of the immune system, or can neutralize its target directly (for example, by inhibiting a part of a microbe that is essential for its invasion and survival). Depending on the antigen, the binding may impede the biological process causing the disease or may activate macrophages to destroy the foreign substance. The ability of an antibody to communicate with the other components of the immune system is mediated via its Fc region (located at the base of the "Y"), which contains a conserved glycosylation site involved in these interactions. The production of antibodies is the main function of the humoral immune system.

Antibodies are secreted by B cells of the adaptive immune system, mostly by differentiated B cells called plasma cells. Antibodies can occur in two physical forms, a soluble form that is secreted from the cell to be free in the blood plasma, and a membrane-bound form that is attached to the surface of a B cell and is referred to as the B-cell receptor (BCR). The BCR is found only on the surface of B cells and facilitates the activation of these cells and their subsequent differentiation into either antibody factories called plasma cells or memory B cells that will survive in the body and remember that same antigen so the B cells can respond faster upon future exposure. In most cases, interaction of the B cell with a T helper cell is necessary to produce full activation of the B cell and, therefore, antibody generation following antigen binding. Soluble antibodies are released into the blood and tissue fluids, as well as many secretions to continue to survey for invading microorganisms.

Antibodies are glycoproteins belonging to the immunoglobulin superfamily. They constitute most of the gamma globulin fraction of the blood proteins. They are typically made of basic structural units—each with two large heavy chains and two small light chains. There are several different types of antibody heavy chains that define the five different types of crystallisable fragments (Fc) that may be attached to the antigen-binding fragments. The five different types of Fc regions allow antibodies to be grouped into five *isotypes*. Each Fc region of a particular antibody isotype is able to bind to its specific Fc Receptor (except for IgD, which is essentially the BCR), thus allowing the antigen-antibody complex to mediate different roles depending on which FcR it binds. The ability of an antibody to bind to its corresponding FcR is further modulated by the structure of the glycan(s) present at conserved sites within its Fc region. The ability of antibodies to bind to FcRs helps to direct the appropriate immune response for each different type of foreign object they encounter. For example, IgE is responsible for an allergic response consisting of mast cell degranulation and histamine release. IgE's Fab paratope binds to allergic antigen, for example house dust mite particles, while its Fc region binds to Fc receptor ε. The allergen-IgE-FcRε interaction mediates allergic signal transduction to induce conditions such as asthma.

Though the general structure of all antibodies is very similar, a small region at the tip of the protein is extremely variable, allowing millions of antibodies with slightly different tip structures, or antigen-binding sites, to exist. This region is known as the *hypervariable region*. Each of these variants can bind to a different antigen. This enormous diversity of antibody paratopes on the antigen-binding fragments allows the immune system to recognize an equally wide variety of antigens. The large and diverse population of antibody paratope is generated by random recombination events of a set of gene segments that encode different antigen-binding sites (or *paratopes*), followed by random mutations in this area of the antibody gene, which create further diversity. This recombinational process that produces clonal antibody paratope diversity is called V(D)J or VJ recombination. Basically, the antibody paratope is polygenic, made up of three genes, V, D, and J. Each paratope locus is also polymorphic, such that during antibody production, one allele of V, one of D, and one of J is chosen. These gene segments are then joined together using random genetic recombination to produce the paratope. The regions where the genes are randomly recombined together is the hyper variable region used to recognise different antigens on a clonal basis.

Antibody genes also re-organize in a process called class switching that changes the one type of heavy chain Fc fragment to another, creating a different isotype of the antibody that retains the antigen-specific variable region. This allows a single antibody to be used by different types of Fc receptors, expressed on different parts of the immune system.

The first use of the term "antibody" occurred in a text by Paul Ehrlich. The term Antikörper (the German word for antibody) "Experimental Studies on Immunity", published in October 1891, which states that, "if two substances give rise to two different Antikörper, then they themselves must be different". However, the term was not accepted immediately and several other terms for antibody were proposed; these included Immunkörper, Amboceptor, Zwischenkörper, substance sensibilisatrice, copula, Desmon, philocytase, fixateur, and Immunisin. The word antibody has formal analogy to the word antitoxin and a similar concept to Immunkörper (immune body in English). As such, the original construction of the word contains a logical flaw; the antitoxin is something directed against a toxin, while the antibody is a body directed against something.

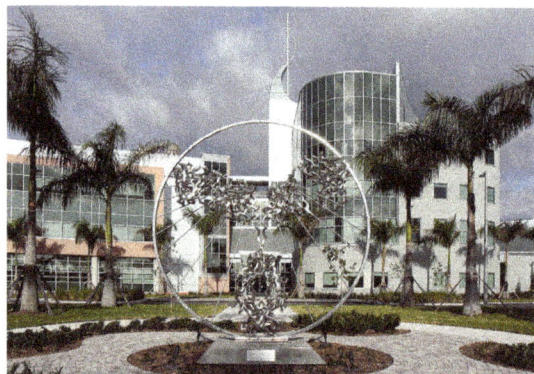

Angel of the West by Julian Voss-Andreae is a sculpture based on the antibody structure.

Created for the Florida campus of the Scripps Research Institute, the antibody is placed into a ring referencing Leonardo da Vinci's *Vitruvian Man* thus highlighting the similarity of the antibody and the human body.

The study of antibodies began in 1890 when Kitasato Shibasaburō described antibody activity against diphtheria and tetanus toxins. Kitasato put forward the theory of humoral immunity, proposing that a mediator in serum could react with a foreign antigen. His idea prompted Paul Ehrlich to propose the side-chain theory for antibody and antigen interaction in 1897, when he hypothesized that receptors (described as "side-chains") on the surface of cells could bind specifically to toxins – in a "lock-and-key" interaction – and that this binding reaction is the trigger for the production of antibodies. Other researchers believed that antibodies existed freely in the blood and, in 1904, Almroth Wright suggested that soluble antibodies coated bacteria to label them for phagocytosis and killing; a process that he named opsoninization.

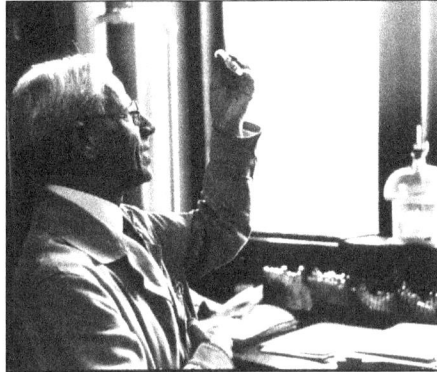

Michael Heidelberger

In the 1920s, Michael Heidelberger and Oswald Avery observed that antigens could be precipitated by antibodies and went on to show that antibodies are made of protein. The biochemical properties of antigen-antibody-binding interactions were examined in more detail in the late 1930s by John Marrack. The next major advance was in the 1940s, when Linus Pauling confirmed the lock-and-key theory proposed by Ehrlich by showing that the interactions between antibodies and antigens depend more on their shape than their chemical composition. In 1948, Astrid Fagreaus discovered that B cells, in the form of plasma cells, were responsible for generating antibodies.

Further work concentrated on characterizing the structures of the antibody proteins. A major advance in these structural studies was the discovery in the early 1960s by Gerald Edelman and Joseph Gally of the antibody light chain, and their realization that this protein is the same as the Bence-Jones protein described in 1845 by Henry Bence Jones. Edelman went on to discover that antibodies are composed of disulfide bond-linked heavy and light chains. Around the same time, antibody-binding (Fab) and antibody tail (Fc) regions of IgG were characterized by Rodney Porter. Together, these scientists deduced the structure and complete amino acid sequence of IgG, a feat for which they were jointly awarded the 1972 Nobel Prize in Physiology or Medicine. The Fv fragment was prepared and characterized by David Givol. While most of these early studies focused on IgM and IgG, other immunoglobulin isotypes were identified in the 1960s: Thomas Tomasi discovered secretory antibody (IgA); David S. Rowe and John L. Fahey discovered IgD; and Kimishige Ishizaka and Teruko Ishizaka discovered IgE and showed it was a class of antibodies involved in allergic reactions. In a landmark series of experiments beginning in 1976, Susumu Tonegawa showed that genetic material can rearrange itself to form the vast array of available antibodies.

Forms

The membrane-bound form of an antibody may be called a surface immunoglobulin (sIg) or a membrane immunoglobulin (mIg). It is part of the B cell receptor (BCR), which allows a B cell to detect when a specific antigen is present in the body and triggers B cell activation. The BCR is composed of surface-bound IgD or IgM antibodies and associated Ig-α and Ig-β heterodimers, which are capable of signal transduction. A typical human B cell will have 50,000 to 100,000 antibodies bound to its surface. Upon antigen binding, they cluster in large patches, which can exceed 1 micrometer in diameter, on lipid rafts that isolate the BCRs from most other cell signaling receptors.

These patches may improve the efficiency of the cellular immune response. In humans, the cell surface is bare around the B cell receptors for several hundred nanometers, which further isolates the BCRs from competing influences.

Antibody–antigen Interactions

The antibody's paratope interacts with the antigen's epitope. An antigen usually contains different epitopes along its surface arranged discontinuously, and dominant epitopes on a given antigen are called determinants.

Antibody and antigen interact by spatial complementarity (lock and key). The molecular forces involved in the Fab-epitope interaction are weak and non-specific – for example electrostatic forces, hydrogen bonds, hydrophobic interactions, and van der Waals forces. This means binding between antibody and antigen is reversible, and the antibody's affinity towards an antigen is relative rather than absolute. Relatively weak binding also means it is possible for an antibody to cross-react with different antigens of different relative affinities.

Often, once an antibody and antigen bind, they become an immune complex, which functions as a unitary object and can act as an antigen in its own right, being countered by other antibodies. Similarly, haptens are small molecules that provoke no immune response by themselves, but once they bind to proteins, the resulting complex or hapten-carrier adduct is antigenic.

Isotypes

Antibodies can come in different varieties known as isotypes or classes. In placental mammals there are five antibody isotypes known as IgA, IgD, IgE, IgG, and IgM. They are each named with an "Ig" prefix that stands for immunoglobulin (a name sometimes used interchangeably with antibody) and differ in their biological properties, functional locations and ability to deal with different antigens, as depicted in the table. The different suffixes of the antibody isotypes denote the different types of heavy chains the antibody contains, with each heavy chain class named alphabetically: α (alpha), γ (gamma), δ (delta), ε (epsilon), and μ (mu). This gives rise to IgA, IgG, IgD, IgE, and IgM, respectively.

Antibody isotypes of mammals			
Class	Subclass	Description	Antibody complexes
IgA	2	Found in mucosal areas, such as the gut, respiratory tract and urogenital tract, and prevents colonization by pathogens. Also found in saliva, tears, and breast milk.	
IgD	1	Functions mainly as an antigen receptor on B cells that have not been exposed to antigens. It has been shown to activate basophils and mast cells to produce antimicrobial factors.	Monomer IgD, IgE, IgG
IgE	1	Binds to allergens and triggers histamine release from mast cells and basophils, and is involved in allergy. Also protects against parasitic worms.	Dimer IgA
IgG	4	In its four forms, provides the majority of antibody-based immunity against invading pathogens. The only antibody capable of crossing the placenta to give passive immunity to the fetus.	Pentamer IgM
IgM	1	Expressed on the surface of B cells (monomer) and in a secreted form (pentamer) with very high avidity. Eliminates pathogens in the early stages of B cell-mediated (humoral) immunity before there is sufficient IgG.	

The antibody isotype of a B cell changes during cell development and activation. Immature B cells, which have never been exposed to an antigen, express only the IgM isotype in a cell surface bound form. The B lymphocyte, in this ready-to-respond form, is known as a "naive B lymphocyte." The naive B lymphocyte expresses both surface IgM and IgD. The co-expression of both of these immunoglobulin isotypes renders the B cell ready to respond to antigen. B cell activation follows engagement of the cell-bound antibody molecule with an antigen, causing the cell to divide and differentiate into an antibody-producing cell called a plasma cell. In this activated form, the B cell starts to produce antibody in a secreted form rather than a membrane-bound form. Some daughter cells of the activated B cells undergo isotype switching, a mechanism that causes the production of antibodies to change from IgM or IgD to the other antibody isotypes, IgE, IgA, or IgG, that have defined roles in the immune system.

Antibody isotypes not found in mammals		
Class	Types	Description
IgY		Found in birds and reptiles; related to mammalian IgG.
IgW		Found in sharks and skates; related to mammalian IgD.

Structure

Antibodies are heavy (~150 kDa) globular plasma proteins. The size of an antibody molecule is about 10 nm. They have sugar chains (glycans) added to conserved amino acid residues. In other words, antibodies are glycoproteins. The attached glycans are critically important to the structure and function of the antibody. Among other things the expressed glycans can modulate an antibody's affinity for its corresponding FcR(s).

The basic functional unit of each antibody is an immunoglobulin (Ig) monomer (containing only one Ig unit); secreted antibodies can also be dimeric with two Ig units as with IgA, tetrameric with four Ig units like teleost fish IgM, or pentameric with five Ig units, like mammalian IgM.

The variable parts of an antibody are its V regions, and the constant part is its C region.

Immunoglobulin Domains

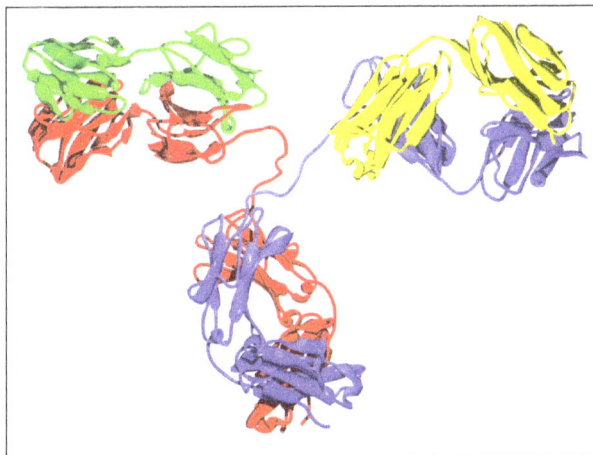

Several immunoglobulin domains make up the two heavy chains (red and blue) and the two light chains (green and yellow) of an antibody. The immunoglobulin domains are composed of between 7 (for constant domains) and 9 (for variable domains) β-strands.

The Ig monomer is a "Y"-shaped molecule that consists of four polypeptide chains; two identical heavy chains and two identical light chains connected by disulfide bonds. Each chain is composed of structural domains called immunoglobulin domains. These domains contain about 70–110 amino acids and are classified into different categories (for example, variable or IgV, and constant or IgC) according to their size and function. They have a characteristic immunoglobulin fold in which two beta sheets create a "sandwich" shape, held together by interactions between conserved cysteines and other charged amino acids.

Heavy Chain

There are five types of mammalian Ig heavy chain denoted by the Greek letters: α, δ, ε, γ, and μ. The type of heavy chain present defines the *class* of antibody; these chains are found in IgA, IgD, IgE, IgG, and IgM antibodies, respectively. Distinct heavy chains differ in size and composition; α and γ contain approximately 450 amino acids, whereas μ and ε have approximately 550 amino acids.

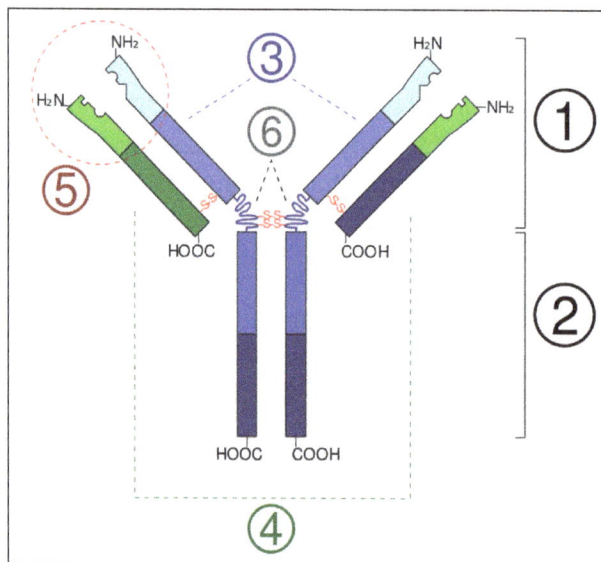

In figure:

1. Fab region.

2. Fc region.

3. Heavy chain (blue) with one variable (V_H) domain followed by a constant domain (C_H1), a hinge region, and two more constant (C_H2 and C_H3) domains.

4. Light chain (green) with one variable (V_L) and one constant (C_L) domain.

5. Antigen binding site (paratope).

6. Hinge regions.

Each heavy chain has two regions, the constant region and the variable region. The constant region is identical in all antibodies of the same isotype, but differs in antibodies of different isotypes. Heavy chains γ, α and δ have a constant region composed of three tandem (in a line) Ig domains, and a hinge region for added flexibility; heavy chains μ and ε have a constant region composed of four immunoglobulin domains. The variable region of the heavy chain differs in antibodies produced by different B cells, but is the same for all antibodies produced by a single B cell or B cell clone. The variable region of each heavy chain is approximately 110 amino acids long and is composed of a single Ig domain.

Light Chain

In mammals there are two types of immunoglobulin light chain, which are called lambda (λ) and kappa (κ). A light chain has two successive domains: one constant domain and one variable domain. The approximate length of a light chain is 211 to 217 amino acids. Each antibody contains two light chains that are always identical; only one type of light chain, κ or λ, is present per antibody in mammals. Other types of light chains, such as the iota (ι) chain, are found in other vertebrates like sharks (Chondrichthyes) and bony fishes (Teleostei).

CDRs, Fv, Fab and Fc Regions

Different parts of an antibody have different functions. Specifically, the "arms" (which are generally identical) contain sites that can bind to specific molecules, enabling recognition of specific antigens. This region of the antibody is called the *Fab (fragment, antigen-binding) region*. It is composed of one constant and one variable domain from each heavy and light chain of the antibody. The paratope at the amino terminal end of the antibody monomer is shaped by the variable domains from the heavy and light chains. The variable domain is also referred to as the F_V region and is the most important region for binding to antigens. To be specific, variable loops of β-strands, three each on the light (V_L) and heavy (V_H) chains are responsible for binding to the antigen. These loops are referred to as the complementarity determining regions (CDRs). The structures of these CDRs have been clustered and classified by Chothia et al. and more recently by North et al. and Nikoloudis et al. In the framework of the immune network theory, CDRs are also called idiotypes. According to immune network theory, the adaptive immune system is regulated by interactions between idiotypes.

The base of the Y plays a role in modulating immune cell activity. This region is called the Fc (Fragment, crystallizable) region, and is composed of two heavy chains that contribute two or three constant domains depending on the class of the antibody. Thus, the Fc region ensures that each antibody generates an appropriate immune response for a given antigen, by binding to a specific class of Fc receptors, and other immune molecules, such as complement proteins. By doing this, it mediates different physiological effects, including recognition of opsonized particles (binding to FcγR), lysis of cells (binding to complement), and degranulation of mast cells, basophils, and eosinophils (binding to FcεR).

The Fab region of the antibody determines antigen specificity while the Fc region of the antibody determines the antibody's class effect. Since only the constant domains of the heavy chains make up the Fc region of an antibody, the classes of heavy chain in antibodies determine their class effects. Possible classes of heavy chains in antibodies include alpha, gamma, delta, epsilon, and mu, and they define the antibody's isotypes IgA, G, D, E, and M, respectively. This infers different isotypes of antibodies have different class effects due to their different Fc regions binding and activating different types of receptors. Possible class effects of antibodies include: Opsonisation, agglutination, haemolysis, complement activation, mast cell degranulation, and neutralisation (though this class effect may be mediated by the Fab region rather than the Fc region). It also implies that Fab-mediated effects are directed at microbes or toxins, whilst Fc mediated effects are directed at effector cells or effector molecules.

Function

The main categories of antibody action include the following:

- Neutralisation, in which neutralizing antibodies block parts of the surface of a bacterial cell or virion to render its attack ineffective.

- Agglutination, in which antibodies "glue together" foreign cells into clumps that are attractive targets for phagocytosis.

- Precipitation, in which antibodies "glue together" serum-soluble antigens, forcing them to precipitate out of solution in clumps that are attractive targets for phagocytosis.

- Complement activation (fixation), in which antibodies that are latched onto a foreign cell encourage complement to attack it with a membrane attack complex, which leads to the following:

    o Lysis of the foreign cell.

    o Encouragement of inflammation by chemotactically attracting inflammatory cells.

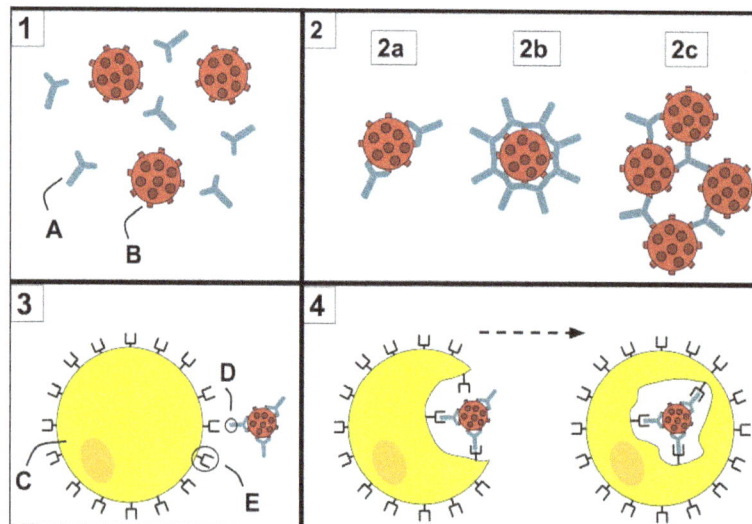

Antibodies (A) and pathogens (B) free roam in the blood. 2) The antibodies bind to pathogens, and can do so in different formations such as: opsonization (2a), neutralisation (2b), and agglutination (2c). 3) A phagocyte (C) approaches the pathogen, and the Fc region (D) of the antibody binds to one of the Fc receptors (E) of the phagocyte. 4) Phagocytosis occurs as the pathogen is ingested.

Activated B cells differentiate into either antibody-producing cells called plasma cells that secrete soluble antibody or memory cells that survive in the body for years afterward in order to allow the immune system to remember an antigen and respond faster upon future exposures.

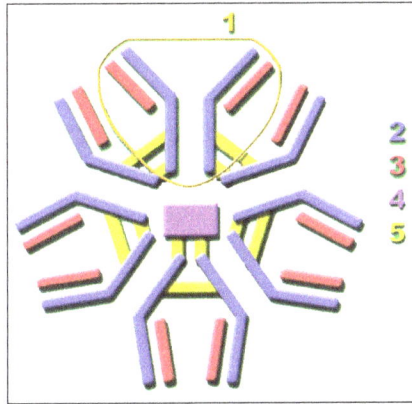

The secreted mammalian IgM has five Ig units. Each Ig unit (labeled 1) has two epitope binding Fab regions, so IgM is capable of binding up to 10 epitopes.

At the prenatal and neonatal stages of life, the presence of antibodies is provided by passive immunization from the mother. Early endogenous antibody production varies for different kinds of antibodies, and usually appear within the first years of life. Since antibodies exist freely in the bloodstream, they are said to be part of the humoral immune system. Circulating antibodies are produced by clonal B cells that specifically respond to only one antigen (an example is a virus capsid protein fragment). Antibodies contribute to immunity in three ways: They prevent pathogens from entering or damaging cells by binding to them; they stimulate removal of pathogens by macrophages and other cells by coating the pathogen; and they trigger destruction of pathogens by stimulating other immune responses such as the complement pathway. Antibodies will also trigger vasoactive amine degranulation to contribute to immunity against certain types of antigens (helminths, allergens).

Activation of Complement

Antibodies that bind to surface antigens (for example, on bacteria) will attract the first component of the complement cascade with their Fc region and initiate activation of the "classical" complement system. This results in the killing of bacteria in two ways. First, the binding of the antibody and complement molecules marks the microbe for ingestion by phagocytes in a process called opsonization; these phagocytes are attracted by certain complement molecules generated in the complement cascade. Second, some complement system components form a membrane attack complex to assist antibodies to kill the bacterium directly (bacteriolysis).

Activation of Effector Cells

To combat pathogens that replicate outside cells, antibodies bind to pathogens to link them together, causing them to agglutinate. Since an antibody has at least two paratopes, it can bind more than one antigen by binding identical epitopes carried on the surfaces of these antigens. By coating the pathogen, antibodies stimulate effector functions against the pathogen in cells that recognize their Fc region.

Those cells that recognize coated pathogens have Fc receptors, which, as the name suggests, interact with the Fc region of IgA, IgG, and IgE antibodies. The engagement of a particular antibody with the Fc receptor on a particular cell triggers an effector function of that cell; phagocytes will phagocytose, mast cells and neutrophils will degranulate, natural killer cells will release cytokines and cytotoxic molecules; that will ultimately result in destruction of the invading microbe. The activation of natural killer cells by antibodies initiates a cytotoxic mechanism known as antibody-dependent cell-mediated cytotoxicity (ADCC) – this process may explain the efficacy of monoclonal antibodies used in biological therapies against cancer. The Fc receptors are isotype-specific, which gives greater flexibility to the immune system, invoking only the appropriate immune mechanisms for distinct pathogens.

Natural Antibodies

Humans and higher primates also produce "natural antibodies" that are present in serum before viral infection. Natural antibodies have been defined as antibodies that are produced without any previous infection, vaccination, other foreign antigen exposure or passive immunization. These antibodies can activate the classical complement pathway leading to lysis of enveloped virus particles long before the adaptive immune response is activated. Many natural antibodies are directed against the disaccharide galactose α(1,3)-galactose (α-Gal), which is found as a terminal sugar on glycosylated cell surface proteins, and generated in response to production of this sugar by bacteria contained in the human gut. Rejection of xenotransplantated organs is thought to be, in part, the result of natural antibodies circulating in the serum of the recipient binding to α-Gal antigens expressed on the donor tissue.

Immunoglobulin Diversity

Virtually all microbes can trigger an antibody response. Successful recognition and eradication of many different types of microbes requires diversity among antibodies; their amino acid composition varies allowing them to interact with many different antigens. It has been estimated that humans generate about 10 billion different antibodies, each capable of binding a distinct epitope of an antigen. Although a huge repertoire of different antibodies is generated in a single individual, the number of genes available to make these proteins is limited by the size of the human genome. Several complex genetic mechanisms have evolved that allow vertebrate B cells to generate a diverse pool of antibodies from a relatively small number of antibody genes.

Domain Variability

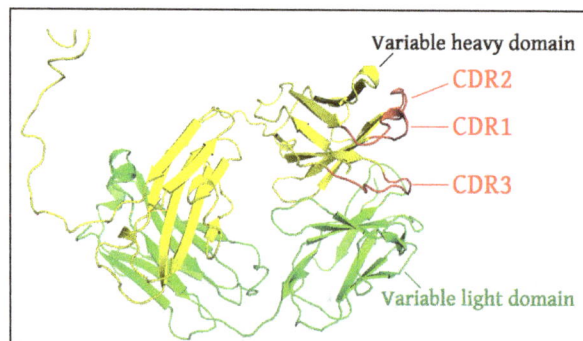

The complementarity determining regions of the heavy chain are shown in red (PDB: 1IGT).

The chromosomal region that encodes an antibody is large and contains several distinct gene loci for each domain of the antibody—the chromosome region containing heavy chain genes (IGH@) is found on chromosome 14, and the loci containing lambda and kappa light chain genes (IGL@ and IGK@) are found on chromosomes 22 and 2 in humans. One of these domains is called the variable domain, which is present in each heavy and light chain of every antibody, but can differ in different antibodies generated from distinct B cells. Differences, between the variable domains, are located on three loops known as hypervariable regions (HV-1, HV-2 and HV-3) or complementarity determining regions (CDR1, CDR2 and CDR3). CDRs are supported within the variable domains by conserved framework regions. The heavy chain locus contains about 65 different variable domain genes that all differ in their CDRs. Combining these genes with an array of genes for other domains of the antibody generates a large cavalry of antibodies with a high degree of variability. This combination is called V(D)J recombination.

V(D)J Recombination

Somatic recombination of immunoglobulins, also known as *V(D)J recombination*, involves the generation of a unique immunoglobulin variable region. The variable region of each immunoglobulin heavy or light chain is encoded in several pieces—known as gene segments (subgenes). These segments are called variable (V), diversity (D) and joining (J) segments. V, D and J segments are found in Ig heavy chains, but only V and J segments are found in Ig light chains. Multiple copies of the V, D and J gene segments exist, and are tandemly arranged in the genomes of mammals. In the bone marrow, each developing B cell will assemble an immunoglobulin variable region by randomly selecting and combining one V, one D and one J gene segment (or one V and one J segment in the light chain). As there are multiple copies of each type of gene segment, and different combinations of gene segments can be used to generate each immunoglobulin variable region, this process generates a huge number of antibodies, each with different paratopes, and thus different antigen specificities. The rearrangement of several subgenes (i.e. V2 family) for lambda light chain immunoglobulin is coupled with the activation of microRNA miR-650, which further influences biology of B-cells.

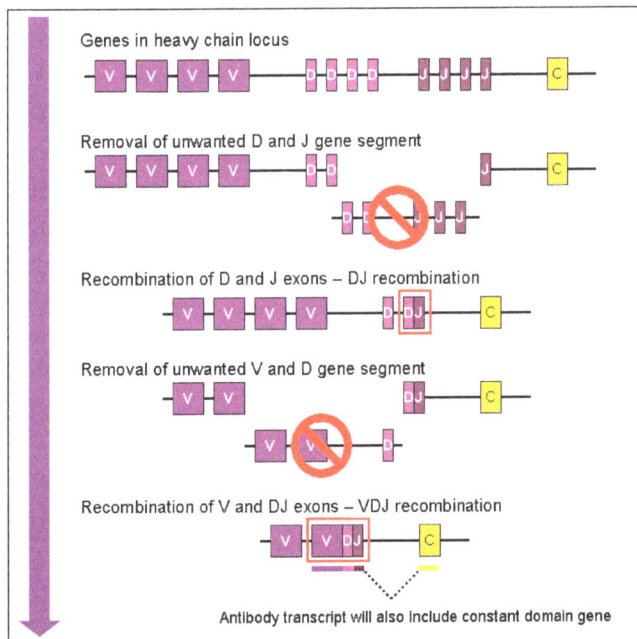

Simplified overview of V(D)J recombination of immunoglobulin heavy chains.

RAG proteins play an important role with V(D)J recombination in cutting DNA at a particular region. Without the presence of these proteins, V(D)J recombination would not occur.

After a B cell produces a functional immunoglobulin gene during V(D)J recombination, it cannot express any other variable region (a process known as allelic exclusion) thus each B cell can produce antibodies containing only one kind of variable chain.

Somatic Hypermutation and Affinity Maturation

Following activation with antigen, B cells begin to proliferate rapidly. In these rapidly dividing cells, the genes encoding the variable domains of the heavy and light chains undergo a high rate of point mutation, by a process called *somatic hypermutation* (SHM). SHM results in approximately one nucleotide change per variable gene, per cell division. As a consequence, any daughter B cells will acquire slight amino acid differences in the variable domains of their antibody chains.

This serves to increase the diversity of the antibody pool and impacts the antibody's antigen-binding affinity. Some point mutations will result in the production of antibodies that have a weaker interaction (low affinity) with their antigen than the original antibody, and some mutations will generate antibodies with a stronger interaction (high affinity). B cells that express high affinity antibodies on their surface will receive a strong survival signal during interactions with other cells, whereas those with low affinity antibodies will not, and will die by apoptosis. Thus, B cells expressing antibodies with a higher affinity for the antigen will outcompete those with weaker affinities for function and survival allowing the average affinity of antibodies to increase over time. The process of generating antibodies with increased binding affinities is called *affinity maturation*. Affinity maturation occurs in mature B cells after V(D)J recombination, and is dependent on help from helper T cells.

Class Switching

Isotype or class switching is a biological process occurring after activation of the B cell, which allows the cell to produce different classes of antibody (IgA, IgE, or IgG). The different classes of antibody, and thus effector functions, are defined by the constant (C) regions of the immunoglobulin heavy chain. Initially, naive B cells express only cell-surface IgM and IgD with identical antigen binding regions. Each isotype is adapted for a distinct function; therefore, after activation, an antibody with an IgG, IgA, or IgE effector function might be required to effectively eliminate an antigen. Class switching allows different daughter cells from the same activated B cell to produce antibodies of different isotypes. Only the constant region of the antibody heavy chain changes during class switching; the variable regions, and therefore antigen specificity, remain unchanged. Thus the progeny of a single B cell can produce antibodies, all specific for the same antigen, but with the ability to produce the effector function appropriate for each antigenic challenge. Class switching is triggered by cytokines; the isotype generated depends on which cytokines are present in the B cell environment.

Class switching occurs in the heavy chain gene locus by a mechanism called class switch recombination (CSR). This mechanism relies on conserved nucleotide motifs, called *switch (S) regions*, found in DNA upstream of each constant region gene (except in the δ-chain). The DNA strand is broken by the activity of a series of enzymes at two selected S-regions. The variable domain exon is rejoined through a process called non-homologous end joining (NHEJ) to the desired constant region (γ, α or ε). This process results in an immunoglobulin gene that encodes an antibody of a different isotype.

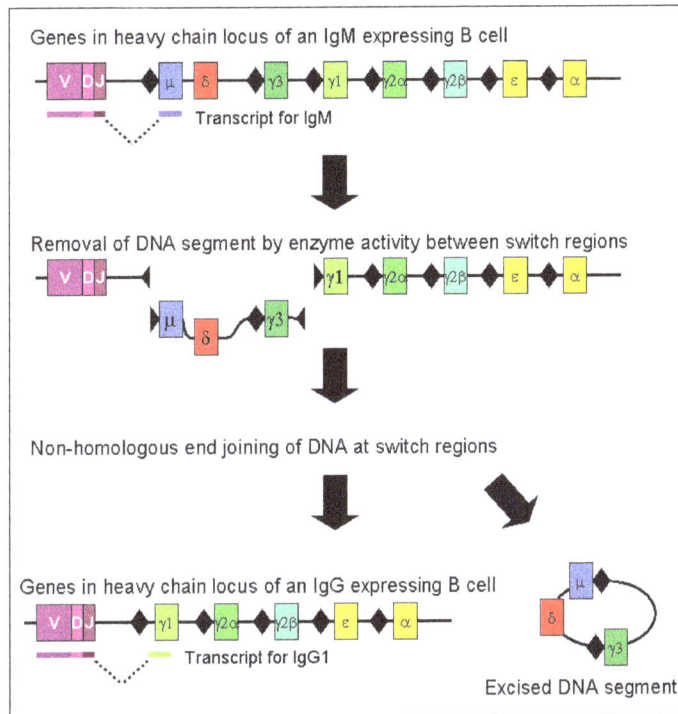

Mechanism of class switch recombination that allows isotype switching in activated B cells.

Specificity Designations

An antibody can be called monospecific if it has specificity for the same antigen or epitope, or bispecific if they have affinity for two different antigens or two different epitopes on the same antigen. A group of antibodies can be called polyvalent (or unspecific) if they have affinity for various antigens or microorganisms. Intravenous immunoglobulin, if not otherwise noted, consists of a variety of different IgG (polyclonal IgG). In contrast, monoclonal antibodies are identical antibodies produced by a single B cell.

Asymmetrical Antibodies

Heterodimeric antibodies, which are also asymmetrical and antibodies, allow for greater flexibility and new formats for attaching a variety of drugs to the antibody arms. One of the general formats for a heterodimeric antibody is the "knobs-into-holes" format. This format is specific to the heavy chain part of the constant region in antibodies. The "knobs" part is engineered by replacing a small amino acid with a larger one. It fits into the "hole", which is engineered by replacing a large amino acid with a smaller one. What connects the "knobs" to the "holes" are the disulfide bonds between each chain. The "knobs-into-holes" shape facilitates antibody dependent cell mediated cytotoxicity. Single chain variable fragments (scFv) are connected to the variable domain of the heavy and light chain via a short linker peptide. The linker is rich in glycine, which gives it more flexibility, and serine/threonine, which gives it specificity. Two different scFv fragments can be connected together, via a hinge region, to the constant domain of the heavy chain or the constant domain of the light chain. This gives the antibody bispecificity, allowing for the binding specificities of two different antigens. The "knobs-into-holes" format enhances heterodimer formation but doesn't suppress homodimer formation.

To further improve the function of heterodimeric antibodies, many scientists are looking towards artificial constructs. Artificial antibodies are largely diverse protein motifs that use the functional strategy of the antibody molecule, but aren't limited by the loop and framework structural constraints of the natural antibody. Being able to control the combinational design of the sequence and three-dimensional space could transcend the natural design and allow for the attachment of different combinations of drugs to the arms.

Heterodimeric antibodies have a greater range in shapes they can take and the drugs that are attached to the arms don't have to be the same on each arm, allowing for different combinations of drugs to be used in cancer treatment. Pharmaceuticals are able to produce highly functional bispecific, and even multispecific, antibodies. The degree to which they can function is impressive given that such a change of shape from the natural form should lead to decreased functionality.

Medical Applications

Disease Diagnosis

Detection of particular antibodies is a very common form of medical diagnostics, and applications such as serology depend on these methods. For example, in biochemical assays for disease diagnosis, a titer of antibodies directed against Epstein-Barr virus or Lyme disease is estimated from the blood. If those antibodies are not present, either the person is not infected or the infection occurred a very long time ago, and the B cells generating these specific antibodies have naturally decayed.

In clinical immunology, levels of individual classes of immunoglobulins are measured by nephelometry (or turbidimetry) to characterize the antibody profile of patient. Elevations in different classes of immunoglobulins are sometimes useful in determining the cause of liver damage in patients for whom the diagnosis is unclear. For example, elevated IgA indicates alcoholic cirrhosis, elevated IgM indicates viral hepatitis and primary biliary cirrhosis, while IgG is elevated in viral hepatitis, autoimmune hepatitis and cirrhosis.

Autoimmune disorders can often be traced to antibodies that bind the body's own epitopes; many can be detected through blood tests. Antibodies directed against red blood cell surface antigens in immune mediated hemolytic anemia are detected with the Coombs test. The Coombs test is also used for antibody screening in blood transfusion preparation and also for antibody screening in antenatal women.

Practically, several immunodiagnostic methods based on detection of complex antigen-antibody are used to diagnose infectious diseases, for example ELISA, immunofluorescence, Western blot, immunodiffusion, immunoelectrophoresis, and magnetic immunoassay. Antibodies raised against human chorionic gonadotropin are used in over the counter pregnancy tests.

New dioxaborolane chemistry enables radioactive fluoride (^{18}F) labeling of antibodies, which allows for positron emission tomography (PET) imaging of cancer.

Disease Therapy

Targeted monoclonal antibody therapy is employed to treat diseases such as rheumatoid arthritis, multiple sclerosis, psoriasis, and many forms of cancer including non-Hodgkin's lymphoma, colorectal cancer, head and neck cancer and breast cancer.

Some immune deficiencies, such as X-linked agammaglobulinemia and hypogammaglobulinemia, result in partial or complete lack of antibodies. These diseases are often treated by inducing a short term form of immunity called passive immunity. Passive immunity is achieved through the transfer of ready-made antibodies in the form of human or animal serum, pooled immunoglobulin or monoclonal antibodies, into the affected individual.

Prenatal Therapy

Rh factor, also known as Rh D antigen, is an antigen found on red blood cells; individuals that are Rh-positive (Rh+) have this antigen on their red blood cells and individuals that are Rh-negative (Rh−) do not. During normal childbirth, delivery trauma or complications during pregnancy, blood from a fetus can enter the mother's system. In the case of an Rh-incompatible mother and child, consequential blood mixing may sensitize an Rh- mother to the Rh antigen on the blood cells of the Rh+ child, putting the remainder of the pregnancy, and any subsequent pregnancies, at risk for hemolytic disease of the newborn.

Rho(D) immune globulin antibodies are specific for human RhD antigen. Anti-RhD antibodies are administered as part of a prenatal treatment regimen to prevent sensitization that may occur when a Rh-negative mother has a Rh-positive fetus. Treatment of a mother with Anti-RhD antibodies prior to and immediately after trauma and delivery destroys Rh antigen in the mother's system from the fetus. It is important to note that this occurs before the antigen can stimulate maternal B cells to "remember" Rh antigen by generating memory B cells. Therefore, her humoral immune system will not make anti-Rh antibodies, and will not attack the Rh antigens of the current or subsequent babies. Rho(D) Immune Globulin treatment prevents sensitization that can lead to Rh disease, but does not prevent or treat the underlying disease itself.

Research Applications

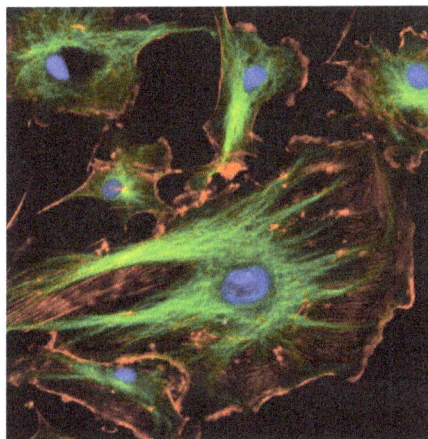

Immunofluorescence image of the eukaryotic cytoskeleton. Microtubules as shown in green, are marked by an antibody conjugated to a green fluorescing molecule, FITC.

Specific antibodies are produced by injecting an antigen into a mammal, such as a mouse, rat, rabbit, goat, sheep, or horse for large quantities of antibody. Blood isolated from these animals contains polyclonal antibodies—multiple antibodies that bind to the same antigen—in the serum, which can now be called antiserum. Antigens are also injected into chickens for generation of polyclonal antibodies in egg yolk. To obtain antibody that is specific for a single epitope of an antigen, antibody-secreting lymphocytes are isolated from the animal and immortalized by fusing them with a cancer cell line. The fused cells are called hybridomas, and will continually grow and secrete antibody in culture. Single hybridoma cells are isolated by dilution cloning to generate cell clones that all produce the same antibody; these antibodies are called monoclonal antibodies. Polyclonal and monoclonal antibodies are often purified using Protein A/G or antigen-affinity chromatography.

In research, purified antibodies are used in many applications. Antibodies for research applications can be found directly from antibody suppliers, or through use of a specialist search engine. Research antibodies are most commonly used to identify and locate intracellular and extracellular proteins. Antibodies are used in flow cytometry to differentiate cell types by the proteins they express; different types of cell express different combinations of cluster of differentiation molecules on their surface, and produce different intracellular and secretable proteins. They are also used in immunoprecipitation to separate proteins and anything bound to them (co-immunoprecipitation) from other molecules in a cell lysate, in Western blot analyses to identify proteins separated by electrophoresis, and in immunohistochemistry or immunofluorescence to examine protein expression in tissue sections or to locate proteins within cells with the assistance of a microscope. Proteins can also be detected and quantified with antibodies, using ELISA and ELISpot techniques.

Antibodies used in research are some of the most powerful, yet most problematic reagents with a tremendous number of factors that must be controlled in any experiment including cross reactivity, or the antibody recognizing multiple epitopes and affinity, which can vary widely depending on experimental conditions such as pH, solvent, state of tissue etc. Multiple attempts have been made to improve both the way that researchers validate antibodies and ways in which they report on antibodies. Researchers using antibodies in their work need to record them correctly in order to allow their research to be reproducible (and therefore tested, and qualified by other researchers). Less than half of research antibodies referenced in academic papers can be easily identified.

Structure Prediction and Computational Antibody Design

The importance of antibodies in health care and the biotechnology industry demands knowledge of their structures at high resolution. This information is used for protein engineering, modifying the antigen binding affinity, and identifying an epitope, of a given antibody. X-ray crystallography is one commonly used method for determining antibody structures. However, crystallizing an antibody is often laborious and time-consuming. Computational approaches provide a cheaper and faster alternative to crystallography, but their results are more equivocal, since they do not produce empirical structures. Online web servers such as Web Antibody Modeling (WAM) and Prediction of Immunoglobulin Structure (PIGS) enables computational modeling of antibody variable regions. Rosetta Antibody is a novel antibody FV region structure prediction server, which incorporates sophisticated techniques to minimize CDR loops and optimize the relative orientation of the light and heavy chains, as well as homology models that predict successful docking of antibodies with their unique antigen.

The ability to describe the antibody through binding affinity to the antigen is supplemented by information on antibody structure and amino acid sequences for the purpose of patent claims. Several methods have been presented for computational design of antibodies based on the structural bioinformatics studies of antibody CDRs.

There are a variety of methods used to sequence an antibody including Edman degradation, cDNA, etc.; albeit one of the most common modern uses for peptide/protein identification is liquid chromatography coupled with tandem mass spectrometry (LC-MS/MS). High volume antibody sequencing methods require computational approaches for the data analysis, including de novo sequencing directly from tandem mass spectra and database search methods that use existing protein sequence databases. Many versions of shotgun protein sequencing are able to increase the coverage by utilizing CID/HCD/ETD fragmentation methods and other techniques, and they have achieved substantial progress in attempt to fully sequence proteins, especially antibodies. Other methods have assumed the existence of similar proteins, a known genome sequence, or combined top-down and bottom up approaches. Current technologies have the ability to assemble protein sequences with high accuracy by integrating de novo sequencing peptides, intensity, and positional confidence scores from database and homology searches.

Antibody Mimetic

Antibody mimetics are organic compounds, like antibodies, that can specifically bind antigens. They are usually artificial peptides or proteins with a molar mass of about 3 to 20 kDa. Nucleic acids and small molecules are sometimes considered antibody mimetics, but not artificial antibodies, antibody fragments and fusion proteins are composed from these. Common advantages over antibodies are better solubility, tissue penetration, stability towards heat and enzymes, and comparatively low production costs. Antibody mimetics such as the Affimer and the DARPin have being developed and commercialised as research, diagnostic and therapeutic agents.

Antigen

In immunology, antigens (Ag) are structures (aka substances) specifically bound by antibodies (Ab) or a cell surface version of Ab ~ B cell antigen receptor (BCR). The term antigen originally described a structural molecule that binds specifically to an antibody only in the form of native antigen. It was expanded later to refer to any molecule or a linear molecular fragment after processing the native antigen that can be recognized by T-cell receptor (TCR). BCR and TCR are both highly variable antigen receptors diversified by somatic V(D)J recombination. Both T cells and B cells are cellular components of adaptive immunity. The Ag abbreviation stands for an antibody generator.

Antigens are "targeted" by antibodies. Each antibody is specifically produced by the immune system to match an antigen after cells in the immune system come into *contact* with it; this allows a precise identification or matching of the antigen and the initiation of a tailored response. The antibody is said to "match" the antigen in the sense that it can bind to it due to an adaptation in a region of the antibody; because of this, many different antibodies are produced, each able to bind a different antigen while sharing the same basic structure. In most cases, an adapted antibody can only react to and bind one specific antigen; in some instances, however, antibodies may cross-react and bind more than one antigen.

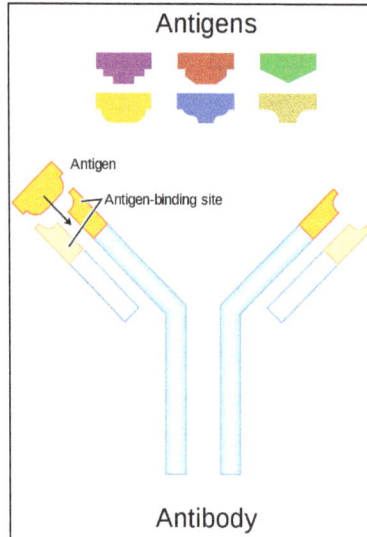

An illustration that shows how antigens induce the immune system response by interacting with an antibody that matches the antigen's molecular structure.

Also, an antigen is a molecule that binds to Ag-specific receptors, but cannot necessarily induce an immune response in the body by itself. Antigens are usually proteins, peptides (amino acid chains) and polysaccharides (chains of monosaccharides/simple sugars) but lipids and nucleic acids become antigens only when combined with proteins and polysaccharides. In general, saccharides and lipids (as opposed to peptides) qualify as antigens but not as immunogens since they cannot elicit an immune response on their own. Furthermore, for a peptide to induce an immune response (activation of T-cells by antigen-presenting cells) it must be a large enough size, since peptides too small will also not elicit an immune response.

The antigen may originate from within the body ("self-antigen") or from the external environment ("non-self"). The immune system is supposed to identify and attack "non-self" invaders from the outside world or modified/harmful substances present in the body and usually does not react to self-antigens under normal homeostatic conditions due to negative selection of T cells in the thymus.

Vaccines are examples of antigens in an immunogenic form, which are intentionally administered to a recipient to induce the memory function of adaptive immune system toward the antigens of the pathogen invading that recipient.

Terminology

- Epitope – The distinct surface features of an antigen, its antigenic determinant. Antigenic molecules, normally "large" biological polymers, usually present surface features that can act as points of interaction for specific antibodies. Any such feature constitutes an epitope. Most antigens have the potential to be bound by multiple antibodies, each of which is specific to one of the antigen's epitopes. Using the "lock and key" metaphor, the antigen can be seen as a string of keys (epitopes) each of which matches a different lock (antibody). Different antibody idiotypes, each have distinctly formed complementarity determining regions.

- Allergen – A substance capable of causing an allergic reaction. The (detrimental) reaction may result after exposure via ingestion, inhalation, injection, or contact with skin.

- Superantigen – A class of antigens that cause non-specific activation of T-cells, resulting in polyclonal T-cell activation and massive cytokine release.

- Tolerogen – A substance that invokes a specific immune non-responsiveness due to its molecular form. If its molecular form is changed, a tolerogen can become an immunogen.

- Immunoglobulin-binding protein – Proteins such as protein A, protein G, and protein L that are capable of binding to antibodies at positions outside of the antigen-binding site. While antigens are the "target" of antibodies, immunoglobulin-binding proteins "attack" antibodies.

- T-dependent antigen – Antigens that require the assistance of T cells to induce the formation of specific antibodies.

- T-independent antigen – Antigens that stimulate B cells directly.

- Immunodominant antigens – Antigens that dominate (over all others from a pathogen) in their ability to produce an immune response. T cell responses typically are directed against a relatively few immunodominant epitopes, although in some cases (e.g., infection with the malaria pathogen Plasmodium spp.) it is dispersed over a relatively large number of parasite antigens.

Antigen presenting cells present antigens in the form of peptides on histocompatibility molecules. The T cell selectively recognize the antigens; depending on the antigen and the type of the histocompatibility molecule, different types of T cells will be activated. For T Cell Receptor (TCR) recognition, the peptide must be processed into small fragments inside the cell and presented by a major histocompatibility complex (MHC). The antigen cannot elicit the immune response without the help of an immunologic adjuvant. Similarly, the adjuvant component of vaccines plays an essential role in the activation of the innate immune system.

An immunogen is an antigen substance (or adduct) that is able to trigger a humoral (innate) or cell-mediated immune response. It first initiates an innate immune response, which then causes the activation of the adaptive immune response. An antigen binds the highly variable immunoreceptor products (B cell receptor or T cell receptor) once these have been generated. Immunogens are those antigens, termed immunogenic, capable of inducing an immune response.

At the molecular level, an antigen can be characterized by its ability to bind to an antibody's variable Fab region. Different antibodies have the potential to discriminate among specific epitopes present on the antigen surface. A hapten is a small molecule that changes the structure of an antigenic epitope. In order to induce an immune response, it needs to be attached to a large carrier molecule such as a protein (a complex of peptides). Antigens are usually carried by proteins and polysaccharides, and less frequently, lipids. This includes parts (coats, capsules, cell walls, flagella, fimbriae, and toxins) of bacteria, viruses, and other microorganisms. Lipids and nucleic acids are antigenic only when combined with proteins and polysaccharides. Non-microbial non-self antigens can include pollen, egg white and proteins from transplanted tissues and organs or on the surface of transfused blood cells.

Exogenous Antigens

Exogenous antigens are antigens that have entered the body from the outside, for example, by inhalation, ingestion or injection. The immune system's response to exogenous antigens is often subclinical. By endocytosis or phagocytosis, exogenous antigens are taken into the antigen-presenting cells (APCs) and processed into fragments. APCs then present the fragments to T helper cells (CD4+) by the use of class II histocompatibility molecules on their surface. Some T cells are specific for the peptide: MHC complex. They become activated and start to secrete cytokines, substances that activate cytotoxic T lymphocytes (CTL), antibody-secreting B cells, macrophages and other particles.

Some antigens start out as exogenous, and later become endogenous (for example, intracellular viruses). Intracellular antigens can be returned to circulation upon the destruction of the infected cell.

Endogenous Antigens

Endogenous antigens are generated within normal cells as a result of normal cell metabolism, or because of viral or intracellular bacterial infection. The fragments are then presented on the cell surface in the complex with MHC class I molecules. If activated cytotoxic CD8+ T cells recognize them, the T cells secrete various toxins that cause the lysis or apoptosis of the infected cell. In order to keep the cytotoxic cells from killing cells just for presenting self-proteins, the cytotoxic cells (self-reactive T cells) are deleted as a result of tolerance (negative selection). Endogenous antigens include xenogenic (heterologous), autologous and idiotypic or allogenic (homologous) antigens. Sometimes antigens are part of the host itself in an autoimmune disease.

Autoantigens

An autoantigen is usually a normal protein or protein complex (and sometimes DNA or RNA) that is recognized by the immune system of patients suffering from a specific autoimmune disease. Under normal conditions, these antigens should not be the target of the immune system, but in autoimmune diseases, their associated T cells are not deleted and instead attack.

Neoantigens

Neoantigens are those that are entirely absent from the normal human genome. As compared with nonmutated self-antigens, neoantigens are of relevance to tumor control, as the quality of the T cell pool that is available for these antigens is not affected by central T cell tolerance. Technology to systematically analyze T cell reactivity against neoantigens became available only recently.

Viral Antigens

For virus-associated tumors, such as cervical cancer and a subset of head and neck cancers, epitopes derived from viral open reading frames contribute to the pool of neoantigens.

Tumor Antigens

Tumor antigens are those antigens that are presented by MHC class I or MHC class II molecules on the surface of tumor cells. Antigens found only on such cells are called tumor-specific antigens (TSAs) and generally result from a tumor-specific mutation. More common are antigens that are presented by tumor cells and normal cells, called tumor-associated antigens (TAAs). Cytotoxic T lymphocytes that recognize these antigens may be able to destroy tumor cells.

Tumor antigens can appear on the surface of the tumor in the form of, for example, a mutated receptor, in which case they are recognized by B cells.

For human tumors without a viral etiology, novel peptides (neo-epitopes) are created by tumor-specific DNA alterations.

Process

A large fraction of human tumor mutations are effectively patient-specific. Therefore, neoantigens may also be based on individual tumor genomes. Deep-sequencing technologies can identify mutations within the protein-coding part of the genome (the exome) and predict potential neoantigens. In mice models, for all novel protein sequences, potential MHC-binding peptides were predicted. The resulting set of potential neoantigens was used to assess T cell reactivity. Exome–based analyses were exploited in a clinical setting, to assess reactivity in patients treated by either tumor-infiltrating lymphocyte (TIL) cell therapy or checkpoint blockade. Neoantigen identification was successful for multiple experimental model systems and human malignancies.

The false-negative rate of cancer exome sequencing is low—i.e.: the majority of neoantigens occur within exonic sequence with sufficient coverage. However, the vast majority of mutations within expressed genes do not produce neoantigens that are recognized by autologous T cells.

As of 2015 mass spectrometry resolution is insufficient to exclude many false positives from the pool of peptides that may be presented by MHC molecules. Instead, algorithms are used to identify the most likely candidates. These algorithms consider factors such as the likelihood of proteasomal processing, transport into the endoplasmic reticulum, affinity for the relevant MHC class I alleles and gene expression or protein translation levels.

The majority of human neoantigens identified in unbiased screens display a high predicted MHC binding affinity. Minor histocompatibility antigens, a conceptually similar antigen class are also correctly identified by MHC binding algorithms. Another potential filter examines whether the mutation is expected to improve MHC binding. The nature of the central TCR-exposed residues of MHC-bound peptides is associated with peptide immunogenicity.

Nativity

A native antigen is an antigen that is not yet processed by an APC to smaller parts. T cells cannot bind native antigens, but require that they be processed by APCs, whereas B cells can be activated by native ones.

Antigenic Specificity

Antigenic specificity is the ability of the host cells to recognize an antigen specifically as a unique molecular entity and distinguish it from another with exquisite precision. Antigen specificity is due primarily to the side-chain conformations of the antigen. It is measurable and need not be linear or of a rate-limited step or equation.

Antigen Presentation

In order to be capable of engaging the key elements of adaptive immunity (specificity, memory, diversity, self/nonself discrimination), antigens have to be processed and presented to immune cells. Antigen presentation is mediated by MHC class I molecules, and the class II molecules found on the surface of antigen-presenting cells (APCs) and certain other cells.

MHC class I and class II molecules are similar in function: they deliver short peptides to the cell surface allowing these peptides to be recognised by CD8+ (cytotoxic) and CD4+ (helper) T cells, respectively. The difference is that the peptides originate from different sources – endogenous, or intracellular, for MHC class I; and exogenous, or extracellular for MHC class II. There is also so called cross-presentation in which exogenous antigens can be presented by MHC class I molecules. Endogenous antigens can also be presented by MHC class II when they are degraded through autophagy.

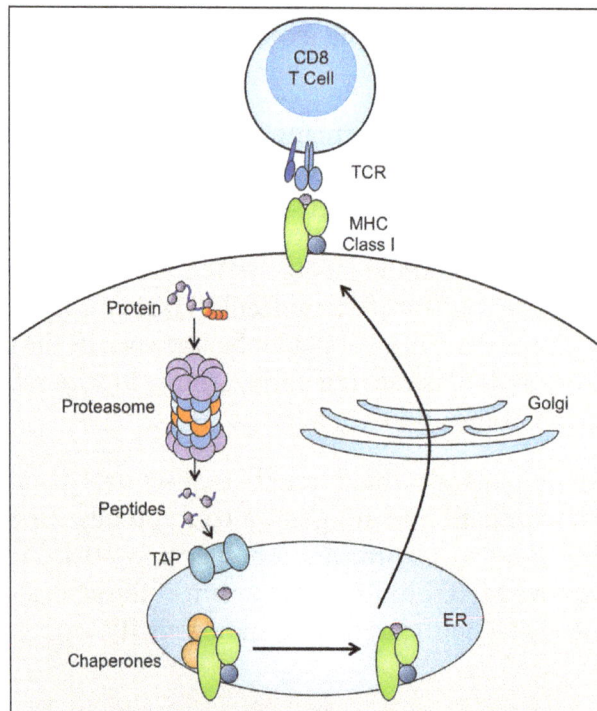

The MHC class I antigen-presentation pathway.

MHC Class I Presentation

MHC class I molecules are expressed by all nucleated cells. MHC class I molecules are assembled in the endoplasmic reticulum (ER) and consist of two types of chain – a polymorphic heavy chain and a chain called β2-microglobulin. The heavy chain is stabilised by the chaperone calnexin, prior to association with the β2-microglobulin. Without peptides, these molecules are stabilised by chaperone proteins: calreticulin, Erp57, protein disulfide isomerase (PDI) and tapasin. The complex of TAP, tapasin, MHC class I, ERp57 and calreticulin is called the peptide-loading complex (PLC). Tapasin interacts with the transport protein TAP (transporter associated with antigen presentation) which translocates peptides from the cytoplasm into the ER. Prior to entering the ER, peptides are derived from the degradation of proteins, which can be of viral- or self origin. Degradation of proteins is mediated by cytosolic- and nuclear proteasomes, and the resulting peptides are translocated into the ER by means of TAP. TAP translocates peptides of 8 –16 amino acids and they may require additional trimming in the ER before binding to MHC class I molecules. This is possibly due to the presence of ER aminopeptidase (ERAAP) associated with antigen processing.

It should be noted that 30–70% of proteins are immediately degraded after synthesis (they are called DRiPs – defective ribosomal products, and they are the result of defective transcription or translation). This process allows viral peptides to be presented very quickly – for example, influenza virus can be recognised by T cells approximately 1.5 hours post-infection. When peptides bind to MHC class I molecules, the chaperones are released and peptide–MHC class I complexes leave the ER for presentation at the cell surface. In some cases, peptides fail to associate with MHC class I and they have to be returned to the cytosol for degradation. Some MHC class I molecules never bind peptides and they are also degraded by the ER-associated protein degradation (ERAD) system.

There are different proteasomes that generate peptides for MHC class-I presentation: 26S proteasome, which is expressed by most cells; the immunoproteasome, which is expressed by many immune cells; and the thymic-specific proteasome expressed by thymic epithelial cells.

Antigen Presentation

On the surface of a single cell, MHC class I molecules provide a readout of the expression level of up to 10,000 proteins. This array is interpreted by cytotoxic T lymphocytes and Natural Killer cells, allowing them to monitor the events inside the cell and detect infection and tumorigenesis.

MHC class I complexes at the cell surface may dissociate as time passes and the heavy chain can be internalised. When MHC class I molecules are internalised into the endosome, they enter the MHC class-II presentation pathway. Some of the MHC class I molecules can be recycled and present endosomal peptides as a part of a process which is called cross-presentation.

The usual process of antigen presentation through the MHC I molecule is based on an interaction between the T-cell receptor and a peptide bound to the MHC class I molecule. There is also an interaction between the CD8+ molecule on the surface of the T cell and non-peptide binding regions on the MHC class I molecule. Thus, peptide presented in complex with MHC class I can only be recognised by CD8+ T cells. This interaction is a part of so-called 'three-signal activation model', and actually represents the first signal. The next signal is the interaction between CD80/86 on the APC and CD28 on the surface of the T cell, followed by a third signal – the production of cytokines by the APC which fully activates the T cell to provide a specific response.

MHC Class I Polymorphism

Human MHC class I molecules are encoded by a series of genes – HLA-A, HLA-B and HLA-C (HLA stands for 'Human Leukocyte Antigen', which is the human equivalent of MHC molecules found in most vertebrates). These genes are highly polymorphic, which means that each individual has his/her own HLA allele set. The consequences of these polymorphisms are differential susceptibilities to infection and autoimmune diseases that may result from the high diversity of peptides that can bind to MHC class I in different individuals. Also, MHC class I polymorphisms make it virtually impossible to have a perfect tissue match between donor and recipient, and thus are responsible for graft rejection.

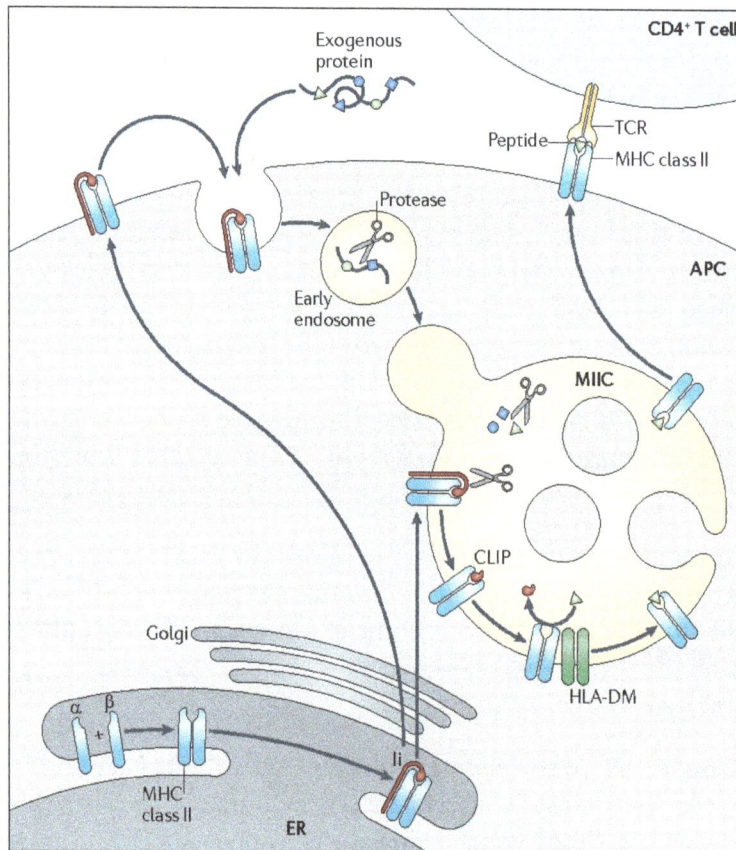

The MHC class II antigen-presentation pathway.

MHC Class II Presentation

MHC class II molecules are expressed by APCs, such as dendritic cells (DC), macrophages and B cells (and, under IFNγ stimuli, by mesenchymal stromal cells, fibroblasts and endothelial cells, as well as by epithelial cells and enteric glial cells). MHC class II molecules bind to peptides that are derived from proteins degraded in the endocytic pathway. MHC class II complexes consists of α- and β-chains that are assembled in the ER and are stabilised by invariant chain (Ii). The complex of MHC class II and Ii is transported through the Golgi into a compartment which is termed the MHC class II compartment (MIIC). Due to acidic pH, proteases cathepsin S and cathepsin L are activated and digest Ii, leaving a residual class II-associated Ii peptide (CLIP) in the peptide-binding groove of the MHC class II. Later, the CLIP is exchanged for an antigenic peptide derived from a protein degraded in the endosomal pathway. This process requires the chaperone HLA-DM, and, in the case of B cells, the HLA-DO molecule. MHC class II molecules loaded with foreign peptide are then transported to the cell membrane to present their cargo to CD4+ T cells. Thereafter, the process of antigen presentation by means of MHC class II molecules basically follows the same pattern as for MHC class I presentation.

As opposed to MHC class I, MHC class II molecules do not dissociate at the plasma membrane. The mechanisms that control MHC class II degradation have not been established yet, but MHC class II molecules can be ubiquitinised and then internalised in an endocytic pathway.

MHC Class II Polymorphism

Like the MHC class I heavy chain, human MHC class II molecules are encoded by three polymorphic genes: HLA-DR, HLA-DQ and HLA-DP. Different MHC class II alleles can be used as genetic markers for several autoimmune diseases, possibly owing to the peptides that they present.

Immunoglobulin Class Switching

Immunoglobulin class switching, also known as isotype switching, isotypic commutation or class-switch recombination (CSR), is a biological mechanism that changes a B cell's production of immunoglobulin from one type to another, such as from the isotype IgM to the isotype IgG. During this process, the constant-region portion of the antibody heavy chain is changed, but the variable region of the heavy chain stays the same (the terms "variable" and "constant" refer to changes or lack thereof between antibodies that target different epitopes). Since the variable region does not change, class switching does not affect antigen specificity. Instead, the antibody retains affinity for the same antigens, but can interact with different effector molecules.

Mechanism

Class switching occurs after activation of a mature B cell via its membrane-bound antibody molecule (or B cell receptor) to generate the different classes of antibody, all with the same variable domains as the original antibody generated in the immature B cell during the process of V(D)J recombination, but possessing distinct constant domains in their heavy chains.

Naïve mature B cells produce both IgM and IgD, which are the first two heavy chain segments in the immunoglobulin locus. After activation by antigen, these B cells proliferate. If these activated B cells encounter specific signaling molecules via their CD40 and cytokine receptors (both modulated by T helper cells), they undergo antibody class switching to produce IgG, IgA or IgE antibodies. During class switching, the constant region of the immunoglobulin heavy chain changes but the variable regions, and therefore antigenic specificity, stay the same. This allows different daughter cells from the same activated B cell to produce antibodies of different isotypes or subtypes (e.g. IgG1, IgG2 etc.).

The order of the heavy chain exons are as follows:

- μ - IgM

- δ - IgD

- γ_3 - IgG3

- γ_1 - IgG1

- α_1 - IgA1

- γ_2 - IgG2

- γ_4 - IgG4

- ε - IgE

- α_2 - IgA2

Class switching occurs by a mechanism called class switch recombination (CSR) binding. Class switch recombination is a biological mechanism that allows the class of antibody produced by an activated B cell to change during a process known as isotype or class switching. During CSR, portions of the antibody heavy chain locus are removed from the chromosome, and the gene segments surrounding the deleted portion are rejoined to retain a functional antibody gene that produces antibody of a different isotype. Double-stranded breaks are generated in DNA at conserved nucleotide motifs, called switch (S) regions, which are upstream from gene segments that encode the constant regions of antibody heavy chains; these occur adjacent to all heavy chain constant region genes with the exception of the δ-chain. DNA is nicked and broken at two selected S-regions by the activity of a series of enzymes, including Activation-Induced (Cytidine) Deaminase (AID), uracil DNA glycosylase and apyrimidic/apurinic (AP)-endonucleases. The intervening DNA between the S-regions is subsequently deleted from the chromosome, removing unwanted μ or δ heavy chain constant region exons and allowing substitution of a γ, α or ε constant region gene segment. The free ends of the DNA are rejoined by a process called non-homologous end joining (NHEJ) to link the variable domain exon to the desired downstream constant domain exon of the antibody heavy chain. In the absence of non-homologous end joining, free ends of DNA may be rejoined by an alternative pathway biased toward microhomology joins. With the exception of the μ and δ genes, only one antibody class is expressed by a B cell at any point in time. While class switch recombination is mostly a deletional process, rearranging a chromosome in "cis", it can also occur (in 10 to 20% of cases, depending upon the Ig class) as an inter-chromosomal translocation mixing immunoglobulin heavy chain genes from both alleles.

Cytokines Responsible for Class Switching

T cell cytokines modulate class switching in mouse and human. These cytokines may have suppressive effect on production of IgM.

Gene Regulatory Sequences Responsible for Class Switching

In addition to the highly repetitive structure of the target S regions, the process of class switching needs S regions to be first transcribed and spliced out of the immunoglobulin heavy chain transcripts (where they lie within introns). Chromatin remodeling, accessibility to transcription and to AID and synapsis of broken S regions are under the control of a large super-enhancer, located downstream the more distal Calpha gene, the 3' regulatory region (3'RR). In some occasions, the 3'RR super-enhancer can itself be targeted by AID and undergo DNA breaks and junction with Sµ, which then deletes the Ig heavy chain locus and defines locus suicide recombination (LSR).

Table: Class switching in mouse								
T cells	Cytokines	Immunoglobulin classes						
		IgG1	IgG2a	IgG2b	IgG3	IgG4	IgE	IgA
Th2	IL-4	↑	↓	↓	↓	↓	↑	
	IL-5					↑		
Th1	IFNγ	↓	↑	↓	↑	↓	↓	
Treg	TGFβ			↑	↓	↑		
	IL-10				↑			

Table: Class switching in human							
T cells	Cytokines	Immunoglobulin classes					
		IgG1	IgG2	IgG3	IgG4	IgA	IgE
Th2	IL-4	↑		↓	↑		↑
	IL-5					↑	
Th1	IFNγ	↓		↑			↓
Treg	TGFβ			↓		↑	
	IL-10	↑		↑			

Immune Repertoire

The immune repertoire, is defined as, the number of different sub-types an organism's immune system makes, of any of the 6 key types of protein, either immunoglobulin or T cell receptor.

In most vertebrates, immune systems have 6 key types of proteins, which help the immune system recognise viruses, germs, etc. The 6 main types are: Immunoglobulins (2), and T cell receptors (4). Immunoglobulin proteins consist of 2 parts, a light chain and a heavy chain. T cell receptors come in 4 types, labelled alpha, beta, gamma and delta.

In an organism, each of the 6 types of protein, in fact consists of a large number of sub-types, all differing slightly from each other. In one organism, There can be tens of thousands, or millions of different sub types of each of the 6. The differences are not obvious, and require complex research to detect, e.g. DNA sequencing, or antigen binding tests.

Every day, we are exposed to a wide range of disease causing organisms. thus, how well our immune system is able to detect them—depends on how many sub types of the proteins, it is able to produce. An immune system that produces a wide variety, will likely have one or two subtypes that recognise any germ we are exposed to. An immune system that produces just a few, will likely miss or "not see" certain germs or viruses—and these could then go on, unchallenged, to cause disease.

Immune repertoire is defined, as the number of sub-types that exist in an organism's immune system, of one or other of the 6 key types of proteins, in a certain "compartment" of the immune system (i.e. a certain set of cells from the immune system).

Size of Immune Repertoire

A few researchers have measured immune repertoires for humans, but as the task until recently was technically difficult, it was seldom attempted. Estimates will depend on the precise type or 'compartment' of immune cells studied; and the protein studied.

1. Pasqual et al. JEM publication showed that the expected billions of combinations were over-estimated. The authors described the genetic spatio temporal rule which governs the TCR locus rearrangements and were able to demonstrate for the first time that the V(D)J rearrangements are not random, hence resulting in a smaller V(D)J diversity.

2. Dare et al. estimated repertoire for TCR gamma genes, in CD8+CD45RO$^+$ memory T cells in blood, as 40,000–100,000 sub-types, in 3 healthy young adults. In healthy older adults, (over 75) they found smaller repertoires, being 3,600; 5,500; 14,000 and 97,000.

3. Artsila et al. estimated repertoire for TCR alpha and TCR beta in CD4+/CD8+ T-cells, as approx 100,000.

Immune Repertoire Generation

1. The repertoire is generated, by immune system cells (lymphocytes) cutting a bit of DNA from 2 or 3 parts of the genome, and joining them together in different combinations. Each part of the genome, has only a few different pieces of DNA that can be used. But the different combinations of these, give a massive range of total sequences.

2. Following that, the repertoire is edited. Cells whose protein would cause an immune reaction with the body, are removed. Cells which actually detect an invading organism, become more numerous. And cells with new types, may be added.

Factors affecting Immune Repertoire

1. Age: The immune system develops over life, as stem cells mature, and generate their own maybe unique, gene sequences.

2. What diseases you are exposed to: When exposed to a disease, your body can create further sub types of proteins that recognise the virus, and thus fine tune the immune response. Also after the disease is gone, cells which recognised it, tend to hang around in the body.

3. Immune memory: Generally after one has had a disease, the cells whose genes recognise the disease, are allowed to persist for many years in the body.

4. Old age: There is some evidence, that cells with existing subtypes die off, and are not replaced by new subtypes.

5. Genetic disease primary immunodeficiency: A few genetic diseases, people don't have the genes for the 6 immune proteins; or don't have the genes to do the splicing. Thus they can't generate the immune repertoire, or have a reduced one.

6. Treatments that seriously affect the immune system e.g. bone marrow transplant and cancer treatment: In these your entire bone marrow—[which is the source of the immune system]—is wiped out, to clear the body of cancer (which can often spread to the marrow). After that you get a transplant in of cancer-free marrow, from a donor, or from yourself when you were in remission. These basically have to re-generate the immune repertoire again.

Measuring Immune Repertoire

There is an interesting mathematical problem—if a set of objects consists of a large number of sub types—how does one count how many sub types there are? For instance, if you have a bag of balls, and they come in a range of colours—how can you work out, how many different colours there are in the bag?

Where there are only a few colours—say 4—it's easy. You just keep examining balls, one at a time, until you are happy you've seen all the colours. The same old ones keep coming up time and time again. And you just count the different types.

Where there are say 30–50 different colours—it is more difficult. A large number of balls need examining, and comparing one to another. Anyone who has ever tried collecting say football cards, knows that in order to be sure you have seen all of them—you need to open a very great number of packs.

Where there could be say several thousand colour types—the problem of finding out how many types there are, becomes challenging. Sampling and sorting and counting types—becomes difficult, involve a lot of work.

Yet this is the problem encountered in some areas of biology. For instance, health of an ecosystem, might depend on presence of thousands of species. An immune system's ability to detect disease, might require hundreds of thousands of different types of cells.

Approaches

For immune systems, there are four approaches:

1. Use a low-resolution technique to catalogue cell types, and use that as an index of overall repertoire. In ecology, the analogy would be cataloguing animals at the genus level, rather than species. This assumes diversity of one, reflects diversity of the other. It can pick up severe losses in diversity, large enough to knock out whole classes of things. It is perhaps less able to show, when the number of different things in a class is reduced.

2. Look at a lot of individual cells, and count or estimate the total number of sub types that must be present. Thus if you look at 100 cells and find 50 subtypes—then look at another 100 cells, and are now up to 60 subtypes—and then another 100 cells, and are now up to 65 there is a mathematical approach that predicts the total number of subtypes present. In the past, it took a tremendous amount of effort to obtain DNA sequences from the genes; this is now becoming easier with "next generation " sequencing, where it is possible to sequence tens of thousands of these genes, from a blood sample, simultaneously, for a few hundred dollars.

3. Look at a few sub types, work out how common each is, and thus work out the total number of sub types you expect. Thus if you find 1 makes up a hundredth of the immune system—you might expect the immune system to consist of 100 subtypes.

4. Clinical tests to assess presence of the normal range of cell types. If one type is entirely missing—say B-lymphocytes—then an entire subset of the immune repertoire may be missing.

Need for Immune Repertoire

1. The problem is interesting, of developing methods to count numbers of sub-types present—when there are a great many sub types.

2. The actual size, is the key test of one of the basic theories in immunology, namely MacFarlane Burnet's theory of clonal selection. This theory—now some decades old—postulated that the immune system had to include a very large number of sub types. That number, until recently, has not been measured directly.

3. Numerous treatments are coming into use, which affect the immune system—there is a need to measure repertoire, to monitor these effects. And also to develop treatments, to increase repertoire, e.g. using cytokines as drugs.

4. If a persons immune repertoire is low—say as a result of a cancer treatment which as a side effect, knocks out their immune system—they'll be unusually susceptible to diseases. In fact, one of the limiting factors, in developing cancer treatment, is this—it means patients have to be nursed carefully for some time in sterile environments until the immune system recovers. And if they are unlucky enough to get infected while the immune system is down—the infections can be life-threatening. Any way to make the immune system recover faster, would be useful.

5. Other areas of biology, also involve great variety and diversity. E.g. in a square km of rainforest, there may be several hundred species of trees, or insects. A litre of ocean water, may contain a high diversity of plankton plants and animals. A cubic cm of soil, will contain many different types of bacteria and fungi. High diversity, is a key characteristic of all these.

6. It may be useful, to have methods to measure these large numbers, to put a number on diversity, for its own sake, so we have a better idea how large the diversity is. Also, to use as bench marks. A fall from 1000 species to 10, we can readily detect. A fall from 1000 species to 500, is also a significant change—but the methods to detect this change, would be extremely complex.

7. Research on the immune system repertoire, may develop methods of sampling and statistics, to directly assess diversity in ecology. It may be that this too, is best approached, through genetic markers and high throughput sequencing—rather than more traditional taxonomy.

Future Developments

Next generation sequencing may have a large impact. This can obtain thousands of DNA sequences, from different genes, quickly, at the same time, relatively cheaply. Thus it may be possible, to take a large sample of cells from someones immune system, and look quickly at the range of sub-types present in the sample. The ability to obtain data quickly from tens or hundreds of thousands of cells, one cell at a time, should provide a good idea, of the size of the person's immune repertoire.

These large-scale adaptive immune receptor repertoire sequencing (AIRR-seq) data require specialized bioinformatics pipelines to be analyzed effectively. Many computational tools are being developed for this purpose. The Immcantation framework provide a start-to-finish analytical ecosystem for high-throughput AIRR-seq data analysis. The AIRR Community is community-driven organization that is organizing and coordinating stakeholders in the use of next-generation sequencing technologies to study immune repertoires. In 2017, the AIRR Community published recommendations for a minimal set of metadata that should be used to describe an AIRR-seq data set when published and deposited in a public repository.

Original Antigenic Sin

Original antigenic sin, also known as the Hoskins effect, refers to the propensity of the body's immune system to preferentially utilize immunological memory based on a previous infection when a second slightly different version of that foreign entity (e.g. a virus or bacterium) is encountered. This leaves the immune system "trapped" by the first response it has made to each antigen, and unable to mount potentially more effective responses during subsequent infections. The phenomenon of original antigenic sin has been described in relation to influenza virus, dengue fever, human immunodeficiency virus (HIV), and to several other viruses.

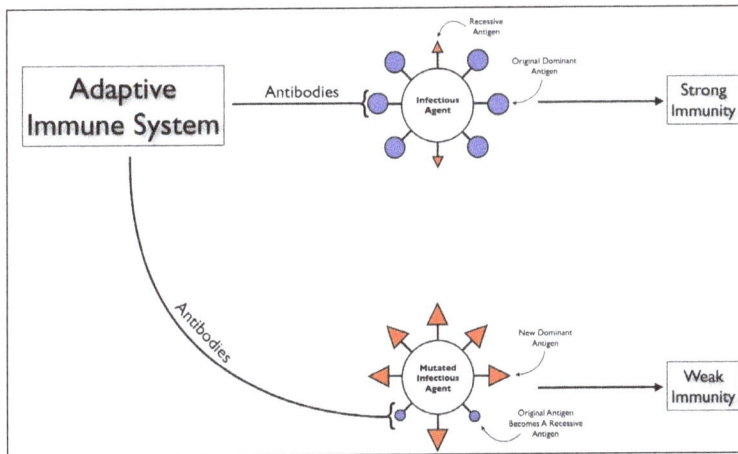

In figure, the original antigenic sin: When the body first encounters an infection it produces effective antibodies against its dominant antigens and thus eliminates the infection. But when it encounters the same infection, at a later evolved stage, with a new dominant antigen, with the original antigen now being recessive, the immune system will still produce the former antibodies against this old "now recessive antigen" and not develop new antibodies against the new dominant one, this results in the production of ineffective antibodies and thus a weak immunity.

This phenomenon was first described in 1960 by Thomas Francis, Jr. in the article "On the Doctrine of Original Antigenic Sin". It is named by analogy to the theological concept of original sin. According to Thomas Francis, who originally described the idea, and cited by Richard Krause:

"The antibody of childhood is largely a response to dominant antigen of the virus causing the first type A influenza infection of the lifetime. The imprint established by the original virus infection governs the antibody response thereafter. This we have called the Doctrine of the Original Antigenic Sin."

In B Cells

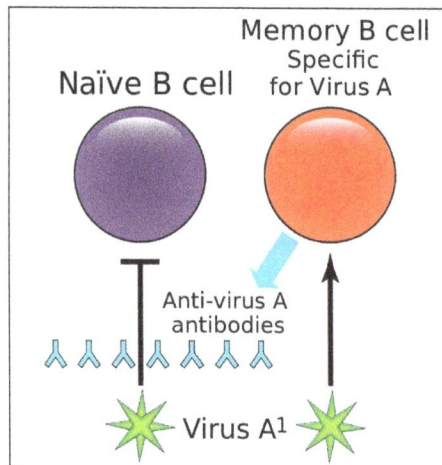

In figure, a high affinity memory B cell, specific for Virus A, is preferentially activated by a new strain, Virus A^1, to produce antibodies that ineffectively bind to the A^1 strain. The presence of these antibodies inhibits activation of a naive B cell that produces more effective antibodies against Virus A^1. This effect leads to a diminished immune response against Virus A^1, and heightens the potential for serious infection.

During a primary infection, long-lived memory B cells are generated, which remain in the body, and provide protection from subsequent infections. These memory B cells respond to specific epitopes on the surface of viral proteins in order to produce antigen-specific antibodies, and are able to respond to infection much faster than B cells are able to respond to novel antigens. This effect shortens the amount of time required to clear subsequent infections.

Between primary and secondary infections, or following vaccination, a virus may undergo antigenic drift, in which the viral surface proteins (the epitopes) are altered through natural mutation, allowing the virus to escape the immune system. When this happens, the altered virus preferentially reactivates previously activated high-affinity memory B cells and spur antibody production. However, the antibodies produced by these B cells generally ineffectively bind to the altered epitopes. In addition, these antibodies inhibit the activation of higher-affinity naive B cells that *would* be able to make more effective antibodies to the second virus. This leads to a less effective immune response and recurrent infections may take longer to clear.

Original antigenic sin is of particular importance in the application of vaccines. In dengue fever, the effect of original antigenic sin has important implications for vaccine development. Once a response against a dengue virus serotype has been established, it is unlikely that vaccination against a second will be effective, implying that balanced responses against all four virus serotypes have to be established with the first vaccine dose. However, in 2015, a new class of highly potent, neutralizing antibodies that is effective against all four virus serotypes has been isolated, bringing hope for the development of a universal dengue vaccine.

The specificity and the quality of the immune response against novel strains of influenza is often diminished in individuals who are repeatedly immunized (by vaccination or recurrent infections). However, the impact of antigenic sin on protection has not been well established, and appears to differ with each infectious agent vaccine, geographic location, and age. Researchers found reduced antibody responses to the 2009 pandemic H1N1 influenza vaccine in individuals who had been vaccinated against the seasonal A/Brisbane/59/2007 (H1N1) within the previous three months.

In Cytotoxic T Cells

A similar phenomenon has been described in cytotoxic T cells (CTL). It has been demonstrated that during the secondary infection by a different strain of dengue virus, the CTLs prefer to release cytokines instead of causing lysis of cell. As a result, the production of these cytokines are thought to increase vascular permeability and exacerbate the damage of endothelial cells.

Several groups have attempted to design vaccines for HIV and hepatitis C based on induction of cytotoxic (CTL) responses. The finding that CTL may be biased by original antigenic sin, may help to explain the limited effectiveness of these vaccines. Viruses like HIV are highly variable and undergo mutation frequently, and thus, due to original antigenic sin, HIV infection induced by viruses that express slightly different epitopes (than those in a viral vaccine) would fail to be controlled by the vaccine. In fact, the vaccine might make the infection even worse, by "trapping" the immune response into the first, ineffective, response it made against the virus.

Immunological Synapse

The molecular interactions underlying regulation of the immune response take place in a nano-scale gap between T cells and antigen presenting cells, termed the immunological synapse. If these interactions are regulated appropriately, the host is defended against a wide range of pathogens and deranged host cells. If these interactions are dis-regulated, the host is susceptible to pathogens or tumor escape at one extreme and autoimmunity at the other. Treatments targeting the synapse have helped to establish immunotherapy as a mainstream element in cancer treatment. This Masters primer will cover the basics of the immunological synapse and some of the applications to tumor immunology.

T cell dependent immune responses protect the host from cancer, but also participate in destructive autoimmunity. TCR engagement leads to suppression of T-cell locomotion, formation of a specialized junction, and T-cell polarization. This combination of a specialized junction, cell polarization, and positional stability bears a striking similarity to the classical synapse of the nervous system. T cells can also integrate signals through the antigen receptor during migration, and we have referred to this type of mobile, antigen recognition structure as a kinapse. The immunological synapse or kinapse integrates three broad categories of receptors: antigen (TCR), adhesion, and costimulatory/checkpoint. The organization of these receptors in the interface impacts how they function in a way that cannot be predicted without this spatial and temporal information. The text book picture of antigen recognition across a ~15 nm gap between a T cell and an antigen-presenting cell (APC) provides the justification for why the immune system needs a synapse or kinapse. Adhesion molecules, identified first by function with blocking antibodies and then by expression cloning, provide the energy needed to pull cells together, allowing sustained antigen recognition and precise execution of effector functions. Finally, co-stimulatory and checkpoint receptors alter the functional outcome of immunological synapse formation substantially and can also influence the synapse-kinapse balance. To date, immunotherapies targeting checkpoint receptors have provided the most promise.

Immunological Synapse Models

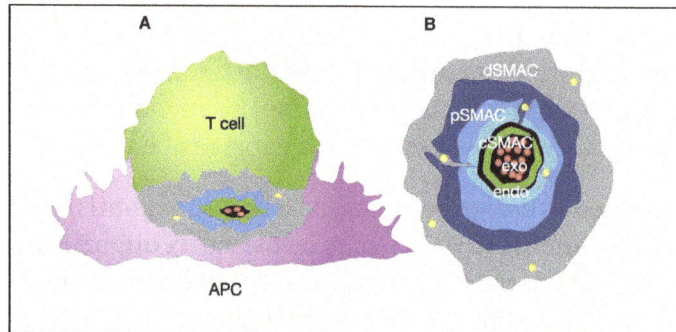

Model immunological synapse- A. Scanning electron micrograph of T cell interacting with an antigen presenting cells to provide scale for contact area only. B and C. Elevated and front on view of model for synapse focusing on interface. Color code- black- F-actin lamellipodium, blue- LFA-1-ICAM-1 adhesion, red- TCR-MHC antigen recognition and green- CD28-CD80 costim SMACs are labelled.

Determining how antigen recognition, adhesion, and co-stimulation/checkpoint receptors come together in the immunological synapse or kinapse required visualization of the close interface between the T cell and the APC. Two major approaches dominated the efforts at molecular analysis. Top down analysis of T cell-APC pairs utilizing immunofluorescence and bottom up approaches of applying purified molecules to substrates have both contributed to our understanding of the immunological synapse. Reconstitution methods based on fluid supported lipid bilayers (SLB), in which the purified molecules are combined in a laterally mobile form, have been effective in recreating the organization of the immunological synapse formed with live T cells. The canonical organization of the immune synapse is a bull's eye structure with a central TCR-MHC (major histocompatibility complex) interaction cluster surrounded by a ring of LFA-1-ICAM-1 adhesion and a distal ring that includes the transmembrane tyrosine phosphatase CD45 Kupfer referred to these radially symmetric compartments as supramolecular activation clusters. The segregation of TCR-MHC interactions from LFA-1-ICAM-1 interactions was a confirmation of the working model formulated by Springer in 1990 that, based on their sizes, the TCR-MHC interactions would need to segregate laterally from the LFA-1-ICAM-1 interactions. This is a stereotypical response of helper, cytotoxic, and regulatory T cells. The SMACs of a stable synapse correspond to polarized compartments in a kinase. T cells and dendritic cells (DC) have a more complex organization of similar compartments, perhaps due to the intricate topology of DCs.

T-cell Antigen Receptor

TCR interaction with MHC-peptide complexes controls the specificity of the immune response and the source of antigens in both cellular and humoral responses. TCR genes undergo rearrangement similar to that of antibody genes. T cells with subunits encoded by the α and β genes make up the classical diverse repertoire of naïve T cells that can respond to pathogens and tumors. T cells with subunits encoded by the γ and δ genes include specialized cells that are not MHC-restricted. The complete TCR on the cell surface is composed of two highly diversified antigen recognition subunits that are essentially unique for each T cell, either αβ or γδ, in a non-covalent complex with non-polymorphic CD3ε–CD3δ, CD3ε–CD3γ and CD3ζ–CD3ζ dimers. The entire complex is critical for surface expression and signal transduction, but it lacks any intrinsic catalytic activity. Instead the TCR complex has 10 immunotyrosine activation motifs (ITAM) with paired tyrosine residues that when phosphorylated can recruit the non-receptor tyrosine kinase Zeta-Associated Protein of 70 kDa.

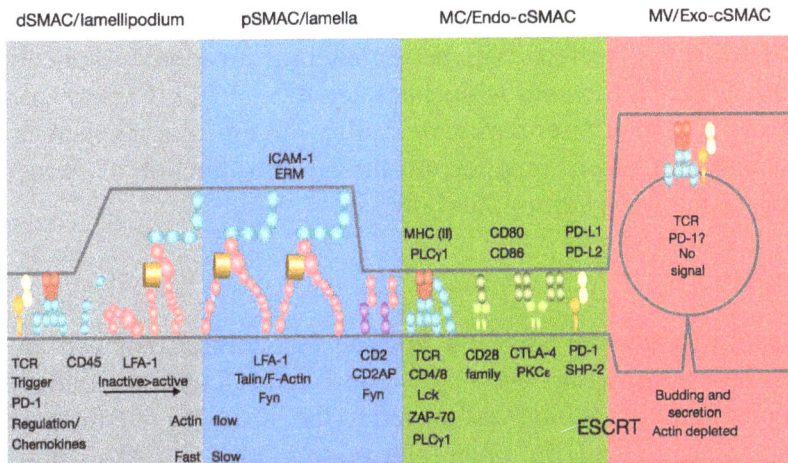

Figure: SMACs and representative receptor classes in immunological synapse.

While it was recognized by 1975 that cell-surface expressed gene products of the highly polymorphic MHC were required to "restrict" T cell recognition of antigen, the full molecular picture of how antigenic peptides bound to MHC was not clear until the crystal structure of an MHC molecule was solved in 1987. There are two distinct types of MHC that control antigen recognition - one set of genes for cytotoxic T cells that bind endogenously synthesized cytoplasmic peptides generated by the proteosome (class I), and a distinct set of genes for helper T cells that bind exogenous antigens taken into the cell by endocytosis (class II). The process of cross-presentation or cross-dressing allows specialized APCs needed for T-cell priming to present exogenous antigens through the class I pathway, which is likely critical for anti-cancer cellular immunity. MHC class II molecules can also engage in signaling. Other MHC-like molecules present non-peptide antigenic structures. These include CD1d presentation of glycolipids to invariant natural killer T cells and MR1 presentation of bacterial metabolites to mucosa-associated invariant T (MAIT) cells. These innate-like T cells may have utility in immune response to tumors.

Conventional αβ T cells are marked by different coreceptors, CD8 and CD4. CD8 binds to non-polymorphic elements of MHC class I, and CD4 to that of MHC class II. In T-cell development, thymocytes rearrange TCR genes and test receptors for interaction with self-peptides on MHC. Strong interactions lead to apoptosis or, for a limited number of clones, the generation of actively suppressive thymic regulatory T (Treg) cells, which are important in tumor immunology as their formation of immunological synapses can suppress antitumor responses in part by destabilizing T-effector immunological synapses. Differences in signaling between conventional αβ T cells and Tregs offer therapeutic opportunities to push the balance toward regulation in autoimmunity and towards responsiveness in cancer therapy. A weaker recognition process is required for thymocyte survival, and this is thought to bias the TCR repertoire toward recognition of MHC with either CD4 or CD8. This weak self-recognition is thought to set the stage for foreign peptide recognition by providing the T cell with weak recognition of the peptide flanking, polymorphic α–helices of the MHC proteins, and also provides survival signals to mature T cells. It is still debated whether the germ-line-encoded TCR are evolutionarily biased to recognize MHC molecules in a certain preferred orientation, or if the germ-line TCR repertoire has an antibody-like lack of bias and entirely learns to recognize MHC molecules in the thymus.

In a tumor context antigen recognition can enhance or inhibit responses. The classical tumor-infiltrating lymphocyte (TIL) is a CD8 cytotoxic T cell that can directly kill tumor cells, and the infiltration of tumors by CD8 T cells correlates with better outcome for some tumors. Antigen-presenting cells in tumors can include CD11c⁺ cells with characteristics of DCs. Cancer vaccines are an effort to promote the expansion and differentiation of T cells with antitumor specificity in a therapeutic setting. T-cell specificity can also be engineered through introduction of chimeric antigen receptors into patient cells in adoptive immunotherapy.

Adhesion Receptors

Adhesion molecules are critical for sensitive antigen recognition required for tumor rejection. Strategies based on immunizing mice with cytotoxic T cell (CTL) lines followed by selection for monoclonal antibodies (mAb) that block killing led to the discovery of lymphocyte function-associated antigen-1 (now CD11a/CD18, but often referred to as LFA-1), LFA-2 (now CD2), and LFA-3 (now CD58).

CD2 and CD58 define a heterophilic adhesion receptor pair. CD2 and CD58 are members of the immunoglobulin (Ig) superfamily and are similar in size to the TCR and MHC-peptide complex, suggesting that CD2 may cooperate very closely with the TCR. CD2 and CD58 are members of the signaling lymphocyte activation molecule (SLAM) family. Most other SLAM family members are homophilic (they mediate adhesion by binding between products of the same gene) that interact through their cytoplasmic domain with SLAM-associated protein (SAP), which links to the tyrosine kinase Fyn. SLAM family members are required for particular interactions between thymocytes in the development of certain specialized T-cell lineages and for early T cell-B cell interactions required for germinal center formation.

LFA-1 is a heterodimer with a unique α subunit that shares a β subunit with 3 other cell-surface heterodimers, each of which has an α subunit with a distinct expression pattern. Functional screening for mAbs that block LFA-1-dependent aggregation after immunization with B cells from LFA-1-deficient patients identified the first LFA-1 ligand, intercellular adhesion molecule-1 (ICAM-1 or CD54). LFA-1 is a member of the integrin family and ICAM-1 is a member of the Ig superfamily. The intercellular link formed by the interaction of LFA-1 with ICAM-1 is much longer than that with the TCR and it was suggested that the TCR-MHC and LFA-1-ICAM-1 interactions would need to segregate laterally in the interface, the first prediction on the structure of the immunological synapse. ICAM-2, a second ligand for LFA-1 was cloned from an endothelial cell library, is also an Ig superfamily member. A third ligand, ICAM-3, was later defined by functional blocking in a screen in which ICAM-1 and ICAM-2 were blocked. T cells express other adhesion molecules including additional integrins. An important aspect of the integrin ligands is that they are expressed on all nucleated cells and can be further induced, in the case of ICAM-1, by exposure of stromal cells to inflammatory cytokines including tumor necrosis factor (TNF), interleukin-1β, or interferon-γ (IFNγ). A complication of the therapeutic use of anti-LFA-1 mAbs is that LFA-1 is important for interactions with endothelial cells and as such is important for optimal localization of cells, in addition to immunological synapse formation. Anti-LFA-1 mAbs were approved for treatment of psoriasis, but the therapeutic window between reduction of disease and increased vulnerability to infection was too small. There are activating Abs to LFA-1, but the affinity of LFA-1 for ICAMs is optimized to allow rapid leukocyte migration, and constitutively active LFA-1 is defective in mediating migration, contraindicating LFA-1 affinity enhancement as a therapeutic strategy.

While adhesion molecules are diverse in structure, both integrins and the SLAM family signal through the Src family kinase Fyn rather than Lck, which is the primary partner for antigen and costimulatory receptors. Another common feature is that both LFA-1 and CD2 engage ligands in the periphery of the immunological synapse, even though the CD2–CD58 interactions are the correct size to co-localize with TCR in the center.

Costimulation

Costimulatory receptors have minimal signaling or adhesive activity on their own, but can enhance adhesion and signaling locally when combined with other stimuli, primarily through the TCR. Costimulatory receptors were predicted as a corollary of the clonal selection model in which T cells must be able to attenuate their responses to harmless foreign proteins from the environment that are not present in the thymus and could drive inappropriate immune responses if not checked by some mechanism for extrathymic tolerance. Pathogens or tumors would need to up-regulate costimulation to drive a T cell to respond, and incorporation of costimulatory ligands directly into tumor cells has been implemented in tumor vaccines. Activation of mature T cells in the absence of costimulation leads to a second round of clonal deletion that protects the host against immune responses to harmless environmental antigens. Schwartz and Jenkins discovered that antigen recognition with sub-optimal costimulation could induce a state of non-responsiveness that they referred to as anergy.

The archetypal costimulator is CD28, which is an Ig superfamily member with a homodimeric structure and a cytoplasmic domain lacking enzymatic activity but containing motifs that recruit and activate Lck and indirectly, protein kinase C (PKC)-θ, an important PKC isoform in T cells that contributes to the activation of NF-κB transcription factors and promotes IL2 production. The activity of CD28 is dependent upon the up-regulation of B7-1 (CD80) and B7-2 (CD86) on APCs and the interaction in an immunological synapse. Both CD80 and CD86 are upregulated on DCs by stimulation through maturation signals delivered by toll-like receptors (TLR) and inflammatory cytokines. This is a critical link between innate and adaptive immunity, and the potential of some tumors to grow without inducing expression of costimulatory ligands may allow them to tolerize tumor-specific T cells.

The inducible T cell costimulator (ICOS, CD278) is a second Ig-superfamily costimulatory system. In contrast to CD28, it is not expressed on naïve T cells, but is upregulated following T cell activation and binds Ligand of ICOS (LICOS, CD275). LICOS is expressed prominently on dendritic cells and B cells, but can be induced on stromal cells by inflammatory cytokines. ICOS is critical for germinal center reactions where it ability to activate phosphatidylinsolitol-3 kinase is particularly important. In the context of cancer immunotherapy, ICOS costimulation promotes Th17 differentiation in CD4 T cells, which is an effective response mode for some solid tumors.

The other large costimulatory receptors are members of the TNF receptor (TNFR) superfamily including CD27, GITR (CD357), 4-1BB (CD137), and OX40 (CD134). These receptors signal through TNFR-associated factors (TRAF) utilizing K63 ubiquitination to signal through activation of NF-κB2 transcription factors. With the exception of CD27, which is constitutively expressed, these costimulatory receptors are induced on conventional T cells in hours to days following initial activation. Therefore, they are involved in effector and memory functions of T cells following the initial expansion phase. These receptors are also constitutively expressed on Tregs, and this perhaps offers an opportunity to modulate negative regulation in the tumor microenvironment (TME). The last set of costimulatory receptors are members of the lectin-like receptor superfamily that pair non-covalently with DAP10, a disulfide linked heterodimer containing a sequence motif that allows recruitment of phosphatidylinositol-3-kinase, which contributes to activation of the growth-promoting kinase AKT. These receptors, with NKG2D as a prime example, are expressed on CTLs as well as NK cells and promote killing. The counter-receptor for NKG2D are induced by cellular stress and are potentially important in recognition of deranged host cells. However, tumor cells proteolytically shed one of the human counter-receptors, MICA, leading to jamming of this system as an escape mechanism.

There is evidence for combinations of adhesion and costimulatory ligands generating partial signals that can lead to transient formation of ligand-independent immunological synapses. This has been observed with NKG2D in human and mouse CTLs and recently for CD28 in helper T cells. In this context, the upregulation of ICAM-1, CD80, and NKG2D ligands like MICA (human) and Rae-1 (mice) can induce a state of heighten surveillance in inflamed or stressed tissues.

Checkpoint Blockade

Co-inhibitory or checkpoint receptors are a natural complement to the costimulators - they use various negative signaling pathways, often recruiting tyrosine phosphatases, such as SHP1 and SHP2, to attenuate tyrosine kinase cascades or other signaling pathways.

One of the best-defined checkpoint inhibitors is cytotoxic T-lymphocyte antigen-4 (CTLA-4, CD152), which is induced rapidly following T-cell activation. CTLA-4 has a constitutively active internalization motif in its cytoplasmic domain such that it does not accumulate on the cell surface except when ligated in the synapse or when the Y-based internalization motif is phosphorylated. CTLA-4 competes with CD28 for binding to CD80 more potently than for CD86. In Tregs, CTLA-4 is constitutively expressed and coupling to the endocytic pathway leads to the removal of CD80 and CD86 from APCs, which impairs CD28-dependent responses of other T cells. CTLA-4 associates with PKCε in Tregs. Anti-CTLA-4 mAbs are approved for treatment of melanoma. While CTLA-4-deficient mice suffer from fatal immunopatholog, there is a significant therapeutic window in which antitumor effects can be achieved with limited toxicity.

Another checkpoint receptor is programmed cell death-1 (PD-1, CD279). PD-1 binds PD-1 ligand 1 and 2 (PD-L1, CD274 and PD-L2, CD273) and is recruited to the immunological synapse in a manner related to MHC-peptide strength and abundance. PD-1 recruits SHP-2 tyrosine phosphatase and attenuates early TCR signaling upon ligand binding. The impact of PD-1 on immunological synapse stability depends upon the context, with destabilization in autoimmune and delayed-type hypersensitivity, but stabilization in anti-viral responses. Stabilization of the immunological synapse in this context results in an immune paralysis in which the T cell cannot respond nor be released to engage other targets. PD-1 is associated with T-cell exhaustion in chronic viral infection and this mechanism can protect the host from immunopathology related to toxicity of chronic immune responses. However, it can be exploited by pathogens and tumors as an evasion mechanism. Recently mAbs to PD-1 have been approved for treatment of melanoma in Japan and results in melanoma and lung cancer are promising. The ability to predict patient response based on information about the tumor is a significant goal of personalized medicine. Trials are in progress to determine if PD-L1 expression on the tumor predicts patient response. An interesting aspect of PD-1 is that it is expressed on and suppresses the activity of Tregs. Thus, blockade of PD-1 may increase Treg function, suggesting a rationale for combining anti-PD-1 with anti-CTLA-4, the latter suppresses Treg function. Other checkpoint inhibitors include Vista and SIRPα (CD172A).

Hierarchy of Interactions

Antigen, adhesion, and costimulatory/checkpoint receptors are highly interdependent. LFA-1 activity on T cells is increased by TCR signaling in a process referred to as inside-out signaling. This observation leads to a "chicken and egg" problem for initiating TCR signaling in that LFA-1 clearly is important for T-cell sensitivity to antigen, yet, TCR signaling is necessary for activation of LFA-1. A likely solution involves the chemokines in the tissue microenvironment, which stimulate the activity of LFA-1 at the leading edge of T cells and establish a low level of transient LFA-1-dependent adhesion, thus increasing the chances that TCR can detect rare MHC-peptide complexes. Once the TCR is triggered this can further enhance LFA-1 activity and promote formation of an immunological synapse. Increases in LFA-1 affinity are driven by large conformational changes in the heterodimers. Costimulatory receptor CD28 interacts with ligands in a TCR-dependent fashion, with the critical regulatory step being its low expression on quiescent cells, indicating that CD28 only engages its ligand at sites "seeded" by TCR microclusters (MC). One way to consider this is that in the steady state LFA-1-ICAM-1 interactions allow rapid scanning of APC surfaces for TCR-MHC complexes, whose signaling increases LFA-1-dependent adhesion and generates local MCs, which favors the participation of CD2, CD28 and other small adhesion molecules. Some adhesion molecules and costimulatory receptors cooperate in a process called superagonism. Antibody combinations to CD2 monomer or single Abs to CD28 homodimer can induce full T-cell activation in a TCR-dependent manner. The structural basis of these effects is not known, but it appears that in some extreme conditions induced by Abs, the normal process of TCR induction of adhesion/costimulation can operate backwards. It is not clear if this happens physiologically, but the phenomenon may be useful in a clinical setting if it can be controlled and directed.

TCR Microclusters

When TCRs are ligated by MHC-peptide complexes presented on a cell, e.g. anti-CD3 Abs on a solid substrate or MHC-peptide complexes and ICAM-1 on a supported planar bilayer, the first structures that can be visualized at the interface are sub-micron TCR clusters that form in an F-actin-dependent manner. It has been argued that TCRs are pre-clustered on T cells, but the ligand-induced clusters have a number of distinct characteristics. Ligand-induced MCs recruit the src family kinase Lck to the TCR leading to the phosphorylation of ITAMs and the recruitment and activation of ZAP-70. ZAP-70 phosphorylates the membrane-anchored linker of activated T cells (LAT) that recruits phospholipase Cγ (PLCγ) and facilitates its activation by the inducible T-cell kinase (ITK). PLCγ-mediated generation of diacylglycerol and inositol-1,3,5-trisphosphate leads to the activation of Ras, PKC, and calcium ion effector pathways that can account for transcriptional activation of the T-cell growth and regulatory cytokines such as IL2. TCR can use a module including the guanine nucleotide exchange factor Vav that activates Notch to directly control Myc transcription and T-cell proliferation independent of IL2.

Src family kinases Fyn (mentioned in adhesion context) and Lck (dominant kinase down-stream of TCR) are regulated by intramolecular interactions. All Src family kinases have a C-terminal tyrosine (Y505 in Lck) that serves as an intramolecular ligand for its own Src homology 2 (SH2) domain. When the SH2 domain is bound to the C-terminal tyrosine in parallel with a second intramolecular interaction of the Src homology-3 (SH3) domain with the polyproline motif between the kinase domain and the SH2 domain, the kinase is locked in an inhibited state. The C-terminal Src kinase (Csk) mediates this phosphorylation when recruited to membrane-anchored Src substrates in the vicinity of the active Src kinase. This negative feedback is counteracted by the transmembrane tyrosine phosphatase CD45. Selective Csk inhibition results in ligand-independent TCR signaling that synergizes with CD28 signals. CD45 deficiency results in inhibition of TCR signaling. However, CD45 also can reverse activating phosphorylations mediated by Lck and ZAP-70. Interestingly, CD45 is excluded from TCR MCs and this reduction in CD45 density, based on the large size of its extracellular domain, appears to be important in setting the appropriate local level of phosphatase activity for TCR triggering. Any small adhesion system will generate interactions that exclude CD45, so it is unlikely the CD45 exclusion is sufficient for full TCR signaling, but some level of exclusion appears to be necessary.

Supramolecular Activation Clusters

SMACs defined by Kupfer are divided into the central, peripheral, and distal regions, or cSMAC, pSMAC, and dSMAC. Based on analysis of immunological synapse dynamics using the SLB system, dSMAC behaves like the leading lamellipodium of migrating cells in that it undergoes cycles of protrusion and retraction. In contrast, pSMAC is rich in LFA-1 and the integrin to cytoskeletal linker talin, defining it as a lamellum, based on an abrupt change in F-actin dynamics and filament decorations compared to the lamellipodium. Higher resolution imaging has forced a revision of Kupfer's SMAC definitions. First, the active TCR-MHC interactions that lead to signaling in the immunological synapse are concentrated in small MCs that are formed in the dSMAC and move centripetally through the pSMAC to the cSMAC. This traversal of the integrin-rich pSMAC by the smaller TCR is possible because the LFA-1-ICAM-1 interaction also begins in MCs in the dSMAC and consolidates into a reticular network with submicron holes in which the TCR-MHC MCs can be fully segregated. The LFA-1-ICAM-1 reticulum in the pSMAC is continually moving inward, which allows the central transport of the TCR-MHC MCs. While the immunological synapse can be stable for hours, the dSMAC and pSMAC are highly dynamic structures that are completely renewed every few minutes. The second major revision is the structure of the cSMAC. The original cSMAC as defined by Kupfer is a TCR-MHC-rich central structure with accumulation of PKC-θ. We now know that the prominent accumulation of PKC-θ is a signature of CD28-dependent costimulation. Work with SLB containing only ICAM-1 and activating MHC-peptide complexes revealed a very different cSMAC in which TCR-MHC interactions were highly stabilized and signaling was terminated. Further study of bilayers containing ICAM-1, MHC, and CD80 revealed that CD28 and PKC-θ are initially co-localized with TCR in MCs, but on convergence in the cSMAC segregate into a TCR-rich, CD28-deficient zone in which signaling is terminated, and a TCR-poor, CD28-rich region in which CD28-PKC-θ-enhanced TCR signaling continues. Further analysis of the TCR-MHC-rich signal termination zone in the cSMAC revealed that it is composed of TCR-enriched extracellular microvesicles that bud from the plasma membrane and become trapped in a persistent interaction with the MHC in the SLB. The budding process is dependent on tumor-susceptibility gene 101 (TSG101) and the buds are arrested by the expression of dominant negative vacuolar protein sorting 4 (VPS4), implicating the endosomal sorting complexes required for transport (ESCRT) pathway. In T cell-B cell interactions these TCR-enriched extracellular vesicles are collected by the B cell and moved away from the interface.

CD28–CD80 interactions are efficiently sorted away from the bulk of the TCR that is sorted to the extracellular vesicles. Thus, the cSMAC can be divided into two components: the endo-cSMAC in which TCR and CD28 continue to signal and the exo-cSMAC, composed of TCR-enriched extracellular vesicles. We have found that the checkpoint receptor PD-1 is highly enriched in the exo-cSMAC. This would suggest that TCR and PD-1 are closely associated and co-sorted or that PD-1 is ubiquitinated. The TCR-enriched vesicles continue to activate signaling in the B cell through engaging surface MHC molecules, and in the case of MHC class II may be relevant to T-cell help delivery as an active form of exo-TCR. Studies using the SLB system suggest that all T cells engage in this type of vesicle transfer, opening the possibility that helper, cytotoxic and regulatory cells may generate exo-TCR in a carrier that can contain other information, including nucleic acids. Whether exo-TCR plays a role in the TME is an open question. The modular structure of the immunological synapse thus incorporates a lamellipodium (dSMAC), lamellum (pSMAC), TCR MCs, a sorting domain that can enrich CD28-enhanced TCR signaling complexes (endo-cSMAC), and an extracellular compartment of TCR-enriched extracellular vesicles (exo-cSMAC). The exo-cSMAC is a transient compartment that is normally internalized by the APC. When projected into the more complex three-dimensional setting of a T cell-DC interface the lamellipodum, lamellum, and multiple endo-cSMACs remain clearly visible at the interface. It is likely that the multifocal close contacts observed in EM are not MCs, but are multiple, larger endo-cSMAC structures. It has also been proposed that the MCs can manifest as small projections that indent the APC surface, rather than moving laterally. There is also an LFA-1-dependent actin cloud or lamellum that imparts a more three-dimensional aspect to the actin cytoskeleton and this structure incorporate a subset of signaling components. This raises issues of sub-synaptic vesicular components that may also play an important role in signaling.

Directed Secretion: A Synaptic Advantage

A central element of the immunological synapse concept is directed secretion of soluble components into the synaptic cleft. This is fundamental to models of T-cell help and cell-mediated killing of infected cells or tumor cells. A major underlying assumption has been that orientation of the centrioles and Golgi toward the APC reflects directed secretion. This has been challenged by studies using antibody-mediated capture to determine the orientation of secretion. In this case molecules that move through the highly oriented Golgi can be secreted randomly based on manner in which secretory vesicles are transported after leaving the Golgi apparatus. For example, IFNγ was found to undergo directed secretion from helper T cells, but TNF and chemokines were not directed to the synapse. The TCR can be directly delivered to the synapse in vesicles. Cytolytic granules are also directly delivered to a secretory domain near the endo-cSMAC compartment. Recently it has been proposed that the centrosome docking at immunological synapse sets up a de facto primary cilium that enables intraflagellar transport machinery and hedgehog pathway signaling to be implemented in the immunological synapse. Despite this high level of specialization, it has been shown that CTLs may operate in a "quick draw" mode and release cytolytic granules at targets without re-orienting and docking the centrioles to the synapse. NK cells also use more dynamic kinapse in signal integration with tumors, with advantages in the ability to penetrate into the tumor over more stable synaptic interactions.

However, even for NK cells, converting kinapses into synapses with tumor-targeting Abs increase the efficiency of killing. The potential advantage of synapses is the inability to concentrate the cytolytic components on the target surface. Comparison of synaptic versus kinaptic killing in the context of CD8 versus CD4 cytotoxic T cells in vitro suggests that the advantage of forming a stable synapse is about 3-fold. In a murine breast cancer model, anti-CTLA-4 mAbs stimulate motility of activated T cells in the tumor, consistent with other evidence that CTLA-4 engagement could stimulate T-cell motility. Stabilization of activated T-cell interactions through induction of Rae-1, which binds NKG2D on T cells, was required to decrease tumor growth. Antigen recognition processes that lead to stable synapses may be desirable in immunotherapy settings. It will be of great interest to determine the mode of interaction induced by chimeric receptors that combine ITAM and costimulatory signaling in one polypeptide, particularly as conventional synapses with B chronic lymphocytic leukemia cells are defective. Exocytic trafficking in the synapse is likely to be balanced by endocytic trafficking. One manifestation of endocytic processes is trogocytosis, in which one cell "gnaws" off pieces of another cell. In addition to ESCRT-dependent budding to generate TCR-enriched extracellular vesicles, some fraction of TCRs in the cSMAC regions undergoes internalization and can bring MHC from the APC with it. CD8 T cells that capture MHC-peptide from target cells through trogocytosis actually become targets for killing by other CTLs in the culture. What controls the ratio of TCR that is transferred to the APCs in extracellular vesicles versus MHC that is captured by the T cell from the APCs is not known, but both processes are readily detectable across a single immunological synapse. The consequence of exo-TCR transfer for tumor cells is not known. CTLs have been shown to release TCR-positive vesicles at target cells. It is not clear if these are similar to the exo-TCR reported by Choudhuri and colleagues as it is not clear if these exosome-like structures contain recently engaged TCR or were sorted into these structures without prior ligand-engagement through a distinct mechanism of TCR sorting. It may be possible to isolate the vesicles budded from the plasma membrane versus those released from granules and subject these to proteomic analysis and functional testing.

References

- Immune-tolerance, research: niaid.nih.gov, Retrieved 26 July, 2019

- Bieniasz PD (November 2004). "Intrinsic immunity: a front-line defense against viral attack". Nat. Immunol. 5 (11): 1109–15. Doi:10.1038/ni1125. PMID 15496950

- Janeway, Charles; Paul Travers; Mark Walport; Mark Shlomchik (2001). Immunobiology; Fifth Edition. New York and London: Garland Science. ISBN 978-0-8153-4101-7

- Patt H, Bandgar T, Lila A, Shah N (2013). "Management issues with exogenous steroid therapy". Indian Journal of Endocrinology and Metabolism. 17 (Suppl 3): s612–s617. Doi:10.4103/2230-8210.123548. PMC 4046616. PMID 24910822

- Rhoades RA, Pflanzer RG (2002). Human Physiology(5th ed.). Thomson Learning. P. 584. ISBN 978-0-534-42174-8

- Antigen-processing-and-presentation, systems-and-processes, bitesized-immunology, public-information: immunology.org, Retrieved 5 February, 2019

- Animated depictions of how antibodies are used in ELISA assays". Cellular Technology Ltd.—Europe. Archived from the original on 14 June 2011. Retrieved 8 May 2007

- Arstila, TP; Casrouge, A; Baron, V; Even, J; Kanellopoulos, J; Kourilsky, P (1999). "A direct estimate of the human alphabeta T cell receptor diversity". Science. 286 (5441): 958–61. Doi:10.1126/science.286.5441.958. PMID 10542151

Sub-disciplines of Immunology 5

- **Immunoproteomics**
- **Cancer Immunology**
- **Computational Immunology**
- **Immunomics**
- **Psychoneuroimmunology**
- **Reproductive Immunology**
- **Palaeoimmunology**
- **Systems Immunology**
- **Immunotoxicology**

Immunology is a broad field that is divided into various sub-disciplines. Some of them are immunoproteomics, cancer immunology, computational immunology, immunomics, psychoneuroimmunology, systems immunology and Immunotoxicology. All the diverse aspects of these sub-disciplines of immunology have been carefully analyzed in this chapter.

Immunoproteomics

The increase in antibiotic resistance and the shortage of new antimicrobials to prevent difficult bacterial infections underlines the importance of prophylactic therapies to prevent infection by bacterial pathogens. Vaccination has reduced the incidence of many serious diseases, including respiratory bacterial infections. However, there are many pathogens for which no vaccine is available and some vaccines are not effective among all age groups or among immunocompromised individuals. Immunoproteomics is a powerful technique which has been used to identify potential vaccine candidates to protect against pathogenic bacteria. The combination of proteomics with the detection of immunoreactive antigens using serum highlights immunogenic proteins that are expressed during infection. This is particularly useful when patient serum is used as the antigens that promote a humoral response during human infection are identified. Many immunoreactive proteins are common to several unrelated pathogens, however some of these are not always protective in animal immunisation and challenge studies. Furthermore, examples of well-established immunogens, including Bordetella pertussis antigen FHA were not detected in immunoproteomics studies, indicating that this technology may underrepresent the immunoreactive proteins in a pathogen. Although only one step in the pathway towards an efficacious approved vaccine, immunoproteomics is an important technology in the identification of novel vaccine antigens.

The value of vaccination as a means of combating life-threatening and chronic infectious diseases is well established. Many diseases which previously contributed to mortality are now prevented by vaccination. However, according to the WHO, about 1.5 million of deaths among children under five in 2008 were caused by vaccine preventable diseases. In addition many approved vaccines are more effective in young children than in adolescents and adults. Given that infectious diseases are still the leading global cause of morbidity and mortality and when considered in the context of both the rise in antimicrobial resistance and the lack of novel effective antibiotics in the drug development pipeline, the need for more efficacious vaccines for bacterial pathogens cannot be underestimated.

There are several bacterial cell components incorporated into subunit vaccines, LPS, glycoconjugated vaccines, DNA vaccines, protein vaccines, which in addition to live attenuated vaccines and whole killed cell vaccines stimulate the host immune response in a variety of ways. Vaccine studies have often focussed on lipopolysaccharide (LPS) due to its potent stimulation of the immune response; however the antigenic diversity of the O-antigen component of LPS within species has limited the potential of LPS as potential vaccine antigens, for example P. aeruginosa LPS. Many approved vaccines are glycoconjugate in nature (e.g. vaccines for Neisseria meningitidis and Streptococcus pneumoniae) and have proved effective against certain serogroups of pathogens; but they tend to suffer from the same issues with variability across strains. In addition, serotype switching and serotype replacement may undermine their effectiveness in the future. Proteins are often more conserved across bacterial strains and have more potential to protect against several strains of the same bacterial species.

Investigation and harnessing of the host-pathogen response are beneficial to two separate but essential aspects to vaccine development. Exploitation of the human humoral response by determining immunogenic bacterial protein using sera from vaccinated, colonised or recovering individuals has played an important part in identifying novel vaccine antigens. Identification of novel antigens is only part of the process of vaccine development, therefore examination of the host response in adults and in human volunteers at the cellular and humoral response level is also essential in the development of more efficacious vaccines. Protection against certain intracellular pathogens requires a strong cell-mediated immune response driven by polarisation towards a Th1 response; while other extracellular pathogens are best protected by a Th2 response which promotes antibody production and antibody-mediated cell killing. Indeed knowledge of the interactions between pathogens and host cells in vitro is also critical, where the bacterial components that attach to host cells are investigated and elucidated.

Exploiting the Microbial–Host Response to Identify New Antigens

Reno Rappuoli and co-workers pioneered the use of a genomics approach to identify novel antigens against Neisseria meningitidis serogroup B using reverse vaccinology, in the late 1990s. They sequenced the genome of the pathogen, identified proteins which were likely to be surface associated, expressed these in Escherichia coli and administered the 350 proteins to mice to identify those that were immunogenic. The sequencing step of the process took 18 months at the time. The development of genomics since then has meant a rapid expansion in the capabilities to identify new antigens. Over 2,800 bacterial genomes have been completely sequenced at time of writing, a figure which is increasing week on week. This vast bank of information combined with the advances in proteomics, including, the relatively reproducibility and ease of preparing 2-D gels has meant a rapid increase in proteomic analysis of bacterial pathogens which has given insights into mechanisms of bacterial virulence and pathogenesis, adaptation during chronic colonisation and host response. The natural step up to immunoproteomics, whereby 2-D blots are probed with host serum following infection or immunisation has greatly enhanced the identification of potential vaccine candidates, by enabling the discovery of novel proteins that stimulate the humoral host immune system. A key advantage of this approach is that final expressed bacterial proteins are used in the analysis, which have been completely processed and post-translationally modified by the pathogen. Several groups have used this method to discover potential vaccine candidates with varying degrees of success. Different sera have been used in these types of studies which range from using colonised patient sera, convalescent sera, or sera from challenged mice or rabbits. Furthermore, the majority of immunoproteomic studies have focussed on cell surface proteins or outer membrane proteins as this subgroup of bacterial proteins represent the interface for host pathogen interactions and regularly include adhesins. Other groups have examined secreted proteins as they are also primary antigen targets of the host immune response and include many virulence factors. Collectively, their exposure to the host immune system marks these pools of proteins as a rich source of vaccine candidates.

Streptococcus Pneumoniae

Streptococcus pneumoniae is a Gram positive bacterium that is a leading cause of bacterial pneumonia, meningitis and pneumococcal septicaemia. It accounts for 20 to 50% of community acquired pneumonia cases and is the cause of over 820,000 deaths each year in children under five. The seven-valent glycoconjugate pneumococcal vaccine Prevnar 7 has reduced the incidence of invasive pneumococcal disease in children and mortality from this disease; however, it is not optimal for protection in children under two or in immunocompromised patients. Furthermore, there has been serotype replacement and increased incidence of non-vaccine serotypes, including the antimicrobially resistant serotype 19A, which now predominates in some countries. Although the recently approved 10- and 13-valent vaccines target more serotypes and prevent invasive disease in children, there are at least 92 serotypes. This means that identification of protein antigens which are more highly conserved across the species than the capsular polysaccharides may present more effective alternatives.

Immunoproteomics has been used to identify potential immunogenic antigens in S. pneumoniae. Adults develop antibodies to S. pneumoniae during asymptomatic carriage and it has been shown that the antibody response is age dependent. This increase in antibody response to S. pneumoniae proteins which correlated with a reduction in morbidity in children prompted Ling et al., to focus on antigens which showed increased immunogenicity with age of the child. Two-dimensional Western blotting of cell wall fractions from S. pneumoniae probed with sera from healthy children ranging in age from 18 to 42 months or with sera from adults highlighted seventeen immunoreactive proteins. Two of these, both metabolic enzymes, were equally protective against two genetically different strains in a mouse challenge model. While this indicates promise for the proteomic approach to identify protective antigens, the protection obtained was only 36%. Another two antigens identified in this study, 6-phosphogluconate dehydrogenase (6-PGD) and Glutamyl-tRNA synthase were subsequently shown to be involved in adhesion to A549 cells. While both independently protected mice against a lethal challenge, the level of protection was only marginally better than that observed with GAPDH and Fructose-bis-phosphate aldolase. In the case of 6-PGD, immunization also reduced lung and blood colonisation levels by several fold. The latter antigen, glutamyl-tRNA synthase shows promise due its lack of a human orthologue, the former protein has high homology to the human orthologue which could be detrimental to its development as a protective antigen.

A separate proteomic analysis of cell wall proteins identified proteins which were expressed across at least 40 S. pneumoniae serotypes and during animal infection. Five proteins were evaluated in a mouse sepsis model, and although lung bacterial burdens were reduced following individual immunisations with two of the proteins, these did not prolong the survival of mice. More recently, immunoproteomic analysis of the S. pneumoniae secretome also identified antigens which were shown to be immunogenic using immunised rabbit serum. In total 54 proteins were detected, of which only 23 were identified, including several proteins which were known virulence factors, in addition to novel proteins. These have the potential as diagnostic markers in addition to vaccine candidates. Many of these immunogenic proteins had been previously identified in other species and in some cases by Ling et al., e.g., Enolase, ZmpB, serine protease. However, vaccine studies on these have not been reported to date.

Overall, the comparable survival rates following lethal challenge (36 to 40%) for the four separate antigens described above and the lack of improved survival for others may suggest that more knowledge of the specific protective host response to S. pneumoniae is required to optimise further vaccine development. Indeed the finding that four distinct antigens showed very comparable survival rates may be a feature of the animal model used. It is possible that mice are not predictive of the immunological response to S. pneumoniae in humans. This is a key limitation of pre-clinical vaccination studies that must be always considered.

Burkholderia Pseudomallei and other Members of Genus Burkholderia

Burkholderia pseudomallei, the causative agent of melioidosis, is a Gram-negative, intracellular pathogen endemic in Southeast Asia and Northern Australia. The disease is considerably variable in humans ranging from acute septicaemia, pneumonia to chronic or latent infection which can persist and emerge decades later. The bacterium is intrinsically antibiotic resistant and has a mortality rate up to 50%; however despite its significant morbidity and mortality, there is currently no licensed vaccine against this infection. Harding et al., have used serum from convalescent patients to probe 2-D blots of B. pseudomallei OMPs. By biotinylation of the bacteria prior to OMP preparation, they were able to focus solely on surface expressed proteins. They identified nine surface proteins which were immunoreactive, including elongation factor Tu (EF-Tu), polyribonucleotide nucleotidyl transferase and two chaperones, GroEL and DnaK. Among the biotinylated proteins identified were several that would be considered to be cytoplasmic. This highlights a common theme in proteomic analysis, that proteins predicted to be cytoplasmic and without any signal peptide are exposed at the bacterial surface. A later study utilised rabbit serum to probe 2-D blots of membrane proteins and again identified elongation factor Tu (EF-Tu) and DnaK among the immunoreactive proteins of a less virulent related species, B. thailandensis, which shares 94% identity at the amino acid level with B. pseudomallei. EF-Tu was shown to be secreted in outer membrane vesicles (OMVs) which are shed from B. pseudomallei during in vitro growth. Mucosal immunisation of mice with EF-Tu resulted in the generation of antigen specific IgG and IgA, polarised Th1 immune response and significantly reduced the bacterial burden in the lungs following a lethal challenge with B. thailandensis. OMVs are gaining momentum as a potential vaccine platform. These are engineered proteoliposomes which incorporate the vaccine antigen, adjuvant in a particulate carrier. In a later study sub-cutaneous immunisation of mice with purified B. pseudomallei OMVs resulted in protection of 60% of mice against a lethal challenge with high OMV-specific titres, together with T-cell responses and humoral responses which were suggestive of a Th1 cell-mediated immunity. It was not stated whether these purified OMVs contained EF-Tu or what their antigenic composition was.

Immunoscreening of a lambda genomic library with pooled patient serum represents an alternative way of identifying immunoreactive antigens in B. pseudomallei. This functional genomic approach allowed the screening of 5760 open reading frames which were then used to genetically immunise mice. Three clones were selected from an initial screen of 14 serum reactive phagemids, based on their strong reactivity. Serological evaluation of 74 patients showed that 94% of patients were seropositive for one of these proteins, OmpA. B. pseudomallei have several putative OmpA genes, cloning of these resulted in 6 recombinant proteins. Two of these were followed up, Omp3 which clustered with the OmpA of E. coli and Klebsiella pneumonia OmpA following multiple sequence alignment, and Omp7 which was closely related to OmpA of Porphyromonas gingivalis. Subsequent mouse immunisation with these resulted in 50% protection against a lethal challenge for two different recombinant OmpA proteins with the most reactivity with sera from melioidosis patients. When this pilot immunisation study is considered together with the widespread seropositivity for OmpA among convalescent melioidosis patients, it strongly suggest the potential for this antigen as one component of a future multi-valent vaccine against melioidosis. Using a similar approach, Su et al., carried out a genomic survey of B. pseudomallei, screening an expression library with sera from melioidosis patients. Among the 109 proteins identified from seropositive clones, one protein was selected, OMP85, for later study, as it is a highly conserved protein. Intraperitoneal immunisation of mice with this recombinant antigen resulted in 70% protection of mice over 15 days, as opposed to 10% in non-immunised mice in addition to significantly reduced bacterial load in lungs and spleen.

Most recently, protein microarrays have been used to identify immunoreactive proteins with plasma from recovered melioidosis patients or seropositive healthy individuals. Of the antigens identified, seven were more strongly recognised by plasma from recovered individuals over healthy controls. These represented antigens which were previously identified, and/or associated with virulence, including flagellin and flagellar hook associated protein, OmpA and BipB, confirming the capacity for patient serum to identify potential vaccine candidates. Although BipB was previously shown not to prolong survival of challenged mice, antibody levels against OmpA (one of the two OmpAs which was also found to be protective by Hara et al.) were 10-fold higher in patients that had only one episode of melioidosis relative to those with recurrent disease, again indicating that antibodies specific to this protein may be protective. Another closely related pathogen, Burkholderia cepacia is one of 17 closely related species that comprise the Burkholderia cepacia complex.

This group of pathogens are responsible for chronic lung infections in people with cystic fibrosis and other immunocompromised individuals. The secretory proteins of B. cepacia were analysed on 2-D blots probed with serum from immunised mice. One protein in particular showed a 96% homology with a metalloprotease from a B. pseudomallei strain and it was suggested that this could cross-protect against both pathogens. No in vivo challenge experiments were reported.

Overall, investigation of immunoreactive proteins in B. pseudomallei using immunoproteomics or gene expression libraries has already allowed the identification of vaccine candidates to protect against melioidosis, and further identification of additional antigens should allow the development of a multivalent vaccine which will improve protection against B. pseudomallei and eliminate bacterial persistence. Taking both chronic infection and the intracellular lifestyle of B. pseudomallei into consideration, it is evident that there will be significant challenges in the development of an effective vaccine against this agent. A successful vaccine is likely to need the induction of both humoral and cell-mediated immunity for the complete protection against this pathogen.

Cancer Immunology

Cancer immunology is the study of interactions between the immune system and cancer cells, which is a rapid growing field of research that aims to identify biomarkers in cancer immunodiagnosis and to develop innovative cancer immunotherapeutic strategies. The immune response, including the recognition of cancer-specific antigens, is of particular interest in cancer immunology field, which can further drive the development of new vaccines and antibody therapies. It is also well demonstrated that the immune system can recognize the antigenic changes in cancer cell and further develop antibody against these cellular antigens that have been generally called tumor-associated antigens (TAAs). These cancer-associated anti-TAAs autoantibodies might be considered as "reporters" from the immune system, to identify the antigenic changes in cellular proteins involved in the transformation process. There has been a growing interest in using serum autoantibodies against TAAs as biomarkers in cancer immunodiagnosis. The persistence and stability of these antibodies in the serum samples of cancer patients is an advantage over other potential markers, including the TAAs themselves, some of which are released by tumors but are rapidly degraded or cleared after circulating in the serum for a limited time. In recent years, the potential utility of TAA-autoantibody systems as early cancer biomarker tools to monitor therapeutic outcomes or as indicators of disease prognosis has been explored.

Activation of the immune system for therapeutic benefit in cancer has long been a goal in immunology and oncology. The passive cancer immunotherapy has been well established for several decades, and continued advances in antibody and T-cell engineering should further enhance their clinical impact in the years to come. In contrast to these passive immunotherapy strategies, the active cancer immunotherapy has been proved elusive. In the context of advances in the understanding of how tolerance, immunity, and immunosuppression regulate antitumour immune responses together with the advent of targeted therapies, these successes suggest that active immunotherapy represents a path to obtain a durable and long-lasting response in cancer patients. The key to cancer immunodiagnosis and immunotherapy is an improved understanding of the immune response during malignant transformation.

Computational Immunology

In academia, computational immunology is a field of science that encompasses high-throughput genomic and bioinformatics approaches to immunology. The field's main aim is to convert immunological data into computational problems, solve these problems using mathematical and computational approaches and then convert these results into immunologically meaningful interpretations.

The immune system is a complex system of the human body and understanding it is one of the most challenging topics in biology. Immunology research is important for understanding the mechanisms underlying the defense of human body and to develop drugs for immunological diseases and maintain health. Recent findings in genomic and proteomic technologies have transformed the immunology research drastically. Sequencing of the human and other model organism genomes has produced increasingly large volumes of data relevant to immunology research and at the same time huge amounts of functional and clinical data are being reported in the scientific literature and stored in clinical records. Recent advances in bioinformatics or computational biology were helpful to understand and organize these large scale data and gave rise to new area that is called Computational immunology or immunoinformatics.

Computational immunology is a branch of bioinformatics and it is based on similar concepts and tools, such as sequence alignment and protein structure prediction tools. Immunomics is a discipline like genomics and proteomics. It is a science, which specifically combines Immunology with computer science, mathematics, chemistry, and biochemistry for large-scale analysis of immune system functions. It aims to study the complex protein–protein interactions and networks and allows a better understanding of immune responses and their role during normal, diseased and reconstitution states. Computational immunology is a part of immunomics, which is focused on analyzing large scale experimental data.

Computational immunology began over 90 years ago with the theoretic modeling of malaria epidemiology. At that time, the emphasis was on the use of mathematics to guide the study of disease transmission. Since then, the field has expanded to cover all other aspects of immune system processes and diseases.

Tools

A variety of computational, mathematical and statistical methods are available and reported. These tools are helpful for collection, analysis, and interpretation of immunological data. They include text mining, information management, sequence analysis, analysis of molecular interactions, and mathematical models that enable advanced simulations of immune system and immunological processes. Attempts are being made for the extraction of interesting and complex patterns from non-structured text documents in the immunological domain. Such as categorization of allergen cross-reactivity information, identification of cancer-associated gene variants and the classification of immune epitopes.

Immunoinformatics is using the basic bioinformatics tools such as ClustalW, BLAST, and TreeView, as well as specialized immunoinformatics tools, such as EpiMatrix, IMGT/V-QUEST for IG and TR sequence analysis, IMGT/ Collier-de-Perles and IMGT/StructuralQuery for IG variable domain structure analysis. Methods that rely on sequence comparison are diverse and have been applied to analyze HLA sequence conservation, help verify the origins of human immunodeficiency virus (HIV) sequences, and construct homology models for the analysis of hepatitis B virus polymerase resistance to lamivudine and emtricitabine.

There are also some computational models which focus on protein–protein interactions and networks. There are also tools which are used for T and B cell epitope mapping, proteasomal cleavage site prediction, and TAP– peptide prediction. The experimental data is very much important to design and justify the models to predict various molecular targets. Computational immunology tools is the game between experimental data and mathematically designed computational tools.

Applications

Allergies

Allergies, while a critical subject of immunology, also vary considerably among individuals and sometimes even among genetically similar individuals. The assessment of protein allergenic potential focuses on three main aspects: (i) immunogenicity; (ii) cross-reactivity; and (iii) clinical symptoms. Immunogenicity is due to responses of an IgE antibody-producing B cell and/or of a T cell to a particular allergen. Therefore, immunogenicity studies focus mainly on identifying recognition sites of B-cells and T-cells for allergens. The three-dimensional structural properties of allergens control their allergenicity.

The use of immunoinformatics tools can be useful to predict protein allergenicity and will become increasingly important in the screening of novel foods before their wide-scale release for human use. Thus, there are major efforts under way to make reliable broad based allergy databases and combine these with well validated prediction tools in order to enable the identification of potential allergens in genetically modified drugs and foods. Though the developments are on primary stage, the World Health organization and Food and Agriculture Organization have proposed guidelines for evaluating allergenicity of genetically modified foods. According to the Codex alimentarius, a protein is potentially allergenic if it possesses an identity of ≥ 6 contiguous amino acids or $\geq 35\%$ sequence similarity over an 80 amino acid window with a known allergen. Though there are rules, their inherent limitations have started to become apparent and exceptions to the rules have been well reported.

Infectious Diseases and Host Responses

In the study of infectious diseases and host responses, the mathematical and computer models are a great help. These models were very useful in characterizing the behavior and spread of infectious disease, by understanding the dynamics of the pathogen in the host and the mechanisms of host factors which aid pathogen persistence. Examples include Plasmodium falciparum and nematode infection in ruminants.

Much has been done in understanding immune responses to various pathogens by integrating genomics and proteomics with bioinformatics strategies. Many exciting developments in large-scale screening of pathogens are currently taking place. National Institute of Allergy and Infectious Diseases (NIAID) has initiated an endeavor for systematic mapping of B and T cell epitopes of category A-C pathogens. These pathogens include Bacillus anthracis (anthrax), Clostridium botulinum toxin (botulism), Variola major (smallpox), Francisella tularensis (tularemia), viral hemorrhagic fevers, Burkholderia pseudomallei, Staphylococcus enterotoxin B, yellow fever, influenza, rabies, Chikungunya virus etc. Rule-based systems have been reported for the automated extraction and curation of influenza A records.

This development would lead to the development of an algorithm which would help to identify the conserved regions of pathogen sequences and in turn would be useful for vaccine development. This would be helpful in limiting the spread of infectious disease. Examples include a method for identification of vaccine targets from protein regions of conserved HLA binding and computational assessment of cross-reactivity of broadly neutralizing antibodies against viral pathogens. These examples illustrate the power of immunoinformatics applications to help solve complex problems in public health. Immunoinformatics could accelerate the discovery process dramatically and potentially shorten the time required for vaccine development. Immunoinformatics tools have been used to design the vaccine against Dengue virus and Leishmania.

Immune System Function

Using this technology it is possible to know the model behind immune system. It has been used to model T-cell-mediated suppression, peripheral lymphocyte migration, T-cell memory, tolerance, thymic function, and antibody networks. Models are helpful to predicts dynamics of pathogen toxicity and T-cell memory in response to different stimuli. There are also several models which are helpful in understanding the nature of specificity in immune network and immunogenicity.

For example, it was useful to examine the functional relationship between TAP peptide transport and HLA class I antigen presentation. TAP is a transmembrane protein responsible for the transport of antigenic peptides into the endoplasmic reticulum, where MHC class I molecules can bind them and presented to T cells. As TAP does not bind all peptides equally, TAP-binding affinity could influence the ability of a particular peptide to gain access to the MHC class I pathway. Artificial neural network (ANN), a computer model was used to study peptide binding to human TAP and its relationship with MHC class I binding. The affinity of HLA-binding peptides for TAP was found to differ according to the HLA supertype concerned using this method. This research could have important implications for the design of peptide based immuno-therapeutic drugs and vaccines. It shows the power of the modeling approach to understand complex immune interactions.

There exist also methods which integrate peptide prediction tools with computer simulations that can provide detailed information on the immune response dynamics specific to the given pathogen's peptides.

Cancer Informatics

Cancer is the result of somatic mutations which provide cancer cells with a selective growth advantage. Recently it has been very important to determine the novel mutations. Genomics and proteomics techniques are used worldwide to identify mutations related to each specific cancer and their treatments. Computational tools are used to predict growth and surface antigens on cancerous cells. There are publications explaining a targeted approach for assessing mutations and cancer risk. Algorithm CanPredict was used to indicate how closely a specific gene resembles known cancer-causing genes. Cancer immunology has been given so much importance that the data related to it is growing rapidly. Protein–protein interaction networks provide valuable information on tumorigenesis in humans. Cancer proteins exhibit a network topology that is different from normal proteins in the human interactome. Immunoinformatics have been useful in increasing success of tumour vaccination. Recently, pioneering works have been conducted to analyse the host immune system dynamics in response to artificial immunity induced by vaccination strategies. Other simulation tools use predicted cancer peptides to forecast immune specific anticancer responses that is dependent on the specified HLA. These resources are likely to grow significantly in the near future and immunoinformatics will be a major growth area in this domain.

Immunomics

Immunomics is the study of immune system regulation and response to pathogens using genome-wide approaches. With the rise of genomic and proteomic technologies, scientists have been able to visualize biological networks and infer interrelationships between genes and/or proteins; recently, these technologies have been used to help better understand how the immune system functions and how it is regulated. Two thirds of the genome is active in one or more immune cell types and less than 1% of genes are uniquely expressed in a given type of cell. Therefore, it is critical that the expression patterns of these immune cell types be deciphered in the context of a network, and not as an individual, so that their roles be correctly characterized and related to one another. Defects of the immune system such as autoimmune diseases, immunodeficiency, and malignancies can benefit from genomic insights on pathological processes. For example, analyzing the systematic variation of gene expression can relate these patterns with specific diseases and gene networks important for immune functions.

Traditionally, scientists studying the immune system have had to search for antigens on an individual basis and identify the protein sequence of these antigens ("epitopes") that would stimulate an immune response. This procedure required that antigens be isolated from whole cells, digested into smaller fragments, and tested against T- and B-cells to observe T- and B- cell responses. These classical approaches could only visualize this system as a static condition and required a large amount of time and labor.

Immunomics has made this approach easier by its ability to look at the immune system as a whole and characterize it as a dynamic model. It has revealed that some of the immune system's most distinguishing features are the continuous motility, turnover, and plasticity of its constituent cells. In addition, current genomic technologies, like microarrays, can capture immune system gene expression over time and can trace interactions of microorganisms with cells of the innate immune system. New, proteomic approaches, including T-cell and B-cells-epitope mapping, can also accelerate the pace at which scientists discover antibody-antigen relationships.

A host's immune system responds to pathogen invasion by a set of pathogen-specific responses in which many "players" participate; these include antibodies, T-helper cells, cytotoxic T-cells, and many others. Antigen-presenting cells (APC) are capable of internalizing pathogens and displaying a fragment of the antigen – the epitope - with major histocompatibility complexes (MHCs) on the cell surface. T-cell response is initiated when T-cells recognize these displayed epitopes. Only specific peptide sequences from some pathogen-specific antigens are needed to stimulate T-and B-cell responses; that is, the whole pathogenic peptide sequence is not necessary to initiate an immune response. The 'immunome' of a pathogen is described by its set of epitopes, and can be defined by comparing genome sequences and applying immunoinformatic tools.

Ash Alizadeh et al. were some of the first to recognize the potential of cDNA microarrays to define gene expression of immune cells. Their analysis probed gene expression of human B and T lymphocytes during cellular activation and/or stimulation with cytokines, a type of signaling regulatory molecule. Many of the activated genes in stimulated T lymphocytes were known to be involved in the G0/G1 cell cycle transition or encoding for chemokines, signaling molecules involved in inflammatory response. This team was also able to visualize temporal patterns of gene expression during T cell mitogenesis. In the concluding paragraphs of their landmark paper, these scientists state "virtually every corner of immunological research will benefit from cDNA microarray analysis of gene expression," and, thus, heralded the rise of immunomics.

Limited by available microarrays and a non-complete human genome at this point in time, this same set of researchers were motivated to create a specialized microarray that focused on genes preferentially expressed in a given cell type, or known to be functionally important in a given biological process. As a result, they designed the "Lymphochip" cDNA microarray, which contained 13,000 genes and was enriched for genes of importance to the immune system.

Iyer et al.'s 1999 article was another to reveal the importance of applying genomic technologies to immunological research. Although not intending to address any aspect of immunity at the start of their experiment, these researchers observed that the expression profiles of serum-stimulated fibroblasts were far richer than anticipated and suggested an important physiological role for fibroblasts in healing wounds. The serum-induced genes have been associated with processes relevant to wound healing, including genes directly involved in remodeling the clot and extracellular matrix, as well as genes encoding signal proteins for inflammation, the development of new blood vessels, and regrowth of epithelial tissue. Additionally, one of the most significant results of this expression analysis was the discovery of more than 200 previously unknown genes whose expression was temporally regulated during the response of fibroblasts to serum. These results revealed the importance of viewing the immune response as a collaborative physiological program and begged for further study of the immune system as a network, and not just as individual pieces.

In 2006, Moutaftsi et al. demonstrated that epitope-mapping tools could accurately identify the epitopes responsible for 95% of the murine T-cell response to vaccinia virus. Through their work, these scientists introduced the interdisciplinary realm of informatics and immunology while employing genomic, proteomic, and immunological data. The striking success and ease of this method encouraged researchers both to define the immunome of other pathogens, and to measure the breadth and overlap of pathogen immunomes that give rise to immunity. Additionally, it suggested other applications in which epitope-mapping tools could be used including autoimmunity, transplantation, and immunogenicity.

Technologies Used

Immunomic Microarrays

Several types of microarrays have been created to specifically observe the immune system response and interactions. Antibody microarrays use antibodies as probes and antigens as targets. They can be used to directly measure the antigen concentrations for which the antibody probes are specific. Peptide microarrays use antigen peptides as probes and serum antibodies as targets. These can be used for functional immunomic applications to the understanding of autoimmune diseases and allergies, definition of B-cell epitopes, vaccine studies, detection assays, and analysis of antibody specificity. MHC microarrays are the most recent development in immunomic arrays and use peptide-MHC complexes and their co-stimulatory molecules as probes and T-cell populations as targets. Bound T-cells are activated and secrete cytokines, which are captured by specific detection antibodies. This microarray can map MHC-restricted T cell epitopes.

Lymphochip

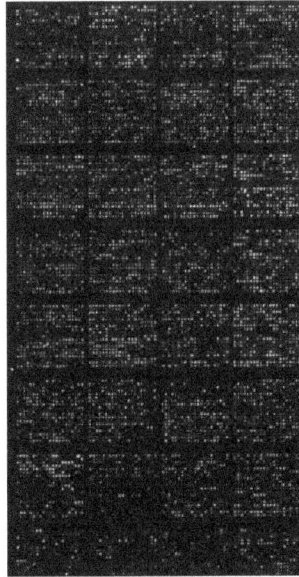

The Lymphochip: A specialized cDNA microarray.

The Lymphochip is a specialized human cDNA microarray enriched for genes related to immune function. 17,853 cDNA clones were taken from three sources. The first set of clones were selected if identified expressed sequence tags (ESTs) were unique or enriched specifically in lymphoid cDNA libraries; these represent ~80% of the Lymphochip clones. The second set of clones was identified during first-generation microarray analysis of immune responses. Finally, 3,183 genes that are known or suspected to have roles in immune function, oncogenesis, apoptosis, cell proliferation, or being open reading frames from pathogenic human viruses were used on the Lymphochip. New genes are frequently being added.

T- and B-cell-epitope Mapping Tools

Epitope mapping identifies the sites of antibodies to which their target antigens bind. In the past, scientists would have to isolate antigens, digest them into smaller fragments, and determine which of these fragments stimulated T- and B- cell responses to define an antibody's epitope. Immunomics harnesses the power of bioinformatics and offers mapping algorithms that accelerate the discovery of epitope sequences. These algorithms are relevant to vaccine design and for characterizing and modifying immune responses in the context of autoimmunity, endocrinology, allergy, transplantation, diagnostics and engineering of therapeutic proteins.

T-cell and B-cell epitope mapping algorithms can computationally predict epitopes based on the genomic sequence of pathogens, without prior knowledge of a protein's structure or function. A series of steps are used to identify epitopes:

- Comparison between virulent and avirulent organisms identify candidate genes that code for epitopes that solicit T-cell responses by looking for sequences that are unique to virulent strains. Additionally, differential microarray technologies can discover pathogen-specific genes that are upregulated during host-interaction and may be relevant for analysis because they are critical to the function of the pathogen.

- Immunoinformatics tools predict regions of these candidate genes that interact with T cells by scanning genome-derived protein sequences of a pathogen.

- These predicted peptides are synthesized and used in in vitro screening against T cells. Recognizing a positive immune response can suggest that this peptide contains an epitope that stimulates immune response in the course of natural infection or disease.

Available Mapping Tools

- EpiMatrix
- TEPITOPE
- Multipred
- MHC Thread
- MHCPred
- NetMHC
- LpPep
- BIMAS

Tetramer Staining by Flow Cytometry

The guiding principle behind flow cytometry is that cells or subcellular particles are tagged with fluorescent probes are passed through a laser beam and sorted by the strength of fluorescence emitted by cells contained in the droplets. MHC [tetramer staining] by flow cytometry identifies and isolates specific T cells based on the binding specificity of their cell surface receptors with fluorescently-tagged MHC-peptide complexes.

Elispot

ELISPOT is a modified version of the ELISA immunoassay and is a common method of monitoring immune responses.

Contributions to Understanding the Immune System

Immunomics has made a considerable impact on the understanding of the immune system by uncovering differences in gene expression profiles of cell types, characterizing immune response, illuminating immune cell lineages and relationship, and establishing gene regulatory networks. Whereas the following list of contributions is not complete, it is meant to demonstrate the broad application of immunomic research and powerful consequences on immunology.

Immune Cell Activation and Differentiation

B Lymphocyte Anergy

Microarrays have discovered gene expression patterns that correlate with antigen-induced activation or anergy in B lymphocytes. Lymphocyte anergy pathways involve induction of some, but not all of the signaling pathways used during lymphocyte activation. For example, NFAT and MAPK/ERK kinase pathways are expressed in anergic (or "tolerant") cell lines, whereas NF-kB and c-Jun N-terminal kinases pathways are not. Of the 300 genes that were altered in expression after antigen-stimulated naïve B cells, only 8 of these genes were regulated in tolerant B cells. Understanding these "tolerance" pathways have important implications for designing immunosuppressive drugs. These gene expression signatures of tolerant B cells could be used during drug screens to probe for compounds that mimic the functional effects of natural tolerance.

Lymphocyte Differentiation

Gene expression profiles during human lymphocyte differentiation has followed mature, naïve B cells from their resting state through germinal center reactions and into terminal differentiation. These studies have shown that germinal center B cells represent a distinct stage in differentiation because the gene expression profile is different from activated peripheral B cells. Although no in vitro culture system has been able to induce resting peripheral B cells to adopt a full germinal center phenotype, these gene expression profiles can be used to measure the success of in vitro cultures in mimicking the germinal center state as they are being developed.

Lymphoid Malignancies

About 9 of every 10 human lymphoid cancers derive from B cells. Distinct immunome-wide expression patterns in a large number of diffuse large cell lymphoma (DLCL)– the most common form of non-Hodgkin's lymphoma – have identified at least two different subtypes in what was previously thought to be a single disease. One subset of these DLCLs shows a similar gene expression pattern to that of normal germinal center B cells and implies that the tumor cell originated from a germinal center B cell. Other surveys of B cell malignancies show that follicular lymphomas share expression features with germinal center B cells, whereas chronic lymphocytic leukemia cells resemble resting peripheral blood lymphocytes. Furthermore, heterogeneity in each of these cell lines also suggest that different subtypes exist within each type of lymphoma, just as it has been shown in DLCL. Such knowledge can be used to direct patients to the most appropriate therapy.

Immune Response

Macrophage Responses to Bacteria

Microarrays have analyzed global responses of macrophages to different microorganisms and have confirmed that these responses sustain and control inflammatory processes, and also kill microorganisms. These independent studies have been able to better describe how macrophages mount attacks against different microorganisms. A "core transcriptional response" was observed to induce 132 genes and repress 59 genes. Induced genes include pro-inflammatory chemokines and cytokines, and their respective receptors. A "pathogen-specific response" was also observed.

Dendritic Response to Pathogen

Dendritic cells (DCs) help macrophages sustain inflammatory processes and participate in the innate immune system response, but can also prime adaptive immunity. Gene expression analyses have shown that DCs can "multi-task" by temporally segregating their different functions. Soon after recognizing an infectious agent, immature DCs transition to a state of early activation via a core response characterized by rapid downregulation of genes involved with pathogen recognition and phagocytosis, upregulation of cytokine and chemokine genes to recruit other immune cells to the side of inflammations; and expression of genes that control migratory capacity. Early activated DCs are enabled to migrate from non-lymphoid tissues to lymph nodes, where they can prime T-cell responses. These early DCs responses are related to innate immunity and consist of the "core transcriptional response" of DCs. Pathogen-specific responses have a stronger influence on the DC's ability to regulate adaptive immunity.

Distinguishing Immune Cell Types

Comparing distinctions between immune cells' overall transcriptional program can generate plots that position each cell type to best reflect its expression profile relative to all other cells and can reveal interesting relationships between cell types. For example, the transcriptional profiles from thymic medullary epithelial immune cells mapped closer to lymphocytes than to other epithelia. This can suggest that a functional interaction exists between these two cells type and requires the sharing of particular transcripts and proteins. When comparing gene expression profiles from cells of the blood system, T-cell and B-cell subsets tightly group with their respective cell types.

By looking at the transcriptional profile of different T-cells, scientists have shown that natural killer T-cells are a close variant of conventional CD4+ T cells, rather than an intermediary cell-type between T cells and natural killer cells. Additionally, DCs, natural killer cells, and B cells are tightly grouped based on their global expression profiles. It may have been expected that B lymphocytes and T lymphocytes would cluster separately from each other, or that natural killer cells would be more closely related to T cells because they share common precursors, cytolytic activity, and similar activation markers. Therefore, immunomics has established relationship between cell lineages that depart from classical views. Additionally, it may better explain the observed plasticity in lymphoid and myeloid cell differentiation because of the considerable overlap between global expression profiles of these different lineages.

Immune Cell Regulatory Networks

Networks represent the broadest level of genetic interactions and aim to link all genes and transcripts in the immunological genome. Cellular phenotypes and differentiation states are ultimately established by the activity of these networks of co-regulated genes. One of the most complete networks in immunology has deciphered regulatory connections among normal and transformed human B cells. This analysis suggests a hierarchical network where a small number of highly connected genes (called "hubs") regulated most interactions. Proto-oncogene MYC emerged as a major hub and highly influential regulator for B cells. Notably, MYC was found to directly control BYSL, a highly conserved, but poorly characterized gene, and is the largest hub in the whole B cell network. This suggests that BYSL encodes an important cellular molecule and a critical effecter of MYC function, and motivates additional studies to elucidate its function. Therefore, using gene expression data to create networks can reveal genes highly influential in immune cell differentiation that pre-genomic technologies had not yet identified.

Practical Applications

Vaccine Development

As quoted by Stefania Bambini and Rino Rappuoli, "New powerful genomics technologies have increased the number of disease that can be addressed by vaccination, and decreased the time for discover research and vaccine development." The availability of complete genome sequences of pathogens in combination with high-throughput genomics technologies have helped to accelerate vaccine development. Reverse vaccinology uses genomic sequences of viral, bacterial, or parasitic pathogens to identify genes potentially encoding genes that promote pathogenesis. The first application of reverse vaccinology identified vaccine candidates against Neisseria meningitidis serogroup B. Computational tools identified 600 putative surface-exposed or secreted proteins from the complete genome sequence of a MenB pathogenic strain, on the basis of sequence features. These putative proteins were expressed in E. coli, purified, and used to immunize mice. Tests using mice immune sera estimated the ability of antibodies to protect against these proteins. The proteins able to solicit a robust immune response were checked for sequence conservation across a panel of meningitides strains and allowed for further selection of antigen able to elicit an immune response against most strains in the panel. On the basis of these antigen sequences, scientists have been able to develop a universal "cocktail" vaccine against Neisseria meninitidis that uses five antigens to promote immunity. Similar approaches have been used for a variety of other human pathogens, such as Streptococcus pneumoniae, Chlamydia pneumoniae, Bacillus anthracis, Porphyromonas gingivalis, Mycobacterium tuberculosis, Helicobacter pylori, amongst others. Additionally, studies have started for the development of vaccines against viruses.

Disease Diagnosis

The inventory of receptors and signal transduction pathways that immune cells use to monitor and defend the body gives rise to signature patterns of altered gene expression in peripheral blood cells that reflect the character of the infection or injury. Therefore, recognizing characteristic expression profiles of peripheral blood cells may be a powerful diagnostic tool by recruiting these cells as "spies" to detect occult diseases or agents that cannot be readily cultured from the host.

For example, cytomegalovirus (CMV) infection of fibroblasts and HTLV-I infection of T lymphocytes revealed distinct gene expression profiles. CMV infection provoked a unique interferon response whereas HTLV-1 infection induced NF-kB target genes. A type of white blood cells have also been tested again bacterial exposures and immunome expression varied based on the type of bacterial strain used.

Monitoring the change of peripheral blood gene expression can also help determine the course of infection and help treat patients with a therapy tailored to their disease stage. This approach has already been used against sepsis – a disease that progresses through a predictable line of events. Changes gene expression signatures may precede clinical exacerbation of symptoms, like in multiple sclerosis, and allow physicians to nip these "flare-ups" in the bud.

Immunological Genome Project

The immune system is a network of genetic and signaling pathways connected by a network of interacting cells. The Immunological Genome Project seeks to generate a complete compendium of protein-coding gene expression for all cell populations in the mouse immune system. It analyzes both steady-state conditions within different cell populations, and in response to genetic and/or environmental perturbations created by natural genetic polymorphism, gene knock-out, gene knock-down by RNAi, or drug treatment. Computational tools to reverse-engineer or predict immune cell regulatory networks use these expression profiles.

By 2008, the ImmGen project involved seven immunology and three computational biology laboratories across the United States and over 200 cell populations involved in the immune system had been identified and described. This consortium has created a data browser to explore the expression patterns of particular genes, networks of co-regulated genes, and genes that can reliably distinguish cell types. Raw data is also accessible from the NCBI's Gene Expression Omnibus.

Psychoneuroimmunology

Psychoneuroimmunology (PNI) is a relatively new field of study that looks at the interactions between your central nervous system (CNS) and your immune system. Researchers know that our CNS and immune system can communicate with each other, but they only recently started to understand how they do it and what it means for our health.

The nerves in your brain and spinal cord make up your CNS, while your immune system is made up of organs and cells that defend your body against infection. Both systems produce small molecules and proteins that can act as messengers between the two systems. In your CNS, these messengers include hormones and neurotransmitters. Your immune system, on the other hand, uses proteins called cytokines to communicate with your CNS.

There's plenty of existing research about the effects of stress on the immune system. Many of these studies focus on the release of cytokines in response to both physical and psychological stress.

A cytokine is a small protein that's released by cells, especially those in your immune system. There are many types of cytokines, but the ones that are generally stimulated by stress are called pro-inflammatory cytokines.

Under normal circumstances, your body releases pro-inflammatory cytokines in response to an infection or injury to help destroy germs or repair tissue. When you're physically or emotionally stressed, your body also releases certain hormones, including epinephrine (adrenaline). These hormones can bind to specific receptors that signal for the production of pro-inflammatory cytokines.

Examples of PNI

Psoriasis

Psoriasis is a great example of how your immune system, CNS, mental health, and stress levels are all intertwined. It's a chronic condition that causes your skin cells to grow too quickly. Your body usually sheds extra skin cells, but if you have psoriasis, these extra cells build up on your skin's surface. This can lead to intense itching and pain.

The overgrowth of skin cells in psoriasis is due to the release of cytokines from your immune system. We know that psychological stress may worsen or trigger episodes of psoriasis. Indeed, people with psoriasis tend to have increased levels of cortisol, a stress hormone.

Your hypothalamus, which is part of your CNS, is responsible for cortisol production. When it senses stressors, it signals your nearby pituitary gland, which signals for cortisol production. This, in turn, can trigger the release of pro-inflammatory cytokines by your immune system. These cytokines then trigger an overgrowth of skin cells.

In addition, people with psoriasis often report having psychological conditions, such as depression, increased stress, and suicidal thoughts. Previous research has linked an increase in cytokine levels with major depression.

There's currently no cure for psoriasis, but new developments in the field of PNI could change this in the future.

Cancer

A 2013 review Trusted Source of many studies exploring the relationship between PNI and cancer found evidence to suggest that:

- Women with genetic risk factors for developing cancer showed immune system abnormalities in response to stress.

- There appears to be a link in people with breast cancer between depression, the quality of social support they have, and immune cell activity.

- People with breast, cervical, or ovarian cancer who reported feeling stressed or lonely had abnormalities in their immune systems.

- Communication between the immune system and brain may impact symptoms that are related to cancer treatment, including fatigue, depression, and difficulty sleeping.

- Stressful experiences and depression may be associated with a poorer survival rate for several types of cancer.

Coronary Artery Disease

A review from 2010 looking at the relationship between stress, immune function, and coronary artery disease echoed other studies suggesting that psychological stress increases the production of pro-inflammatory cytokines.

This increase in pro-inflammatory cytokines is associated with an increase in heart rate and blood pressure. In addition, the production of cytokines by your immune system promotes feelings of sickness or fatigue. According to this review, this reaction isn't immediately harmful. However, long-term stress and cytokine production may contribute to the development of cardiac disease.

Reproductive Immunology

Reproductive immunology refers to a field of medicine that studies interactions (or the absence of them) between the immune system and components related to the reproductive system, such as maternal immune tolerance towards the fetus, or immunological interactions across the blood-testis barrier. The concept has been used by fertility clinics to explain the fertility problems, recurrent miscarriages and pregnancy complications observed when this state of immunological tolerance is not successfully achieved. Immunological therapy is the new up and coming method for treating many cases of previously "unexplained infertility" or recurrent miscarriage.

Between Mother and Fetus

The fact that the embryo's tissue is half foreign and unlike mismatched organ transplant, it is not normally rejected, suggests that the immunological system of the mother plays an important role in pregnancy. The placenta also plays an important part in protecting the embryo for the immune attack from the mother's system. Studies also propose that proteins in semen may help woman's immune system prepare for conception and pregnancy. For example, there is substantial evidence for exposure to partner's semen as prevention for pre-eclampsia, largely due to the absorption of several immune modulating factors present in seminal fluid, such as transforming growth factor beta (TGFβ).

Sperm Cells within a Male

The presence of anti-sperm antibodies in infertile men was first reported in 1954 by Rumke and Wilson. It has been noticed that the number of cases of sperm autoimmunity is higher in the infertile population leading to the idea that autoimmunity could be a cause of infertility. Anti sperm antigen has been described as three immunoglobulin isotopes (IgG, IgA, IgM) each of which targets different part of the spermatozoa. If more than 10% of the sperm are bound to anti-sperm antibodies (ASA), then infertility is suspected. The blood-testis barrier separates the immune system and the developing spermatozoa. The tight junction between the Sertoli cells form the blood-testis barrier but it is usually breached by physiological leakage. Not all sperms are protected by the barrier because spermatogonia and early spermatocytes are located below the junction. They are protected by other means like immunologic tolerance and immunomodulation.

Infertility after anti-sperm antibody binding can be caused by autoagglutination, sperm cytotoxicity, blockage of sperm-ovum interaction, and inadequate motility. Each presents itself depending on the binding site of ASA.

Immunocontraceptive Vaccine

Experiments are undergoing to test the effectiveness of an immunocontraceptive vaccine that inhibits the fusing of spermatozoa to the zona pellucida. This vaccine is currently being tested in animals and hopefully will be an effective contraceptive for humans. Normally, spermatozoa fuse with the zona pellucida surrounding the mature oocyte; the resulting acrosome reaction breaks down the egg's tough coating so that the sperm can fertilize the ovum. The mechanism of the vaccine is injection with cloned ZP cDNA, therefore this vaccine is a DNA based vaccine. This results in the production of antibodies against the ZP, which stop the sperm from binding to the zona pellucida and ultimately from fertilizing the ovum.

Another vaccine in investigation is one against HCG. This immunization would produce antibodies against hCG and TT. Antibodies against hCG would prevent the maintenance of the uterus for a viable pregnancy therefore preventing conception. Another vaccine that is utilized is the peptide β-hCG that is more specific to hCG and a more rapid and effective response occurs in the absence of LH, FSH, and TSH.

Palaeoimmunology

Palaeoimmunology or paleo-immunology ("paleo"=ancient, "immuno"=referring to immunology) is the analysis using histochemical techniques to look at the matrix proteins in historic and pre-historic materials. Modern immunological assays are used to detect the presence of specific antigens in the sample material. Specimens subject to immunoassays have usually been preserved in a way that has prevented biomolecular targets from degrading. This has either been achieved through natural preservative circumstances, such as accelerated fossilization, or through artificial mummification. Regardless of the path taken to achieve this state, preservation has occurred before the denaturing of antigenic targets. The purpose of applying immunological assays to archaeological materials is to better understand the biochemical makeup and composition of these pre-historic samples. Antigenic elements within these materials may reveal information regarding the "life" and "death" of the sample being studied.

Examples of Use

Paleo-immunology encompasses a variety of immunoassays performed on a diverse array of archaeological materials. Paleo-immunology is a new, growing field that is still being properly defined. Examples of paleo-immunology as they appear in peer reviewed literature are as follows:

- The extraction and analysis of collagen peptides from fossilized bones.

- The use of immunofluorescence and immunohistochemical techniques in order to study the proteins of the extracellular matrix found in mummified tissues. This was done to further understand the physiologic and pathologic alterations that can occur in preserved prehistoric tissues.

- A plague dipstick assay was used to detect the presence of plague antigens in medieval French graves. This paleo-immunological assay is also known as a "rapid diagnostic test for the plague" (RDT).

- Enzyme linked immunosorbent assay (ELISA) was used to detect remnant antigenic structures in preserved sauropod eggshells.

- The ParaSight-F test has been used to detect malaria antigens in Egyptian mummies.

Systems Immunology

Systems immunology is a recent research field that, under the larger umbrella of systems biology, aims to study the immune system in the more integrated perspective on how entities and players participate at different system levels to the immune function.

The immune system has been thoroughly analyzed as regards to its components and function by using a very successful "reductionist" approach, but its overall functioning principles cannot easily be predicted by studying the properties of its isolated components because they strongly rely on and arise from the interactions among these numerous constituents. Systems immunology represents a different approach for the integrated comprehension of the immune system structure and function based on complex systems theory, high-throughput techniques, as well as on mathematical and computational tools.

Immunotoxicology

Immunotoxicology has been defined as "the discipline concerned with the study of the events that can lead to undesired effects as a result of interaction of xenobiotics with the immune system. These undesired events may result as a consequence of (1) a direct and/or indirect effect of the xenobiotic (and/or its biotransformation product) on the immune system, or (2) an immunologically based host response to the compound and/or its metabolite(s), or host antigens modified by the compound or its metabolites".

When the immune system acts as a passive target of chemical insults, the result can be decreased resistance to infection and certain forms of neoplasia, or immune disregulation/stimulation that can exacerbate allergy or auto-immunity. In the case that the immune system responds to the antigenic specificity of the xenobiotic or host antigen modified by the compound, toxicity can become manifest as allergies or autoimmune diseases.

Animal models to investigate chemical-induced immune suppression have been developed, and a number of these methods are validated. For testing purposes, a tiered approach is followed to make an adequate selection from the overwhelming number of assays available. Generally, the objective of the first tier is to identify potential immunotoxicants. If potential immunotoxicity is identified, a second tier of testing is performed to confirm and characterize further the changes observed. Third-tier investigations include special studies on the mechanism of action of the compound. Several xenobiotics have been identified as immunotoxicants causing immunosuppression in such studies with laboratory animals.

The database on immune function disturbances in humans by environmental chemicals is limited. The use of markers of immunotoxicity has received little attention in clinical and epidemiological studies to investigate the effect of these chemicals on human health. Such studies have not been performed frequently, and their interpretation often does not permit unequivocal conclusions to be drawn, due for instance to the uncontrolled nature of exposure. Therefore, at present, immunotoxicity assessment in rodents, with subsequent extrapolation to man, forms the basis of decisions regarding hazard and risk.

Hypersensitivity reactions, notably allergic asthma and contact dermatitis, are important occupational health problems in industrialized countries. The phenomenon of contact sensitization was investigated first in the guinea pig. Until recently this has been the species of choice for predictive testing. Many guinea pig test methods are available, the most frequently employed being the guinea pig maximization test and the occluded patch test of Buehler. Guinea pig tests and newer approaches developed in mice, such as ear swelling tests and the local lymph node assay, provide the toxicologist with the tools to assess skin sensitization hazard. The situation with respect to sensitization of the respiratory tract is very different. There are, as yet, no well-validated or widely accepted methods available for the identification of chemical respiratory allergens although progress in the development of animal models for the investigation of chemical respiratory allergy has been achieved in the guinea pig and mouse.

Human data show that chemical agents, in particular drugs, can cause autoimmune diseases. There are a number of experimental animal models of human autoimmune diseases. Such comprise both spontaneous pathology (for example systemic lupus erythematosus in New Zealand Black mice) and autoimmune phenomena induced by experimental immunization with a cross-reactive autoantigen (for example the H37Ra adjuvant induced arthritis in Lewis strain rats). These models are applied in the preclinical evaluation of immunosuppressive drugs. Very few studies have addressed the potential of these models for assessment of whether a xenobiotic exacerbates induced or congenital autoimmunity. Animal models that are suitable to investigate the ability of chemicals to induce autoimmune diseases are virtually lacking. One model that is used to a limited extent is the popliteal lymph node assay in mice. Like the situation in humans, genetic factors play a crucial role in the development of autoimmune disease (AD) in laboratory animals, which will limit the predictive value of such tests.

Immune System

The major function of the immune system is defence against bacteria, viruses, parasites, fungi and neoplastic cells. This is achieved by the actions of various cell types and their soluble mediators in a finely tuned concert. The host defence can be roughly divided into non-specific or innate resistance and specific or acquired immunity mediated by lymphocytes.

Components of the immune system are present throughout the body. The lymphocyte compartment is found within lymphoid organs. The bone marrow and thymus are classified as primary or central lymphoid organs; the secondary or peripheral lymphoid organs include lymph nodes, spleen and lymphoid tissue along secretory surfaces such as the gastrointestinal and respiratory tracts, the so-called mucosa-associated lymphoid tissue (MALT). About half of the body's lymphocytes are located at any one time in MALT. In addition the skin is an important organ for the induction of immune responses to antigens present on the skin. Important in this process are epidermal Langerhans cells that have an antigen-presenting function.

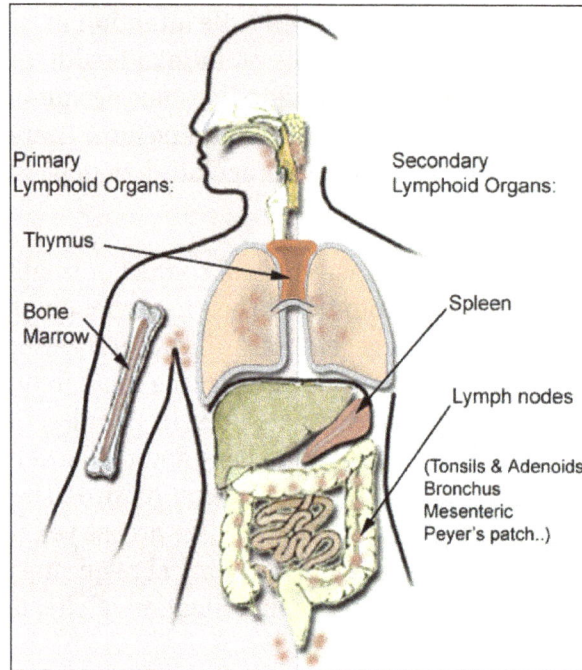

Primary and secondary lymphoid organs and tissues.

Phagocytic cells of the monocyte/macrophage lineage, called the mononuclear phagocyte system (MPS), occur in lymphoid organs and also at extranodal sites; the extranodal phagocytes include Kupffer cells in the liver, alveolar macrophages in the lung, mesangial macrophages in the kidney and glial cells in the brain. Polymorphonuclear leukocytes (PMNs) are present mainly in blood and bone marrow, but accumulate at sites of inflammation.

Non-specific Defence

A first line of defence to micro-organisms is executed by a physical and chemical barrier, such as at the skin, the respiratory tract and the alimentary tract. This barrier is helped by non-specific protective mechanisms including phagocytic cells, such as macrophages and polymorphonuclear leukocytes, which are able to kill pathogens, and natural killer cells, which can lyse tumour cells and virus-infected cells. The complement system and certain microbial inhibitors (e.g., lysozyme) also take part in the non-specific response.

Specific Immunity

After initial contact of the host with the pathogen, specific immune responses are induced. The hallmark of this second line of defence is specific recognition of determinants, so-called antigens or epitopes, of the pathogens by receptors on the cell surface of B- and T-lymphocytes. Following interaction with the specific antigen, the receptor-bearing cell is stimulated to undergo proliferation and differentiation, producing a clone of progeny cells that are specific for the eliciting antigen. The specific immune responses help the non-specific defence presented to the pathogens by stimulating the efficacy of the non-specific responses. A fundamental characteristic of specific immunity is that memory develops. Secondary contact with the same antigen provokes a faster and more vigorous but well-regulated response.

The genome does not have the capacity to carry the codes of an array of antigen receptors sufficient to recognize the number of antigens that can be encountered. The repertoire of specificity develops by a process of gene rearrangements. This is a random process, during which various specificities are brought about. This includes specificities for self components, which are undesirable. A selection process that takes place in the thymus (T cells), or bone marrow (B cells) operates to delete these undesirable specificities.

Normal immune effector function and homeostatic regulation of the immune response is dependent upon a variety of soluble products, known collectively as cytokines, which are synthesized and secreted by lymphocytes and by other cell types. Cytokines have pleiotropic effects on immune and inflammatory responses. Cooperation between different cell populations is required for the immune response—the regulation of antibody responses, the accumulation of immune cells and molecules at inflammatory sites, the initiation of acute phase responses, the control of macrophage cytotoxic function and many other processes central to host resistance. These are influenced by, and in many cases are dependent upon, cytokines acting individually or in concert.

Two arms of specific immunity are recognized—humoral immunity and cell-mediated or cellular immunity:

Humoral immunity: In the humoral arm B-lymphocytes are stimulated following recognition of antigen by cell-surface receptors. Antigen receptors on B-lymphocytes are immunoglobulins (Ig). Mature B cells (plasma cells) start the production of antigen-specific immunoglobulins that act as antibodies in serum or along mucosal surfaces. There are five major classes of immunoglobulins: (1) IgM, pentameric Ig with optimal agglutinating capacity, which is first produced after antigenic stimulation; (2) IgG, the main Ig in circulation, which can pass the placenta; (3) IgA, secretory Ig for the protection of mucosal surfaces; (4) IgE, Ig fixing to mast cells or basophilic granulocytes involved in immediate hypersensitivity reactions and (5) IgD, whose major function is as a receptor on B-lymphocytes.

Cell-mediated immunity: The cellular arm of the specific immune system is mediated by T-lymphocytes. These cells also have antigen receptors on their membranes. They recognize antigen if presented by antigen presenting cells in the context of histocompatibility antigens. Hence, these cells have a restriction in addition to the antigen specificity. T cells function as helper cells for various (including humoral) immune responses, mediate recruitment of inflammatory cells, and can, as cytotoxic T cells, kill target cells after antigen-specific recognition.

Mechanisms of Immunotoxicity

Immunosuppression

Effective host resistance is dependent upon the functional integrity of the immune system, which in turn requires that the component cells and molecules which orchestrate immune responses are available in sufficient numbers and in an operational form. Congenital immunodeficiencies in humans are often characterized by defects in certain stem cell lines, resulting in impaired or absent production of immune cells. By analogy with congenital and acquired human immunodeficiency diseases, chemical-induced immunosuppression may result simply from a reduced number of functional cells. The absence, or reduced numbers, of lymphocytes may have more or less profound effects on immune status. Some immunodeficiency states and severe immunosuppression, as can occur in transplantation or cytostatic therapy, have been associated in particular with increased incidences of opportunistic infections and of certain neoplastic diseases. The infections can be bacterial, viral, fungal or protozoan, and the predominant type of infection depends on the associated immunodeficiency. Exposure to immunosuppressive environmental chemicals may be expected to result in more subtle forms of immunosuppression, which may be difficult to detect. These may lead, for example, to an increased incidence of infections such as influenza or the common cold.

In view of the complexity of the immune system, with the wide variety of cells, mediators and functions that form a complicated and interactive network, immunotoxic compounds have numerous opportunities to exert an effect. Although the nature of the initial lesions induced by many immunotoxic chemicals have not yet been elucidated, there is increasing information available, mostly derived from studies in laboratory animals, regarding the immunobiological changes which result in depression of immune function. Toxic effects might occur at the following critical functions (and some examples are given of immunotoxic compounds affecting these functions):

- Development and expansion of different stem cell populations (benzene exerts immunotoxic effects at the stem cell level, causing lymphocytopenia).

- Proliferation of various lymphoid and myeloid cells as well as supportive tissues in which these cells mature and function (immunotoxic organotin compounds suppress the proliferative activity of lymphocytes in the thymic cortex through direct cytotoxicity; the thymotoxic action of 2,3,7,8-tetrachloro-dibenzo-p-dioxin (TCDD) and related compounds is likely due to an impaired function of thymic epithelial cells, rather than to direct toxicity for thymocytes).

- Antigen uptake, processing and presentation by macrophages and other antigen-presenting cells (one of the targets of 7,12-dimethylbenz(a)anthracene (DMBA) and of lead is antigen presentation by macrophages; a target of ultraviolet radiation is the antigen-presenting Langerhans cell).

- Regulatory function of T-helper and T-suppressor cells (T-helper cell function is impaired by organotins, aldicarb, polychlorinated biphenyls (PCBs), TCDD and DMBA; T-suppressor cell function is reduced by low-dose cyclophosphamide treatment).

- Production of various cytokines or interleukins (benzo(a)pyrene (BP) suppresses interleukin-1 production; ultraviolet radiation alters production of cytokines by keratinocytes).

- Synthesis of various classes of immunoglobulins IgM and IgG is suppressed following PCB and tributyltin oxide (TBT) treatment, and increased after hexachlorobenzene (HCB) exposure).

- Complement regulation and activation (affected by TCDD).

- Cytotoxic T cell function (3-methylcholanthrene (3-MC), DMBA, and TCDD suppress cytotoxic T cell activity).

- Natural killer (NK) cell function (pulmonary NK activity is suppressed by ozone; splenic NK activity is impaired by nickel).

- Macrophage and polymorphonuclear leukocyte chemotaxis and cytotoxic functions (ozone and nitrogen dioxide impair the phagocytic activity of alveolar macrophages).

Allergy

Allergy may be defined as the adverse health effects which result from the induction and elicitation of specific immune responses. When hypersensitivity reactions occur without involvement of the immune system the term pseudo-allergy is used. In the context of immunotoxicology, allergy results from a specific immune response to chemicals and drugs that are of interest. The ability of a chemical to sensitize individuals is generally related to its ability to bind covalently to body proteins. Allergic reactions may take a variety of forms and these differ with respect to both the underlying immunological mechanisms and the speed of the reaction. Four major types of allergic reactions have been recognized: Type I hypersensitivity reactions, which are effectuated by IgE antibody and where symptoms are manifest within minutes of exposure of the sensitized individual. Type II hypersensitivity reactions result from the damage or destruction of host cells by antibody. In this case symptoms become apparent within hours. Type III hypersensitivity, or Arthus, reactions are also antibody mediated, but against soluble antigen, and result from the local or systemic action of immune complexes. Type IV, or delayed-type hypersensitivity, reactions are effected by T-lymphocytes and normally symptoms develop 24 to 48 hours following exposure of the sensitized individual.

The two types of chemical allergy of greatest relevance to occupational health are contact sensitivity or skin allergy and allergy of the respiratory tract.

Contact hypersensitivity: A large number of chemicals are able to cause skin sensitization. Following topical exposure of a susceptible individual to a chemical allergen, a T-lymphocyte response is induced in the draining lymph nodes. In the skin the allergen interacts directly or indirectly with epidermal Langerhans cells, which transport the chemical to the lymph nodes and present it in an immunogenic form to responsive T-lymphocytes. Allergen- activated T-lymphocytes proliferate, resulting in clonal expansion. The individual is now sensitized and will respond to a second dermal exposure to the same chemical with a more aggressive immune response, resulting in allergic contact dermatitis. The cutaneous inflammatory reaction which characterizes allergic contact dermatitis is secondary to the recognition of the allergen in the skin by specific T-lymphocytes. These lymphocytes become activated, release cytokines and cause the local accumulation of other mononuclear leukocytes. Symptoms develop some 24 to 48 hours following exposure of the sensitized individual, and allergic contact dermatitis therefore represents a form of delayed-type hypersensitivity. Common causes of allergic contact dermatitis include organic chemicals (such as 2,4-dinitrochlorobenzene), metals (such as nickel and chromium) and plant products (such as urushiol from poison ivy).

Respiratory hypersensitivity: Respiratory hypersensitivity is usually considered to be a Type I hypersensitivity reaction. However, late phase reactions and the more chronic symptoms associated with asthma may involve cell-mediated (Type IV) immune processes. The acute symptoms associated with respiratory allergy are effected by IgE antibody, the production of which is provoked following exposure of the susceptible individual to the inducing chemical allergen. The IgE antibody distributes systemically and binds, via membrane receptors, to mast cells which are found in vascularized tissues, including the respiratory tract. Following inhalation of the same chemical a respiratory hypersensitivity reaction will be elicited. Allergen associates with protein and binds to, and cross-links, IgE antibody bound to mast cells. This in turn causes the degranulation of mast cells and the release of inflammatory mediators such as histamine and leukotrienes. Such mediators cause bronchoconstriction and vasodilation, resulting in the symptoms of respiratory allergy; asthma and/or rhinitis. Chemicals known to cause respiratory hypersensitivity in man include acid anhydrides (such as trimellitic anhydride), some diisocyanates (such as toluene diisocyanate), platinum salts and some reactive dyes. Also, chronic exposure to beryllium is known to cause hypersensitivity lung disease.

Autoimmunity

Autoimmunity can be defined as the stimulation of specific immune responses directed against endogenous "self" antigens. Induced autoimmunity can result either from alterations in the balance of regulatory T-lymphocytes or from the association of a xenobiotic with normal tissue components such as to render them immunogenic ("altered self"). Drugs and chemicals known to incidentally induce or exacerbate effects like those of autoimmune disease (AD) in susceptible individuals are low molecular weight compounds (molecular weight 100 to 500) that are generally considered to be not immunogenic themselves. The mechanism of AD by chemical exposure is mostly unknown. Disease can be produced directly by means of circulating antibody, indirectly through the formation of immune complexes, or as a consequence of cell-mediated immunity, but likely occurs through a combination of mechanisms. The pathogenesis is best known in immune haemolytic disorders induced by drugs:

- The drug can attach to the red-cell membrane and interact with a drug-specific antibody.

- The drug can alter the red-cell membrane so that the immune system regards the cell as foreign.

- The drug and its specific antibody form immune complexes that adhere to the red-cell membrane to produce injury.

- Red-cell sensitization occurs due to the production of red-cell autoantibody.

A variety of chemicals and drugs, in particular the latter, have been found to induce autoimmune-like responses. Occupational exposure to chemicals may incidentally lead to AD-like syndromes. Exposure to monomeric vinyl chloride, trichloroethylene, perchloroethylene, epoxy resins and silica dust may induce scleroderma-like syndromes. A syndrome similar to systemic lupus erythematosus (SLE) has been described after exposure to hydrazine. Exposure to toluene diisocyanate has been associated with the induction of thrombocytopenic purpura. Heavy metals such as mercury have been implicated in some cases of immune complex glomerulonephritis.

Human Risk Assessment

The assessment of human immune status is performed mainly using peripheral blood for analysis of humoral substances like immunoglobulins and complement, and of blood leukocytes for subset composition and functionality of subpopulations. These methods are usually the same as those used to investigate humoral and cell-mediated immunity as well as nonspecific resistance of patients with suspected congenital immunodeficiency disease. For epidemiological studies (e.g., of occupationally exposed populations) parameters should be selected on the basis of their predictive value in human populations, validated animal models, and the underlying biology of the markers. The strategy in screening for immunotoxic effects after (accidental) exposure to environmental pollutants or other toxicants is much dependent on circumstances, such as type of immunodeficiency to be expected, time between exposure and immune status assessment, degree of exposure and number of exposed individuals. The process of assessing the immunotoxic risk of a particular xenobiotic in humans is extremely difficult and often impossible, due largely to the presence of various confounding factors of endogenous or exogenous origin that influence the response of individuals to toxic damage. This is particularly true for studies which investigate the role of chemical exposure in autoimmune diseases, where genetic factors play a crucial role.

Table: Classification of tests for immune markers.

Test category	Characteristics	Specific tests
Basic-general Should be included with general panels	Indicators of general health and organ system status	Blood urea nitrogen, blood glucose, etc.
Basic-immune Should be included with general panels	General indicators of immune status Relatively low cost Assay methods are standardized among laboratories Results outside reference ranges are clinically interpretable	Complete blood counts Serum IgG, IgA, IgM levels Surface marker phenotypes for major lymphocyte subsets
Focused/reflex Should be included when indicated by clinical findings, suspected exposures, or prior test results	Indicators of specific immune functions/events Cost varies Assay methods are standardized among laboratories Results outside reference ranges are clinically interpretable	Histocompatibility genotype Antibodies to infectious agents Total serum IgE Allergen-specific IgE Autoantibodies Skin tests for hypersensitivity Granulocyte oxidative burst Histopathology (tissue biopsy)
Research Should be included only with control populations and careful study design	Indicators of general or specific immune functions/events Cost varies; often expensive Assay methods are usually not standardized among laboratories Results outside reference ranges are often not clinically interpretable	In vitro stimulation assays Cell activation surface markers Cytokine serum concentrations Clonality assays (anti body, cellular, genetic) Cytotoxicity tests

As adequate human data are seldom available, the assessment of risk for chemical-induced immunosuppression in humans is in the majority of cases based upon animal studies. The identification of potential immunotoxic xenobiotics is undertaken primarily in controlled studies in rodents. In vivo exposure studies present, in this regard, the optimal approach to estimate the immunotoxic potential of a compound. This is due to the multifactoral and complex nature of the immune system and of immune responses. In vitro studies are of increasing value in the elucidation of mechanisms of immunotoxicity. In addition, by investigating the effects of the compound using cells of animal and human origin, data can be generated for species comparison, which can be used in the "parallelogram" approach to improve the risk assessment process. If data are available for three cornerstones of the parallelogram (in vivo animal, and in vitro animal and human) it may be easier to predict the outcome at the remaining cornerstone, that is, the risk in humans.

When assessment of risk for chemical-induced immunosuppression has to rely solely upon data from animal studies, an approach can be followed in the extrapolation to man by the application of uncertainty factors to the no observed adverse effect level (NOAEL). This level can be based on parameters determined in relevant models, such as host resistance assays and in vivo assessment of hypersensitivity reactions and antibody production. Ideally, the relevance of this approach to risk assessment requires confirmation by studies in humans. Such studies should combine the identification and measurement of the toxicant, epidemiological data and immune status assessments.

To predict contact hypersensitivity, guinea pig models are available and have been used in risk assessment since the 1970s. Although sensitive and reproducible, these tests have limitations as they depend on subjective evaluation; this can be overcome by newer and more quantitative methods developed in the mouse. Regarding chemical-induced hypersensitivity induced by inhalation or ingestion of allergens, tests should be developed and evaluated in terms of their predictive value in man. When it comes to setting safe occupational exposure levels of potential allergens, consideration has to be given to the biphasic nature of allergy: the sensitization phase and the elicitation phase. The concentration required to elicit an allergic reaction in a previously sensitized individual is considerably lower than the concentration necessary to induce sensitization in the immunologically naïve but susceptible individual.

As animal models to predict chemical-induced autoimmunity are virtually lacking, emphasis should be given to the development of such models. For the development of such models, our knowledge of chemical-induced autoimmunity in humans should be advanced, including the study of genetic and immune system markers to identify susceptible individuals. Humans that are exposed to drugs that induce autoimmunity offer such an opportunity.

References

- Tong JC, Ren EC (July 2009). "Immunoinformatics: current trends and future directions". Drug Discov. Today. 14 (13–14): 684–9. Doi:10.1016/j.drudis.2009.04.001. PMID 19379830

- Psychoneuroimmunology, health: healthline.com, Retrieved 19 April, 2019

- Sarah A. Robertson; John J. Bromfield & Kelton P. Tremellen (2003). "Seminal 'priming' for protection from pre-eclampsia—a unifying hypothesis". Journal of Reproductive Immunology. 59 (2): 253–265. Doi:10.1016/S0165-0378(03)00052-4. PMID 12896827

- Immunotoxicology, mechanisms, mechanisms-of-toxicity, toxicology: iloencyclopaedia.org, Retrieved 17 May, 2019

- De Groot, AS; et al. (March 2005). "HIV vaccine development by computer assisted design: the GAIA vaccine". Vaccine. 23(17–18): 2136–48. Doi:10.1016/j.vaccine.2005.01.097. PMID 15755584

Immunologic Tests 6

- **Epitope Mapping**

- **Chromatin Immunoprecipitation**

- **Complement Fixation Test**

- **Immunofluorescence**

- **Immunocytochemistry**

- **Skin Allergy Test**

- **Immunoassay**

- **Radioallergosorbent Test**

Immunologic tests are used to detect the presence of substances and pathogens. Some of the common immunologic tests are epitope mapping, chromatin immunoprecipitation, complement fixation test, skin allergy test and radioallergosorbent test. This chapter discusses in detail these types of immunologic tests.

There are immunological tests for many different medical conditions and purposes – for instance, to test for an allergy, to screen for bowel cancer or to find out if a woman is pregnant. They can be used to carry out routine tests in hospitals and laboratories, to do quick tests yourself at home, as well as in family doctors' and specialists' practices.

Certain substances or pathogens (germs) in your body can be detected with the help of immunological techniques. The things that can be detected include viruses, hormones and the blood pigment hemoglobin. The tests take advantage of the body's immune system: In order to fight germs or foreign substances, the immune system produces antibodies. Antibodies are proteins that can bind to a specific germ or substance, just like a key fits into a specific keyhole. They "catch" the germs or substances, neutralize them and attract other immune cells.

The immunological tests used in laboratories are made by producing artificial antibodies that exactly "match" the substance or germ in question. When these antibodies come into contact with a sample of blood, urine or stool, they bind to the matching substance or germ if found in the sample. This reaction shows that the germ or substance is present.

During the Test

As mentioned above, immunological tests contain specific antibodies that bind to the substance or germ that is being looked for. In some tests this reaction is visible to the naked eye. For example, in tests to determine your blood group, the blood coagulates (clumps together) on the test card. In other tests, the reaction has to be made visible using a fluorescent dye or an enzyme.

Immunological tests can generally be divided into rapid tests and laboratory tests.

Laboratory Tests

In laboratory tests, sensitive devices measure the amount of bound antibodies based on the extent of a light or color reaction. The greater the reaction, the more of the substance or germ is present. Laboratory tests take longer than rapid tests but they are also more accurate.

Rapid Test

In rapid tests, the antibodies are usually found on paper strips (test strips), but sometimes glass is used too. Rapid tests are easy to use and provide instant results. But they are not as sensitive as laboratory tests and can't determine exactly how much of the substance or germ is present.

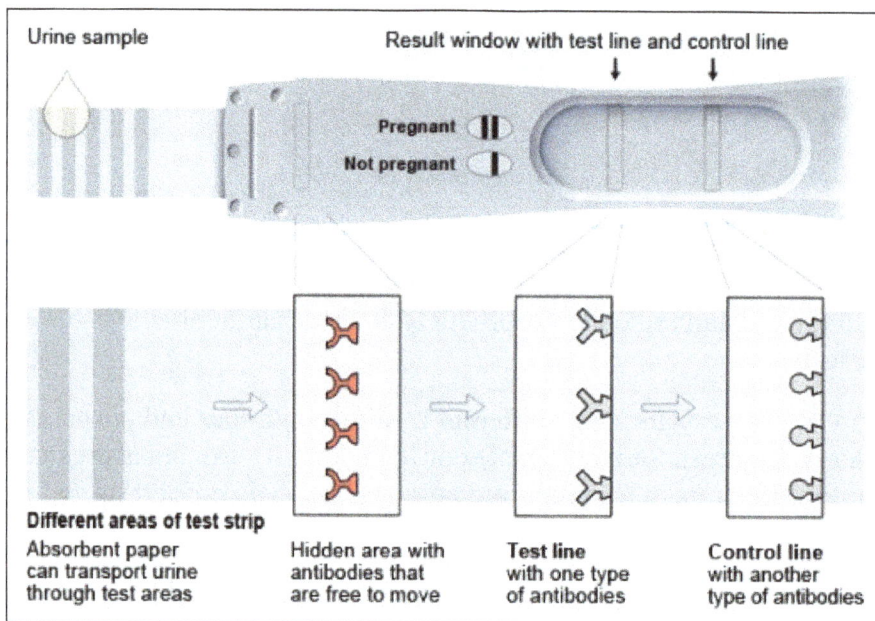

Paper strip for rapid test.

Rapid tests work based on the principle of "lateral flow" (flowing sideways):

When a liquid sample (such as urine) is placed on one end of the test strip, the antibodies on the test strip bind to the substance you are looking for if it is present. Then the liquid slowly moves along the absorbent paper towards the other end of the strip. The antibodies continue to bind to the substance you are looking for, and this reaction causes a change in color. If enough of the liquid sample is used, it flows all the way along the paper strip until it reaches a control line at the other end. If the control line changes color too, the test was carried out properly.

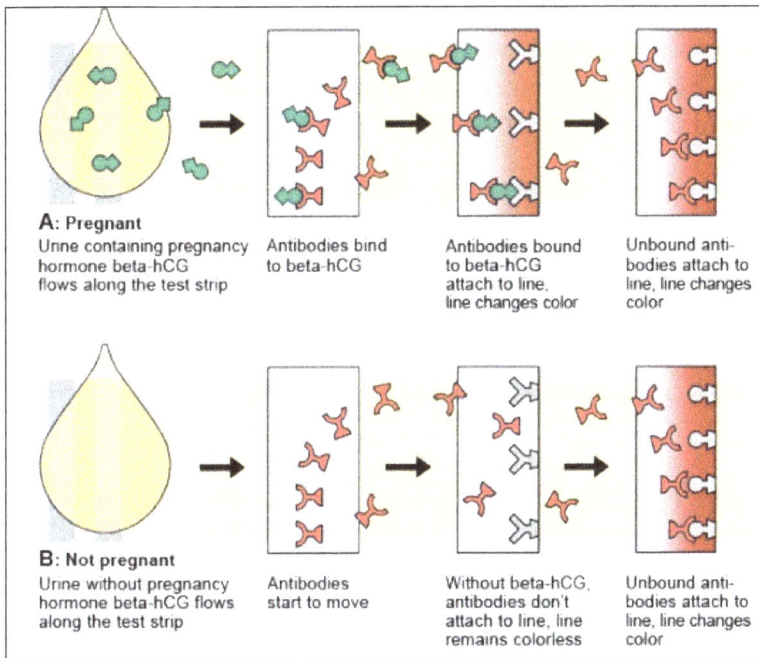

A: Pregnant
Urine containing pregnancy hormone beta-hCG flows along the test strip | Antibodies bind to beta-hCG | Antibodies bound to beta-hCG attach to line, line changes color | Unbound antibodies attach to line, line changes color

B: Not pregnant
Urine without pregnancy hormone beta-hCG flows along the test strip | Antibodies start to move | Without beta-hCG, antibodies don't attach to line, line remains colorless | Unbound antibodies attach to line, line changes color

Paper strip tests: positive and negative reactions.

Immunological Tests Use

Immunological tests are widely used. Their areas of application include:

- Bowel cancer screening: This test looks for the blood pigment hemoglobin, a sign of blood in stool. Blood in stool can be caused by various things, such as hemorrhoids, polyps or even bowel cancer.

- Allergy tests: To detect antibodies against allergy-triggering substances like grass pollen or certain foods.

- Detecting germs causing an infection: If it is thought someone has bacterial tonsillitis or scarlet fever, the test looks for Streptococcus bacteria. In the case of Lyme disease following a tick bite, there are tests that can detect the Borrelia bacteria that cause it, and there are tests that can detect the antibodies to Borrelia bacteria. Immunological tests can also be used to detect viruses. Examples include hepatitis C, HIV or HPV viruses. Pregnant women can have a blood test to find out whether they are protected from (immune to) toxoplasmosis.

- Diagnosing heart attacks and thrombosis: Shortly after a heart attack or if someone has thrombosis , higher levels of a certain protein are found in the blood. These can be detected using an immunological test.

- Urine test: If sugar, blood, proteins or inflammatory cells are found in urine using this rapid test, it could be a sign of diabetes, a urinary tract infection or kidney damage.

- Pregnancy test: Women can use this rapid test to find out whether their urine contains the "pregnancy hormone" beta-hCG.

- Rapid tests for drugs and medication: Immunological tests can also be used to look for recreational drugs such as cannabis, ecstasy and cocaine. Medical drugs that affect the central nervous system can also be detected in this way. These include sleeping pills (benzodiazepines), amphetamines and morphine.

- Determining your blood group: When blood transfusions are done, the person donating the blood and the person receiving the blood have to have the same blood group. Immunological tests can be used to determine the blood groups before a blood transfusion.

Immunological tests can also be used to diagnose congenital or acquired immune diseases, differentiate between different forms of rheumatoid arthritis, or monitor the progression of an existing medical condition, such as certain tumors (in prostate cancer the PSA levels in blood are monitored).

The antibody principle is also applied in doping tests, food hygiene tests, and tests for toxic substances.

Epitope Mapping

Epitope mapping is the process of experimentally identifying the binding site, or "epitope", of an antibody on its target antigen (usually, on a protein). Identification and characterization of antibody binding sites aid in the discovery and development of new therapeutics, vaccines, and diagnostics. Epitope characterization can also help elucidate the mechanism of binding for an antibody and can strengthen intellectual property (patent) protection. Experimental epitope mapping data can be incorporated into robust algorithms to facilitate *in silico* prediction of B-cell epitopes based on sequence and/or structural data.

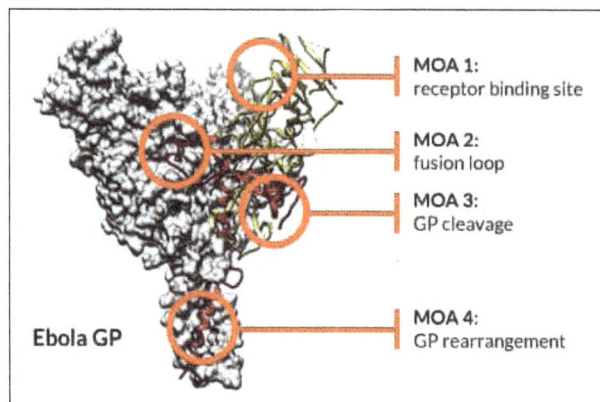

High-resolution epitope maps of antibodies against Ebola glycoprotein (GP), determined using shotgun mutagenesis epitope mapping. Epitope maps provide data for determining mechanism of action (MOA).

Epitopes are generally divided into two classes: linear and conformational. *Linear epitopes* are formed by a continuous sequence of amino acids in a protein. *Conformational epitopes* are composed of amino acids that are discontinuous in the protein sequence but brought together upon three-dimensional protein folding. B-cell epitope mapping studies suggest that most interactions between antigens and antibodies, particularly autoantibodies and protective antibodies (e.g., in vaccines), rely on binding to conformational epitopes.

Importance for Antibody Characterization

By providing information on mechanism of action, epitope mapping is a critical component in therapeutic monoclonal antibody (mAb) development. Epitope mapping can reveal how a mAb exerts its functional effects - for instance, by blocking the binding of a ligand or by trapping a protein in a non-functional state. Many therapeutic mAbs target conformational epitopes that are only present when the protein is in its native (properly folded) state, which can make epitope mapping challenging. Epitope mapping has been crucial to the development of vaccines against prevalent or deadly viral pathogens, such as chikungunya, dengue, Ebola, and Zika viruses, by determining the antigenic elements (epitopes) that confer long-lasting immunization effects.

Complex target antigens, such as membrane proteins (e.g., G protein-coupled receptors [GPCRs]) and multi-subunit proteins (e.g., ion channels) are key targets of drug discovery. Mapping epitopes on these targets can be challenging because of the difficulty in expressing and purifying these complex proteins. Membrane proteins frequently have short antigenic regions (epitopes) that fold correctly only when in the context of a lipid bilayer. As a result, mAb epitopes on these membrane proteins are often conformational and, therefore, are more difficult to map.

Importance for Intellectual Property (IP) Protection

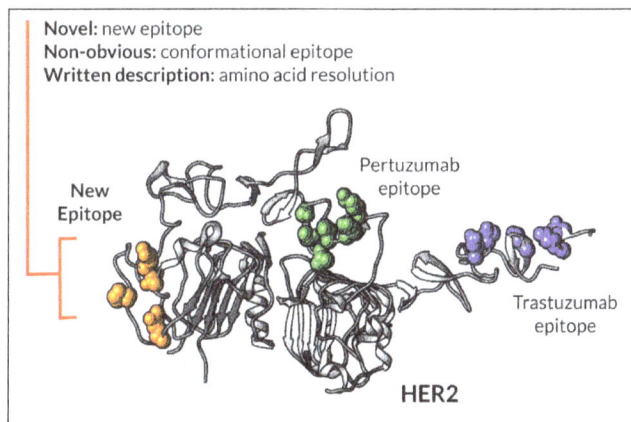

Shotgun mutagenesis epitope mapping of antibodies against HER2 revealed a novel epitope (orange spheres). Epitope maps provide supporting data for intellectual property (patent) claims.

Epitope mapping has become prevalent in protecting the intellectual property (IP) of therapeutic mAbs. Knowledge of the specific binding sites of antibodies strengthens patents and regulatory submissions by distinguishing between current and prior art (existing) antibodies. The ability to differentiate between antibodies is particularly important when patenting antibodies against well-validated therapeutic targets (e.g., PD1 and CD20) that can be drugged by multiple competing antibodies. In addition to verifying antibody patentability, epitope mapping data have been used to support broad antibody claims submitted to the United States Patent and Trademark Office.

Epitope data have been central to several high-profile legal cases involving disputes over the specific protein regions targeted by therapeutic antibodies. In this regard, the Amgen v. Sanofi/Regeneron Pharmaceuticals PCSK9 inhibitor case hinged on the ability to show that both the Amgen and Sanofi/Regeneron therapeutic antibodies bound to overlapping amino acids on the surface of PCSK9.

Methods

There are several methods available for mapping antibody epitopes on target antigens:

- X-ray co-crystallography and cryogenic electron microscopy (cryo-EM). X-ray co-crystallography has historically been regarded as the gold-standard approach for epitope mapping because it allows direct visualization of the interaction between the antigen and antibody. Cryo-EM can similarly provide high-resolution maps of antibody-antigen interactions. However, both approaches are technically challenging, time-consuming, and expensive, and not all proteins are amenable to crystallization. Moreover, these techniques are not always feasible due to the difficulty in obtaining sufficient quantities of correctly folded and processed protein. Finally, neither technique can distinguish key epitope residues (energetic "hot spots") for mAbs that bind to the same group of amino acids.

- Array-based oligo-peptide scanning. Also known as overlapping peptide scan or pepscan analysis, this technique uses a library of oligo-peptide sequences from overlapping and non-overlapping segments of a target protein, and tests for their ability to bind the antibody of interest. This method is fast, relatively inexpensive, and specifically suited to profile epitopes for large numbers of candidate antibodies against a defined target. The epitope mapping resolution depends on the number of overlapping peptides that are used. The main disadvantage of this approach is that it cannot generally be used to obtain conformational epitopes, which are the most relevant epitope type for human therapeutic mAbs. However, one study mapped discontinuous epitopes on CD20 using array-based oligo-peptide scanning, by combining non-adjacent peptide sequences from different parts of the target protein and enforcing conformational rigidity onto this combined peptide (e.g., by using CLIPS scaffolds).

- Site-directed mutagenesis mapping. The molecular biological technique of site-directed mutagenesis (SDM) can be used to enable epitope mapping. In SDM, systematic mutations of amino acids are introduced into the sequence of the target protein. Binding of an antibody to each mutated protein is tested to identify the amino acids that comprise the epitope. This technique can be used to map both linear and conformational epitopes but is labor-intensive and time-consuming, typically limiting analysis to a small number of amino-acid residues.

- High-throughput shotgun mutagenesis epitope mapping. Shotgun mutagenesis is a high-throughput approach for mapping the epitopes of mAbs. The shotgun mutagenesis technique begins with the creation of a mutation library of the entire target antigen, with each clone containing a unique amino acid mutation (typically an alanine substitution). Hundreds of plasmid clones from the library are individually arrayed in 384-well microplates, expressed in human cells, and tested for antibody binding. Amino acids of the target required for antibody binding are identified by a loss of immunoreactivity. These residues are mapped onto structures of the target protein to visualize the epitope. Benefits of high-throughput shotgun mutagenesis epitope mapping include: 1) the ability to identify both linear and conformational epitopes, 2) a shorter assay time than other methods, 3) the presentation of properly folded and post-translationally modified proteins, and 4) the ability to identify key amino acids that drive the energetic interactions (energetic "hot spots" of the epitope).

- Hydrogen–deuterium exchange. This method gives information about the solvent accessibility of various parts of the antigen and antibody, demonstrating reduced solvent accessibility in regions of protein-protein interactions. However, hydrogen-deuterium exchange does not usually provide data at the level of the amino acid.

- Cross-linking-coupled mass spectrometry: Antibody and antigen are bound to a labeled cross-linker, and complex formation is confirmed by high-mass MALDI detection. The binding location of the antibody to the antigen can then be identified by mass spectrometry (MS). The cross-linked complex is highly stable and can be exposed to various enzymatic and digestion conditions, allowing many different peptide options for detection. MS or MS/MS techniques are used to detect the amino-acid locations of the labelled cross-linkers and the bound peptides (both epitope and paratope are determined in one experiment). The key advantage of this technique is the high sensitivity of MS detection, which means that very little material (hundreds of micrograms or less) is needed.

Other methods, such as yeast display, phage display, and limited proteolysis, provide high-throughput monitoring of antibody binding but lack resolution, especially for conformational epitopes.

Chromatin Immunoprecipitation

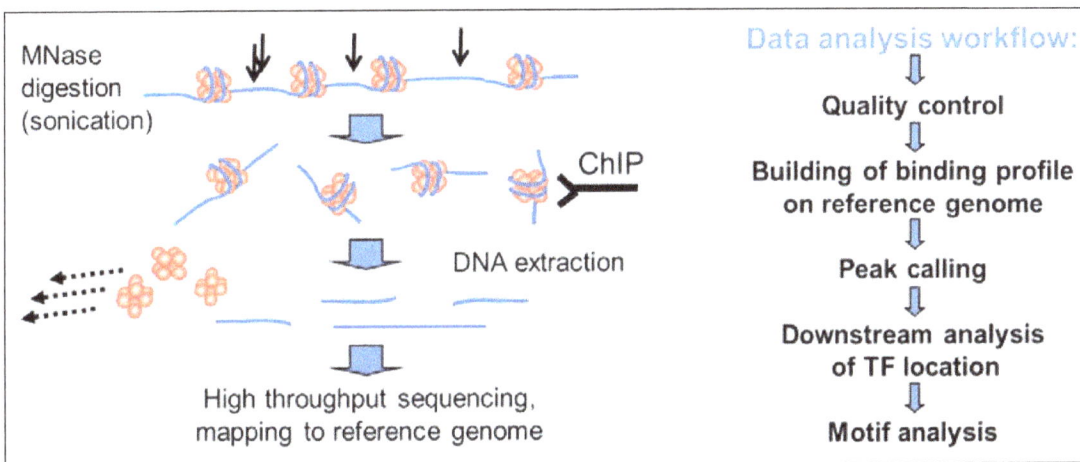

ChIP-sequencing workflow

Chromatin immunoprecipitation (ChIP) is a type of immunoprecipitation experimental technique used to investigate the interaction between proteins and DNA in the cell. It aims to determine whether specific proteins are associated with specific genomic regions, such as transcription factors on promoters or other DNA binding sites, and possibly defining cistromes. ChIP also aims to determine the specific location in the genome that various histone modifications are associated with, indicating the target of the histone modifiers.

Briefly, the conventional method is as follows:

1. DNA and associated proteins on chromatin in living cells or tissues are crosslinked (this step is omitted in Native ChIP).

2. The DNA-protein complexes (chromatin-protein) are then sheared into ~500 bp DNA fragments by sonication or nuclease digestion.

3. Cross-linked DNA fragments associated with the protein(s) of interest are selectively immunoprecipitated from the cell debris using an appropriate protein-specific antibody.

4. The associated DNA fragments are purified and their sequence is determined. Enrichment of specific DNA sequences represents regions on the genome that the protein of interest is associated with *in vivo*.

Typical ChIP

There are mainly two types of ChIP, primarily differing in the starting chromatin preparation. The first uses reversibly cross-linked chromatin sheared by sonication called cross-linked ChIP (XChIP). Native ChIP (NChIP) uses native chromatin sheared by micrococcal nuclease digestion.

Cross-linked ChIP (XChIP)

Cross-linked ChIP is mainly suited for mapping the DNA target of transcription factors or other chromatin-associated proteins, and uses reversibly cross-linked chromatin as starting material. The agent for reversible cross-linking could be formaldehyde or UV light. Then the cross-linked chromatin is usually sheared by sonication, providing fragments of 300 - 1000 base pairs (bp) in length. Mild formaldehyde crosslinking followed by nuclease digestion has been used to shear the chromatin. Chromatin fragments of 400 - 500bp have proven to be suitable for ChIP assays as they cover two to three nucleosomes.

Cell debris in the sheared lysate is then cleared by sedimentation and protein–DNA complexes are selectively immunoprecipitated using specific antibodies to the protein(s) of interest. The antibodies are commonly coupled to agarose, sepharose or magnetic beads. Alternatively, chromatin-antibody complexes can be selectively retained and eluted by inert polymer discs. The immunoprecipitated complexes (i.e., the bead–antibody–protein–target DNA sequence complex) are then collected and washed to remove non-specifically bound chromatin, the protein–DNA cross-link is reversed and proteins are removed by digestion with proteinase K. An epitope-tagged version of the protein of interest, or *in vivo* biotinylation can be used instead of antibodies to the native protein of interest.

The DNA associated with the complex is then purified and identified by polymerase chain reaction (PCR), microarrays (ChIP-on-chip), molecular cloning and sequencing, or direct high-throughput sequencing (ChIP-Seq).

Native ChIP (NChIP)

Native ChIP is mainly suited for mapping the DNA target of histone modifiers. Generally, native chromatin is used as starting chromatin. As histones wrap around DNA to form nucleosomes, they are naturally linked. Then the chromatin is sheared by micrococcal nuclease digestion, which cuts DNA at the length of the linker, leaving nucleosomes intact and providing DNA fragments of one nucleosome (200bp) to five nucleosomes (1000bp) in length.

Thereafter, methods similar to XChIP are used for clearing the cell debris, immunoprecipitating the protein of interest, removing protein from the immunoprecipated complex, and purifying and analyzing the complex-associated DNA.

Comparison of XChIP and NChIP

The major advantage for NChIP is antibody specificity. It is important to note that most antibodies to modified histones are raised against unfixed, synthetic peptide antigens and that the epitopes they need to recognize in the XChIP may be disrupted or destroyed by formaldehyde cross-linking, particularly as the cross-links are likely to involve lysine e-amino groups in the N-terminals, disrupting the epitopes. This is likely to explain the consistently low efficiency of XChIP protocols compare to NChIP.

But XChIP and NChIP have different aims and advantages relative to each other. XChIP is for mapping target sites of transcription factors and other chromatin associated proteins; NChIP is for mapping target sites of histone modifiers.

Table: Advantages and disadvantages of NChIP and XChIP.

	XChIP	NChIP
Advantages	Suitable for transcriptional factors, or any other weakly binding chromatin associated proteins. Applicable to any organisms where native protein is hard to prepare.	Testable antibody specificity Better antibody specificity as target protein naturally intact. Better chromatin and protein recovery efficiency due to better antibody specificity.
Disadvantages	Inefficient chromatin recovery due to antibody target protein epitope disruption May cause false positive result due to fixation of transient proteins to chromatin Wide range of chromatin shearing size due to random cut by sonication.	Usually not suitable for non-histone proteins Nucleosomes may rearrange during digestion.

New ChIP methods

In 1984 John T. Lis and David Gilmour, at the time a graduate student in the Lis lab, used UV irradiation, a zero-length protein-nucleic acid crosslinking agent, to covalently cross-link proteins bound to DNA in living bacterial cells. Following lysis of cross-linked cells and immunoprecipitation of bacterial RNA polymerase, DNA associated with enriched RNA polymerase was hybridized to probes corresponding to different regions of known genes to determine the in vivo distribution and density of RNA polymerase at these genes. A year later they used the same methodology to study distribution of eukaryotic RNA polymerase II on fruit fly heat shock genes. These reports are considered the pioneering studies in the field of chromatin immunoprecipitation. XChIP was further modified and developed by Alexander Varshavsky and co-workers, who examined distribution of histone H4 on heat shock genes using formaldehyde cross-linking. This technique was extensively developed and refined thereafter. NChIP approach was first described by Hebbes et al., 1988, and also been developed and refined quickly. The typical ChIP assay usually take 4–5 days, and require 10^6~ 10^7 cells at least. Now new techniques on ChIP could be achieved as few as 100~1000 cells and complete within one day.

- Bead-free ChIP: This novel method ChIP uses discs of inert, porous polymer functionalized with either Protein A or G in spin columns or microplates. The chromatin-antibody complex is selectively retained by the disc and eluted to obtain enriched DNA for downstream applications such as qPCR and sequencing. The porous environment is specifically designed to maximize capture efficiency and reduce non-specific binding. Due to less manual handling and optimised protocols, ChIP can be performed in 5 hours.

- Carrier ChIP (CChIP): This approach could use as few as 100 cells by adding Drosophila cells as carrier chromatin to reduce loss and facilitate precipitation of the target chromatin. However, it demands highly specific primers for detection of the target cell chromatin from the foreign carrier chromatin background, and it takes two to three days.

- Fast ChIP (qChIP): The fast ChIP assay reduced the time by shortening two steps in a typical ChIP assay: *(i)* an ultrasonic bath accelerates the rate of antibody binding to target proteins—and thereby reduces immunoprecipitation time *(ii)* a resin-based (Chelex-100) DNA isolation procedure reduces the time of cross-link reversal and DNA isolation. However, the fast protocol is suitable only for large cell samples (in the range of 10^6~10^7). Up to 24 sheared chromatin samples can be processed to yield PCR-ready DNA in 5 hours, allowing multiple chromatin factors be probed simultaneously and/or looking at genomic events over several time points.

- Quick and quantitative ChIP (Q²ChIP): The assay uses 100,000 cells as starting material and is suitable for up to 1,000 histone ChIPs or 100 transcription factor ChIPs. Thus many chromatin samples can be prepared in parallel and stored, and Q²ChIP can be undertaken in a day.

- MicroChIP (μChIP): chromatin is usually prepared from 1,000 cells and up to 8 ChIPs can be done in parallel without carriers. The assay can also start with 100 cells, but only suit for one ChIP. It can also use small (1 mm³) tissue biopsies and microChIP can be done within one day.

- Matrix ChIP: This is a microplate-based ChIP assay with increased throughput and simplified the procedure. All steps are done in microplate wells without sample transfers, enabling a potential for automation. It enables 96 ChIP assays for histone and various DNA-bound proteins in a single day.

- Pathology-ChIP (PAT-ChIP): This technique allows ChIP from pathology formalin-fixed and paraffin-embedded tissues and thus the use of pathology archives (even those that are several years old) for epigenetic analyses and the identification of candidate epigenetic biomarkers or targets.

ChIP has also been applied for genome wide analysis by combining with microarray technology (ChIP-on-chip) or second generation DNA-sequencing technology (Chip-Sequencing). ChIP can also combine with paired-end tags sequencing in Chromatin Interaction Analysis using Paired End Tag sequencing (ChIA-PET), a technique developed for large-scale, de novo analysis of higher-order chromatin structures.

Limitations

- Large Scale assays using ChIP is challenging using intact model organisms. This is because antibodies have to be generated for each TF, or, alternatively, transgenic model organisms expressing epitope-tagged TFs need to be produced.

- Researchers studying differential gene expression patterns in small organisms also face problems as genes expressed at low levels, in a small number of cells, in narrow time window.

- ChIP experiments cannot discriminate between different TF isoforms (Protein isoform).

Complement Fixation Test

The complement fixation test is an immunological medical test that can be used to detect the presence of either specific antibody or specific antigen in a patient's serum, based on whether complement fixation occurs. It was widely used to diagnose infections, particularly with microbes that are not easily detected by culture methods, and in rheumatic diseases. However, in clinical diagnostics labs it has been largely superseded by other serological methods such as ELISA and by DNA-based methods of pathogen detection, particularly PCR.

Process

The complement system is a system of serum proteins that react with antigen-antibody complexes. If this reaction occurs on a cell surface, it will result in the formation of trans-membrane pores and therefore destruction of the cell. The basic steps of a complement fixation test are as follows:

- Serum is separated from the patient.

- Patients naturally have different levels of complement proteins in their serum. To negate any effects this might have on the test, the complement proteins in the patient's serum must be destroyed and replaced by a known amount of standardized complement proteins.

    ○ The serum is heated in such a way that all of the complement proteins—but none of the antibodies—within it are destroyed. (This is possible because complement proteins are much more susceptible to destruction by heat than antibodies).

    ○ A known amount of standard complement proteins are added to the serum. (These proteins are frequently obtained from guinea pig serum).

- The antigen of interest is added to the serum.

- Sheep red blood cells (sRBCs) which have been pre-bound to anti-sRBC antibodies are added to the serum. The test is considered negative if the solution turns pink at this point and positive otherwise.

If the patient's serum contains antibodies against the antigen of interest, they will bind to the antigen in step 3 to form antigen-antibody complexes. The complement proteins will react with these complexes and be depleted. Thus when the sRBC-antibody complexes are added in step 4, there will be no complement left in the serum. However, if no antibodies against the antigen of interest are present, the complement will not be depleted and it will react with the sRBC-antibody complexes added in step 4, lysing the sRBCs and spilling their contents into the solution, thereby turning the solution pink.

Testing for Antigen

While detection of antibodies is the more common test format, it is equally possible to test for the presence of antigen. In this case, the patient's serum is supplemented with specific antibody to induce formation of complexes; addition of complement and indicator sRBC is performed as before.

Semi-quantitative Testing

The test can be made quantitative by setting up a series of dilutions of patient serum and determining the highest dilution factor that will still yield a positive CF test. This dilution factor corresponds to the titer.

Immunofluorescence

Immunofluorescence is a technique used for light microscopy with a fluorescence microscope and is used primarily on microbiological samples. This technique uses the specificity of antibodies to their antigen to target fluorescent dyes to specific biomolecule targets within a cell, and therefore allows visualization of the distribution of the target molecule through the sample. The specific region an antibody recognizes on an antigen is called an epitope. There have been efforts in epitope mapping since many antibodies can bind the same epitope and levels of binding between antibodies that recognize the same epitope can vary. Additionally, the binding of the fluorophore to the antibody itself cannot interfere with the immunological specificity of the antibody or the binding capacity of its antigen. Immunofluorescence is a widely used example of immunostaining (using antibodies to stain proteins) and is a specific example of immunohistochemistry (the use of the antibody-antigen relationship in tissues). This technique primarily makes use of fluorophores to visualise the location of the antibodies.

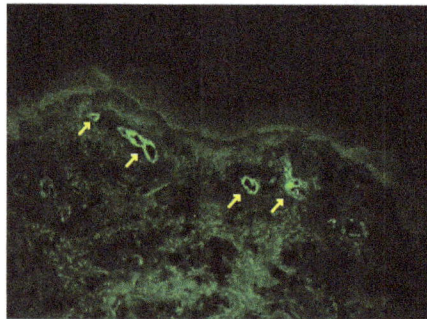

Photomicrograph of a histological section of human skin prepared for direct immunofluorescence using an anti-IgA antibody. The skin is from a patient with Henoch–Schönlein purpura: IgA deposits are found in the walls of small superficial capillaries (yellow arrows). The pale wavy green area on top is the epidermis, the bottom fibrous area is the dermis.

Immunofluorescence can be used on tissue sections, cultured cell lines, or individual cells, and may be used to analyze the distribution of proteins, glycans, and small biological and non-biological molecules. This technique can even be used to visualize structures such as intermediate-sized filaments. If the topology of a cell membrane has yet to be determined, epitope insertion into proteins can be used in conjunction with immunofluorescence to determine structures.

Immunofluorescence can also be used as a "semi-quantitative" method to gain insight into the levels and localization patterns of DNA methylation since it is a more time consuming method than true quantitative methods and there is some subjectivity in the analysis of the levels of methylation. Immunofluorescence can be used in combination with other, non-antibody methods of fluorescent staining, for example, use of DAPI to label DNA. Several microscope designs can be used for analysis of immunofluorescence samples; the simplest is the epifluorescence microscope, and the confocal microscope is also widely used. Various super-resolution microscope designs that are capable of much higher resolution can also be used.

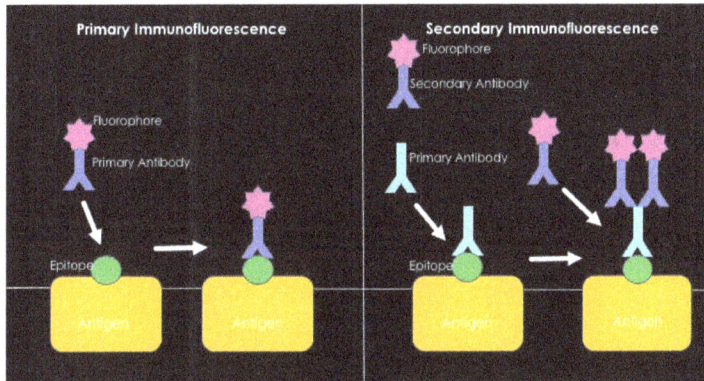

These figures demonstrates the basic mechanism of immunofluorescence. Primary immunofluorescence is depicted on the left, which shows an antibody with a fluorophore group bound to it directly binding to the epitope of the antigen for which it is specific. Once the antibody binds to the epitope, the sample can be viewed under fluorescent microscope to confirm the presence of the antigen in the sample. Conversely, secondary immunofluorescence is depicted to the right, which shows that first an untagged primary antibody binds to the epitope of the antigen in a mechanism similar to the one described above. However, after the primary antibodies have bound to their target, a secondary antibody (tagged with a fluorophore) comes along. This secondary antibody's binding sites are specific for the primary antibody that's already bound to the antigen, and therefore the secondary antibody binds to the primary antibody. This method allows for more fluorophore-tagged antibodies to attach to their target, thus increasing the fluorescent signal during microscopy.

Types

Preparation of Fluorescence

To make fluorochrome-labeled antibodies, a fluorochrome must be conjugated ("tagged") to the antibody. Likewise, an antigen can also be conjugated to the antibody with a fluorescent probe in a technique called fluorescent antigen technique. Staining procedures can apply to both fixed antigen in the cytoplasm or to cell surface antigens on living cells, called "membrane immunofluorescence". It is also possible to label the complement of the antibody-antigen complex with a fluorescent probe. In addition to the element to which fluorescence probes are attached, there are two general classes of immunofluorescence techniques: primary and secondary. The following descriptions will focus primarily on these classes in terms of conjugated antibodies.

There are two classes of immunofluorescence techniques, primary (or direct) and secondary (or indirect).

Primary (Direct)

Primary (direct) immunofluorescence uses a single, primary antibody, chemically linked to a fluorophore. The primary antibody recognizes the target molecule (antigen) and binds to a specific region called the epitope. This is accomplished by a process which manipulates the immune response of organism with adaptive immunity. The attached fluorophore can be detected via fluorescent microscopy, which, depending on the messenger used, will emit a specific wavelength of light once excited. Direct immunofluorescence, although somewhat less common, has notable advantages over the secondary (indirect) procedure. The direct attachment of the messenger to the antibody reduces the number of steps in the procedure, saving time and reducing non-specific background signal. However, some disadvantages do exist in this method. Since the number of fluorescent molecules that can be bound to the primary antibody is limited, direct immunofluorescence is substantially less sensitive than indirect immunofluorescence and may result in false negatives. Direct immunofluorescence also requires the use of much more primary antibody, which is extremely expensive, sometimes running up to $400.00/mL.

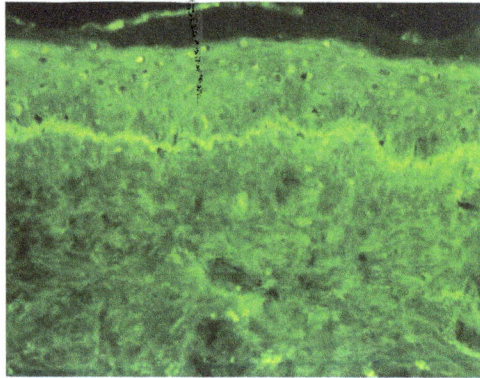

In figure, photomicrograph of a histological section of human skin prepared for direct immunofluorescence using an anti-IgG antibody. The skin is from a patient with systemic lupus erythematosus and shows IgG deposit at two different places: The first is a band-like deposit along the epidermal basement membrane ("lupus band test" is positive). The second is within the nuclei of the epidermal cells (anti-nuclear antibodies).

Secondary (Indirect)

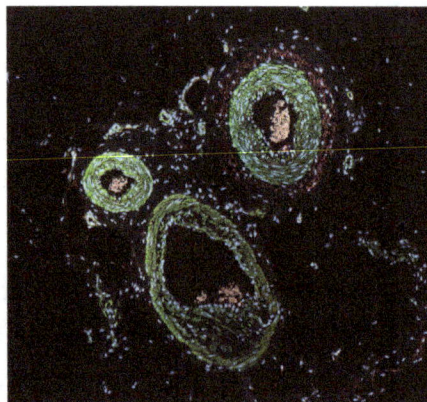

A fluorescent stain for actin in the smooth muscle of the skin.

Secondary (indirect) immunofluorescence uses two antibodies; the unlabeled first (primary) antibody specifically binds the target molecule, and the secondary antibody, which carries the fluorophore, recognizes the primary antibody and binds to it. Multiple secondary antibodies can bind a single primary antibody. This provides signal amplification by increasing the number of fluorophore molecules per antigen. This protocol is more complex and time-consuming than the primary (or direct) protocol above, but allows more flexibility because a variety of different secondary antibodies and detection techniques can be used for a given primary antibody.

This protocol is possible because an antibody consists of two parts, a variable region (which recognizes the antigen) and constant region (which makes up the structure of the antibody molecule). It is important to realize that this division is artificial and in reality the antibody molecule is four polypeptide chains: two heavy chains and two light chains. A researcher can generate several primary antibodies that recognize various antigens (have different variable regions), but all share the same constant region. All these antibodies may therefore be recognized by a single secondary antibody. This saves the cost of modifying the primary antibodies to directly carry a fluorophore.

Different primary antibodies with different constant regions are typically generated by raising the antibody in different species. For example, a researcher might create primary antibodies in a goat that recognize several antigens, and then employ dye-coupled rabbit secondary antibodies that recognize the goat antibody constant region ("rabbit anti-goat" antibodies). The researcher may then create a second set of primary antibodies in a mouse that could be recognized by a separate "donkey anti-mouse" secondary antibody. This allows re-use of the difficult-to-make dye-coupled antibodies in multiple experiments.

Limitations

As with most fluorescence techniques, a significant problem with immunofluorescence is photobleaching. Loss of activity caused by photobleaching can be controlled by reducing or limiting the intensity or time-span of light exposure, by increasing the concentration of fluorophores, or by employing more robust fluorophores that are less prone to bleaching (e.g., Alexa Fluors, Seta Fluors, or DyLight Fluors). Some problems that may arise from this technique include autofluorescence, extraneous undesired specific fluorescence, and nonspecific fluorescence. Autofluorescence includes fluorescence emitted from the sample tissue or cell itself. Extraneous undesired specific fluorescence occurs when a targeted antigen is impure and contains antigenic contaminants. Nonspecific fluorescence involves the loss of a probe's specificity due to fluorophore, from improper fixation, or from a dried out specimen.

Immunofluorescence is only limited to fixed (i.e., dead) cells when structures within the cell are to be visualized because antibodies do not penetrate the cell membrane when reacting with fluorescent labels. Antigenic material must be fixed firmly on the site of its natural localization inside the cell. Intact antibodies can also be too large to dye cancer cells *in vivo*. Their size results in slow tumor penetration and long circulating half-life. Research has been done investigating the use of diabodies to get around this limitation. Proteins in the supernatant or on the outside of the cell membrane can be bound by the antibodies; this allows for living cells to be stained. Depending on the fixative that is being used, proteins of interest might become cross-linked and this could result in either false positive or false negative signals due to non-specific binding.

An alternative approach is using recombinant proteins containing fluorescent protein domains, e.g., green fluorescent protein (GFP). Use of such "tagged" proteins allows determination of their localization in live cells. Even though this seems to be an elegant alternative to immunofluorescence, the cells have to be transfected or transduced with the GFP-tag, and as a consequence they become at least S1 or above organisms that require stricter security standards in a laboratory. This technique involves altering the genetic information of cells.

Advances

Many improvements to this method lie in the improvement of fluorescent microscopes and fluorophores. Super-resolution methods generally refer to a microscope's ability to produce resolution below the Abbe limit (a limit placed on light due to its wavelength). This diffraction limit is about 200-300 nm in the lateral direction and 500-700 nm in the axial direction. This limit is comparable or larger than some structures in the cell, and consequently, this limit prevented scientists from determining details in their structure. Super-resolution in fluorescence, more specifically, refers to the ability of a microscope to prevent the simultaneous fluorescence of adjacent spectrally identical fluorophores. This process effectively sharpens the point-spread function of the microscope. Examples of recently developed super-resolution fluorescent microscope methods include stimulated emission depletion (STED) microscopy, saturated structured-illumination microscopy (SSIM), fluorescence photoactivation localization microscopy (FPALM), and stochastic optical reconstruction microscopy (STORM).

Immunocytochemistry

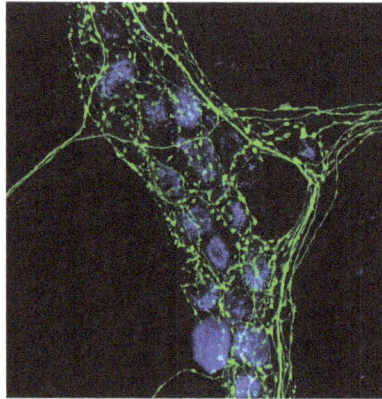

Immunocytochemistry labels individual proteins within cells,
such as TH (green) in the axons of sympathetic autonomic neurons.

Immunocytochemistry (ICC) is a common laboratory technique that is used to anatomically visualize the localization of a specific protein or antigen in cells by use of a specific primary antibody that binds to it. The primary antibody allows visualization of the protein under a fluorescence microscope when it is bound by a secondary antibody that has a conjugated fluorophore. ICC allows researchers to evaluate whether or not cells in a particular sample express the antigen in question. In cases where an immunopositive signal is found, ICC also allows researchers to determine which sub-cellular compartments are expressing the antigen.

Immunocytochemistry vs. Immunohistochemistry

Immunocytochemistry differs from immunohistochemistry in that the former is performed on samples of intact cells that have had most, if not all, of their surrounding extracellular matrix removed. This includes individual cells that have been isolated from a block of solid tissue, cells grown within a culture, cells deposited from suspension, or cells taken from a smear. In contrast, immunohistochemical samples are sections of biological tissue, where each cell is surrounded by tissue architecture and other cells normally found in the intact tissue. Immunocytochemistry is a technique used to assess the presence of a specific protein or antigen in cells (cultured cells, cell suspensions) by use of a specific antibody, which binds to it, thereby allowing visualization and examination under a microscope. It is a valuable tool for the determination of cellular contents from individual cells. Samples that can be analyzed include blood smears, aspirates, swabs, cultured cells, and cell suspensions.

There are many ways to prepare cell samples for immunocytochemical analysis. Each method has its own strengths and unique characteristics so the right method can be chosen for the desired sample and outcome.

Cells to be stained can be attached to a solid support to allow easy handling in subsequent procedures. This can be achieved by several methods: Adherent cells may be grown on microscope slides, coverslips, or an optically suitable plastic support. Suspension cells can be centrifuged onto glass slides (cytospin), bound to solid support using chemical linkers, or in some cases handled in suspension.

Concentrated cellular suspensions that exist in a low-viscosity medium make good candidates for smear preparations. Dilute cell suspensions existing in a dilute medium are best suited for the preparation of cytospins through cytocentrifugation. Cell suspensions that exist in a high-viscosity medium, are best suited to be tested as swab preparations. The constant among these preparations is that the whole cell is present on the slide surface. For any intercellular reaction to take place, immunoglobulin must first traverse the cell membrane that is intact in these preparations. Reactions taking place in the nucleus can be more difficult, and the extracellular fluids can create unique obstacles in the performance of immunocytochemistry. In this situation, permeabilizing cells using detergent (Triton X-100 or Tween-20) or choosing organic fixatives (acetone, methanol, or ethanol) becomes necessary.

Antibodies are an important tool for demonstrating both the presence and the subcellular localization of an antigen. Cell staining is a very versatile technique and, if the antigen is highly localized, can detect as few as a thousand antigen molecules in a cell. In some circumstances, cell staining may also be used to determine the approximate concentration of an antigen, especially by an image analyzer.

Methods

There are many methods to obtain immunological detection on tissues, including those tied directly to primary antibodies or antisera. A direct method involves the use of a detectable tag (e.g., fluorescent molecule, gold particles, etc.,) directly to the antibody that is then allowed to bind to the antigen (e.g., protein) in a cell.

Alternatively, there are many indirect methods. In one such method, the antigen is bound by a primary antibody which is then amplified by use of a secondary antibody which binds to the primary antibody. Next, a tertiary reagent containing an enzymatic moiety is applied and binds to the secondary antibody. When the quaternary reagent, or substrate, is applied, the enzymatic end of the tertiary reagent converts the substrate into a pigment reaction product, which produces a color (many colors are possible; brown, black, red, etc.,) in the same location that the original primary antibody recognized that antigen of interest.

Some examples of substrates used (also known as chromogens) are AEC (3-Amino-9-EthylCarbazole), or DAB (3,3'-Diaminobenzidine). Use of one of these reagents after exposure to the necessary enzyme (e.g., horseradish peroxidase conjugated to an antibody reagent) produces a positive immunoreaction product. Immunocytochemical visualization of specific antigens of interest can be used when a less specific stain like H&E (Hematoxylin and Eosin) cannot be used for a diagnosis to be made or to provide additional predictive information regarding treatment (in some cancers, for example).

Alternatively the secondary antibody may be covalently linked to a fluorophore (FITC and Rhodamine are the most common) which is detected in a fluorescence or confocal microscope. The location of fluorescence will vary according to the target molecule, external for membrane proteins, and internal for cytoplasmic proteins. In this way immunofluorescence is a powerful technique when combined with confocal microscopy for studying the location of proteins and dynamic processes (exocytosis, endocytosis, etc).

Skin Allergy Test

Skin allergy testing or skin prick test is a method for medical diagnosis of allergies that attempts to provoke a small, controlled, allergic response.

Methods

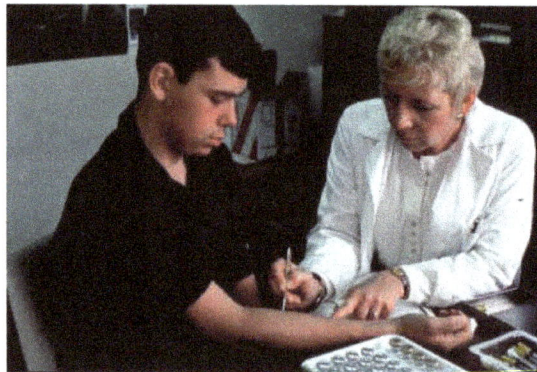

A person receiving a skin allergy test.

A microscopic amount of an allergen is introduced to a patient's skin by various means:

- Skin prick test: Pricking the skin with a needle or pin containing a small amount of the allergen.

- Skin scratch test: A deep dermic scratch is performed with help of the blunt bottom of a lancet.

- Intradermic test: A tiny quantity of allergen is injected under the dermis with a hypodermic syringe.

- Skin scrape Test: A superficial scrape is performed with help of the bovel of a needle to remove the superficial layer of the epidermis.

- Patch test: Applying a patch to the skin, where the patch contains the allergen.

If an immuno-response is seen in the form of a rash, urticaria (hives), or *(worse)* anaphylaxis it can be concluded that the patient has a hypersensitivity (or allergy) to that allergen. Further testing can be done to identify the particular allergen.

The "skin scratch test" as it is called, is not very commonly used due to increased likelihood of infection. On the other hand, the "skin scrape test" is painless, does not leave residual pigmentation and does not have a risk of infection, since it is limited to the superficial layer of the skin.

Some allergies are identified in a few minutes but others may take several days. In all cases where the test is positive, the skin will become raised, red and appear itchy. The results are recorded - larger wheals indicating that the subject is more sensitive to that particular allergen. A negative test does not conclusively rule out an allergy; occasionally, the concentration needs to be adjusted, or the body fails to elicit a response.

Immediate Reactions Tests

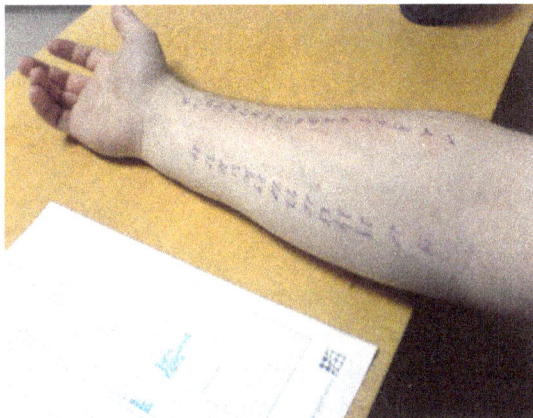

Skin testing on arm.

In the prick, scratch and scrape tests, a few drops of the purified allergen are gently pricked on to the skin surface, usually the forearm. This test is usually done in order to identify allergies to pet dander, dust, pollen, foods or dust mites. Intradermal injections are done by injecting a small amount of allergen just beneath the skin surface. The test is done to assess allergies to drugs like penicillin or bee venom.

To ensure that the skin is reacting in the way it is supposed to, all skin allergy tests are also performed with proven allergens like histamine or glycerin. The majority of people do react to histamine and do not react to glycerin. If the skin does not react appropriately to these allergens then it most likely will not react to the other allergens. These results are interpreted as falsely negative.

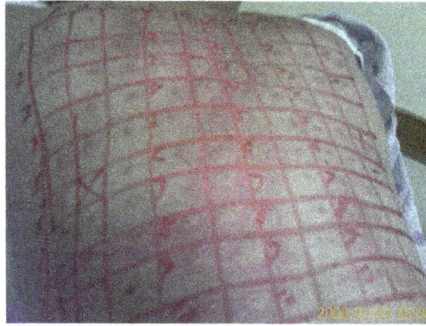

Skin testing on back.

Delayed Reactions Tests

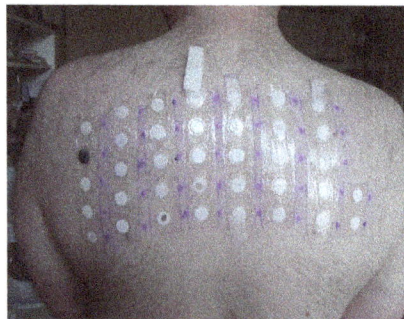

Patch test

The patch test simply uses a large patch which has different allergens on it. The patch is applied onto the skin, usually on the back. The allergens on the patch include latex, medications, preservatives, hair dyes, fragrances, resins and various metals.

Skin End Point Titration

Also called an *intradermal test*, this skin end point titration (SET) uses intradermal injection of allergens at increasing concentrations to measure allergic response. To prevent a severe allergic reaction, the test is started with a very dilute solution. After 10 minutes, the injection site is measured to look for growth of wheal, a small swelling of the skin. Two millimeters of growth in 10 minutes is considered positive. If 2 mm of growth is noted, then a second injection at a higher concentration is given to confirm the response. The end point is the concentration of antigen that causes an increase in the size of the wheal followed by confirmatory whealing. If the wheal grows larger than 13 mm, then no further injection are given since this is considered a major reaction.

Preparation

There are no major preparations required for skin testing. At the first consult, the subject's medical history is obtained and physical examination is performed. All consumers should bring a list of their medications because some may interfere with the testing. Other medications may increase the chance of a severe allergic reaction. Medications that commonly interfere with skin testing include the following:

- Histamine antagonists like Allegra, Claritin, Benadryl, Zyrtec.

- Antidepressants like Amitriptyline, Doxepin.

- Antacid like Tagamet or Zantac.

Consumers who undergo skin testing should know that anaphylaxis can occur anytime. So if any of the following symptoms are experienced, a physician consultation is recommended immediately:

- Low grade Fever.

- Lightheadedness or dizziness.

- Wheezing or Shortness of breath.

- Extensive skin rash.

- Swelling of face, lips or mouth.

- Difficulty swallowing or speaking.

Contraindications

Even though skin testing may seem to be a benign procedure, it does have some risks, including swollen red bumps (hives) which may occur after the test. The hives usually disappear in a few hours after the test. In rare cases they can persist for a day or two. These hives may be itchy and are best treated by applying an over the counter hydrocortisone cream. In very rare cases one may develop a full blown allergic reaction. Physicians who perform skin test always have equipment and medications available in case an anaphylaxis reaction occurs. This is the main reason why consumers should not get skin testing performed at corner stores or by people who have no medical training.

Antihistamines, which are commonly used to treat allergy symptoms, interfere with skin tests, as they can prevent the skin from reacting to the allergens being tested. People who take an antihistamine need either to choose a different form of allergy test or to stop taking the antihistimine temporarily before the test. The period of time needed can range from a day or two to 10 days or longer, depending on the specific medication. Some medications not primarily used as antihistamines, including tricyclic antidepressants, phenothiazine-based antipsychotics, and several kinds of medications used for gastrointestinal disorders, can similarly interfere with skin tests.

People who have severe, generalized skin disease or an acute skin infection should not undergo skin testing, as one needs uninvolved skin for testing. Also, skin testing should be avoided for people at a heightened risk of anaphylactic shock, including people who are known to be highly sensitive to even the smallest amount of allergen.

Besides skin tests, there are blood tests which measure a specific antibody in the blood. The IgE antibody plays a vital role in allergies but its levels in blood do not always correlate with the allergic reaction.

There are many alternative health care practitioners who perform a variety of provocation neutralization tests, but the vast majority of these tests have no validity and have never been proven to work scientifically.

Immunoassay

An immunoassay is a biochemical test that measures the presence or concentration of a macromolecule or a small molecule in a solution through the use of an antibody (usually) or an antigen (sometimes). The molecule detected by the immunoassay is often referred to as an "analyte" and is in many cases a protein, although it may be other kinds of molecules, of different size and types, as long as the proper antibodies that have the adequate properties for the assay are developed. Analytes in biological liquids such as serum or urine are frequently measured using immunoassays for medical and research purposes.

Immunoassays come in many different formats and variations. Immunoassays may be run in multiple steps with reagents being added and washed away or separated at different points in the assay. Multi-step assays are often called separation immunoassays or heterogeneous immunoassays. Some immunoassays can be carried out simply by mixing the reagents and sample and making a physical measurement. Such assays are called homogeneous immunoassays, or less frequently non-separation immunoassays.

The use of a calibrator is often employed in immunoassays. Calibrators are solutions that are known to contain the analyte in question, and the concentration of that analyte is generally known. Comparison of an assay's response to a real sample against the assay's response produced by the calibrators makes it possible to interpret the signal strength in terms of the presence or concentration of analyte in the sample.

Principle

Immunoassays rely on the ability of an antibody to recognize and bind a specific macromolecule in what might be a complex mixture of macromolecules. In immunology the particular macromolecule bound by an antibody is referred to as an antigen and the area on an antigen to which the antibody binds is called an epitope.

In some cases, an immunoassay may use an antigen to detect for the presence of antibodies, which recognize that antigen, in a solution. In other words, in some immunoassays, the analyte may be an antibody rather than an antigen.

In addition to the binding of an antibody to its antigen, the other key feature of all immunoassays is a means to produce a measurable signal in response to the binding. Most, though not all, immunoassays involve chemically linking antibodies or antigens with some kind of detectable label. A large number of labels exist in modern immunoassays, and they allow for detection through different means. Many labels are detectable because they either emit radiation, produce a color change in a solution, fluoresce under light, or can be induced to emit light.

Rosalyn Sussman Yalow and Solomon Berson are credited with the development of the first immunoassays in the 1950s. Yalow accepted the Nobel Prize for her work in immunoassays in 1977, becoming the second American woman to have won the award.

Immunoassays became considerably simpler to perform and more popular when techniques for chemically linked enzymes to antibodies were demonstrated in the late 1960s.

In 1983, Professor Anthony Campbell at Cardiff University replaced radioactive iodine used in immunoassay with an acridinium ester that makes its own light: Chemiluminescence. This type of immunoassay is now used in around 100 million clinical tests every year worldwide, enabling clinicians to measure a wide range of proteins, pathogens and other molecules in blood samples.

By 2012, the commercial immunoassay industry earned US$17,000,000,000 and was thought to have prospects of slow annual growth in the 2 to 3 percent range.

Labels

Immunoassays employ a variety of different labels to allow for detection of antibodies and antigens. Labels are typically chemically linked or conjugated to the desired antibody or antigen.

Enzymes

Possibly one of the most popular labels to use in immunoassays is enzymes. Immunoassays which employ enzymes are referred to as enzyme-linked immunosorbent assays (ELISAs), or sometimes enzyme immunoassays (EIAs).

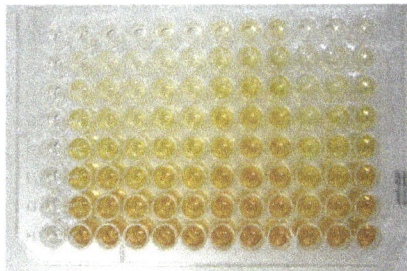

A sandwich ELISA run on a microtitre plate.

Enzymes used in ELISAs include horseradish peroxidase (HRP), alkaline phosphatase (AP) or glucose oxidase. These enzymes allow for detection often because they produce an observable color change in the presence of certain reagents. In some cases these enzymes are exposed to reagents which cause them to produce light or Chemiluminescence.

Radioactive Isotopes

Radioactive isotopes can be incorporated into immunoassay reagents to produce a radioimmunoassay (RIA). Radioactivity emitted by bound antibody-antigen complexes can be easily detected using conventional methods.

RIAs were some of the earliest immunoassays developed, but have fallen out of favor largely due to the difficulty and potential dangers presented by working with radioactivity.

DNA Reporters

A newer approach to immunoassays involves combining real-time quantitative polymerase chain reaction (RT qPCR) and traditional immunoassay techniques. Called real-time immunoquantitative PCR (iqPCR) the label used in these assays is a DNA probe.

Fluorogenic Reporters

Fluorogenic reporters like phycoerythrin are used in a number of modern immunoassays. Protein microarrays are a type of immunoassay that often employ fluorogenic reporters.

Electrochemiluminescent Tags

Some labels work via electrochemiluminescence, in which the label emits detectable light in response to electric current.

Label-free Immunoassays

While some kind of label is generally employed in immunoassays, there are certain kinds of assays which do not rely on labels, but instead employ detection methods that don't require the modification or labeling the components of the assay. Surface plasmon resonance is an example of technique that can detect binding between an unlabeled antibody and antigens. Another demonstrated labeless immunoassay involves measuring the change in resistance on an electrode as antigens bind to it.

Classifications and Formats

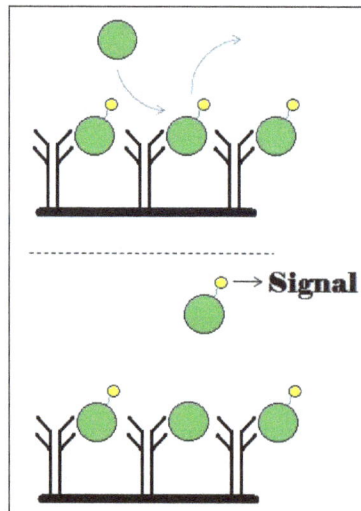

In a competitive, homogeneous immunoassay unlabeled analyte displaces bound labelled analyte, which is then detected or measured.

Immunoassays can be run in a number of different formats. Generally, an immunoassay will fall into one of several categories depending on how it is run.

Competitive, Homogeneous Immunoassays

In a competitive, homogeneous immunoassay, unlabelled analyte in a sample competes with labelled analyte to bind an antibody. The amount of labelled, unbound analyte is then measured. In theory, the more analyte in the sample, the more labelled analyte gets displaced and then measured; hence, the amount of labelled, unbound analyte is proportional to the amount of analyte in the sample.

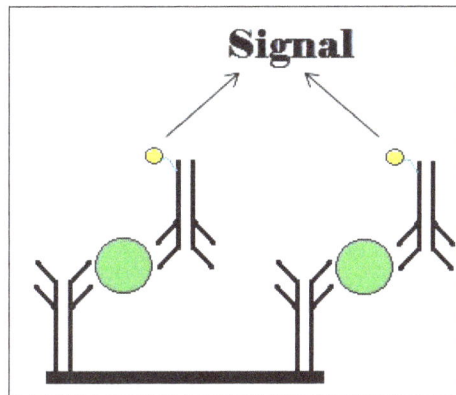

Two-site, noncompetitive immunoassays usually consist of an analyte "sandwiched" between two antibodies. ELISAs are often run in this format.

Competitive, Heterogeneous Immunoassays

As in a competitive, homogeneous immunoassay, unlabelled analyte in a sample competes with labelled analyte to bind an antibody. In the heterogeneous assays, the labelled, unbound analyte is separated or washed away, and the remaining labelled, bound analyte is measured.

One-site, Noncompetitive Immunoassays

The unknown analyte in the sample binds with labelled antibodies. The unbound, labelled antibodies are washed away, and the bound, labelled antibodies are measured. The intensity of the signal is directly proportional to the amount of unknown analyte.

Two-site, Noncompetitive Immunoassays

The analyte in the unknown sample is bound to the antibody site, then the labelled antibody is bound to the analyte. The amount of labelled antibody on the site is then measured. It will be directly proportional to the concentration of the analyte because the labelled antibody will not bind if the analyte is not present in the unknown sample. This type of immunoassay is also known as a sandwich assay as the analyte is "sandwiched" between two antibodies.

Examples

Clinical Tests

A wide range of medical tests are immunoassays, called immunodiagnostics in this context. Many home pregnancy tests are immunoassays, which detect the pregnancy marker human chorionic gonadotropin. Other clinical immunoassays include tests that measure levels of CK-MB to assess heart disease, insulin to assess hypoglycemia, prostate-specific antigen to detect prostate cancer, and some are also used for the detection and/or quantitative measurement of some pharmaceutical compounds.

Sports Anti-doping Analysis

Immunoassays are used in sports anti-doping laboratories to test athletes' blood samples for prohibited recombinant human growth hormone (rhGH, rGH, hGH, GH).

Radioallergosorbent Test

A RAST test or radioallergosorbent test is a way of testing a person's blood to see if they have any allergies. This test checks their blood for specific lgE antibodies to find out what substances they may be allergic to.

Allergies can be a mild annoyance or a life-threatening condition. Allergy tests allow a person to find out what substances they are allergic to so that they can plan ahead and avoid those allergens.

The RAST test is an alternative to the skin prick test. The skin prick test determines how a person's skin reacts to specific allergens.

RAST Test

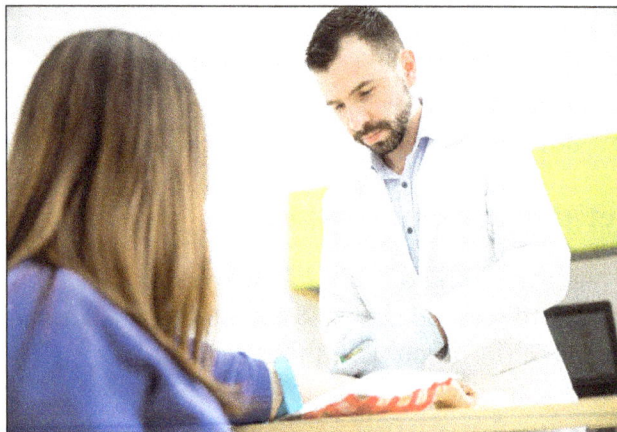

A medical professional will take a blood sample for a RAST test.

The RAST test is a blood test that is used to see if an individual's blood contains antibodies for a specific substance, such as peanuts or pollen. These antibodies are called immunoglobulin E, or IgE antibodies.

If a person's blood contains lgE antibodies that are specific to a certain substance, it means they are allergic to that substance. These antibodies cause the rashes, itching, sneezing, and other symptoms that a person experiences when they come into contact with an allergen.

The name RAST was originally a brand name, but experts say it is now commonly and incorrectly used to describe any lab test for allergens.

According to the Guidelines for the Diagnosis and Management of Food Allergy in the United States, the original RAST test method is now outdated. Instead of RAST tests, a doctor is more likely to order a different blood test called ELISA, which stands for enzyme-linked immunosorbent assay.

RAST Test vs. Skin Test

Different kinds of allergy tests are available, but the most commonly used is a skin or pinprick test.

In a skin test, small amounts of different allergens are placed on an individual's skin, usually with a pinprick. People who are allergic to these substances will develop itchy hives at these sites, while others without allergies will not.

The differences between the skin test and the RAST or ELISA blood tests are as follows:

- Speed of the procedure: Skin tests are faster than blood tests. A skin test can take place in the doctor's office, but in a RAST or ELISA test, the medical professional must send a blood sample to a laboratory for testing.

- Speed of results: Reactions to a skin test typically develop within 15 minutes, whereas it can take between a few days and 2 weeks to get the results of a RAST test.

- Accuracy: Skin tests may be more sensitive than blood tests, though both methods are considered accurate for diagnosing allergies. It may be more difficult to interpret accurately skin test results on people with darker skin, and skin tests may be affected by medications while blood tests are not.

- Safety: Although it is rare, a person can develop a serious reaction to an allergen used in a skin test. There is no risk of this with a blood test, such as RAST or ELISA.

- Cost: A skin test costs less than a RAST or ELISA test to process, which may be a consideration for some people.

In some cases, a person's doctor may recommend a blood test instead of a skin test. These cases can include:

- Testing infants or young children, as blood tests require only one needle prick while skin tests require more.

- Avoiding the risk of a strong allergic reaction to a powerful allergen.

- Allowing individuals to stay on medication that could interfere with a skin test.

- Minimizing the risk of making an existing skin condition, such as psoriasis or eczema, worse.

RAST Test Uses

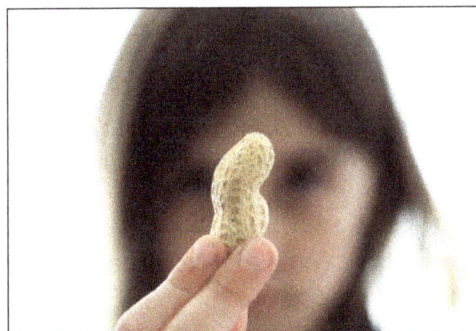

RAST and ELISA can test for pet allergies and food allergies.

Blood tests like RAST and ELISA can test for a range of allergies, including food allergies, drug allergies, seasonal allergies, and pet allergies.

Along with diagnosing current allergies, blood tests can be used as part of the testing and treatment process that doctors use to test the progress of allergies in young children.

The presence and changes of IgE antibodies in the blood help a doctor to determine the progression of allergies, what allergy professionals call the 'allergic march,' that starts in infancy and progresses through childhood.

Doctors tended to avoid skin tests for infants, however. Researchers suggest that using blood testing procedures to diagnose allergies early in a person's life can provide the following benefits:

- The ability to start allergy intervention treatment earlier.

- Avoidance of dangerous reactions to food allergens in infants.

- The potential to prevent the development of asthma.

- A reduction in outbreaks of eczema.

RAST Test Procedure

The RAST test procedure is fairly straightforward and does not require any preparation.

After a person speaks to their doctor, a medical professional will take a blood sample, usually from the individual's arm.

This blood is then sent to a laboratory, where it is subjected to a battery of tests that look for antibodies that have developed in response to specific allergens.

Accuracy of Results

According to Food Allergy Research & Education (FARE), 50–60 percent of blood and skin prick tests will yield some "false positives" for food allergies, meaning the test will show that a person is allergic to something when they are not.

If a blood test finds that a person has antibodies for a specific allergen, it is likely that they have an allergy to the substance, but it is not definite. More tests may be needed.

For example, a RAST test may show that an individual is allergic to a food, such as chickpeas, only because it is in the same family as another food, for example, peanuts, that really do provoke an allergic response.

Also, the level of antibodies in the blood is not necessarily linked to the number of times an individual has been exposed to the allergen or how severe or mild those reactions may have been.

If an individual tests positive for a specific antibody, which is called a positive specific-IgE test, this result indicates that they have probably been exposed to the allergen. But it does not say for sure that the individual is allergic to the substance.

The likelihood of false positive results makes it that much more important for doctors to review RAST test outcomes in the light of an individual's overall medical history, particularly how much exposure they may have had to the allergen in question.

References

- Collas, Philippe. (January 2010). "The Current State of Chromatin Immunoprecipitation". Molecular Biotechnology. 45 (1): 87–100. Doi:10.1007/s12033-009-9239-8. PMID 20077036

- Westwood, Olwyn M. R.; Hay, Frank C., eds. (2001). Epitope Mapping: A Practical Approach. Oxford, Oxfordshire: Oxford University Press. ISBN 978-0-19-963652-5

- C. Vaman Rao (2005). Immunology: a textbook. Alpha Science Int'l Ltd. Pp. 112–. ISBN 978-1-84265-255-8. Retrieved 3 December 2010

- Deng, X; Storz, U; Doranz, BJ (2018). "Enhancing antibody patent protection using epitope mapping information". Mabs. 10 (2): 204–9. Doi:10.1080/19420862.2017.1402998. PMC 5825199. PMID 29120697

- Diaspro, Alberto; van, Zandvoort, Marc A. M. J. (2016-11-03). Super-resolution imaging in biomedicine. ISBN 9781482244359. OCLC 960719686

- Yetisen A. K. (2013). "Paper-based microfluidic point-of-care diagnostic devices". Lab on a Chip. 13 (12): 2210–2251. Doi:10.1039/C3LC50169H. PMID 23652632

- Rall JE. Solomon A. Berson. In "Biographical Memoirs". National Academy of Sciences 1990;59:54-71. ISBN 0-309-04198-8. Fulltext

PERMISSIONS

All chapters in this book are published with permission under the Creative Commons Attribution Share Alike License or equivalent. Every chapter published in this book has been scrutinized by our experts. Their significance has been extensively debated. The topics covered herein carry significant information for a comprehensive understanding. They may even be implemented as practical applications or may be referred to as a beginning point for further studies.

We would like to thank the editorial team for lending their expertise to make the book truly unique. They have played a crucial role in the development of this book. Without their invaluable contributions this book wouldn't have been possible. They have made vital efforts to compile up to date information on the varied aspects of this subject to make this book a valuable addition to the collection of many professionals and students.

This book was conceptualized with the vision of imparting up-to-date and integrated information in this field. To ensure the same, a matchless editorial board was set up. Every individual on the board went through rigorous rounds of assessment to prove their worth. After which they invested a large part of their time researching and compiling the most relevant data for our readers.

The editorial board has been involved in producing this book since its inception. They have spent rigorous hours researching and exploring the diverse topics which have resulted in the successful publishing of this book. They have passed on their knowledge of decades through this book. To expedite this challenging task, the publisher supported the team at every step. A small team of assistant editors was also appointed to further simplify the editing procedure and attain best results for the readers.

Apart from the editorial board, the designing team has also invested a significant amount of their time in understanding the subject and creating the most relevant covers. They scrutinized every image to scout for the most suitable representation of the subject and create an appropriate cover for the book.

The publishing team has been an ardent support to the editorial, designing and production team. Their endless efforts to recruit the best for this project, has resulted in the accomplishment of this book. They are a veteran in the field of academics and their pool of knowledge is as vast as their experience in printing. Their expertise and guidance has proved useful at every step. Their uncompromising quality standards have made this book an exceptional effort. Their encouragement from time to time has been an inspiration for everyone.

The publisher and the editorial board hope that this book will prove to be a valuable piece of knowledge for students, practitioners and scholars across the globe.

INDEX

www.ingramcontent.com/pod-product-compliance
Lightning Source LLC
Chambersburg PA
CBHW082049190326
41458CB00010B/3487